Sleep-Related Epilepsy and Electroencephalography

Guest Editors

MADELEINE M. GRIGG-DAMBERGER, MD
NANCY FOLDVARY-SCHAEFER, DO, MS

SLEEP MEDICINE CLINICS

www.sleep.theclinics.com

March 2012 • Volume 7 • Number 1

SAUNDERS an imprint of ELSEVIER, Inc.

W.B. SAUNDERS COMPANY
A Division of Elsevier Inc.

1600 John F. Kennedy Boulevard • Suite 1800 • Philadelphia, PA 19103-2899

http://www.sleep.theclinics.com

SLEEP MEDICINE CLINICS Volume 7, Number 1
March 2012, ISSN 1556-407X, ISBN-13: 978-1-4557-3933-2

Editor: Katie Hartner
Developmental Editor: Donald E. Mumford

Sleep Medicine Clinics (ISSN 1556-407X) is published quarterly by Elsevier Inc., 360 Park Avenue South, New York, NY 10010-1710. Months of issue are March, June, September and December. Business and Editorial Offices: 1600 John F. Kennedy Blvd., Ste. 1800, Philadelphia, PA 19103-2899. Customer Service Office: 3251 Riverport Lane, Maryland Heights, MO 63043. Periodicals postage paid at New York, NY and additional mailing offices. Subscription prices are $174.00 per year (US individuals), $86.00 (US residents), $368.00 (US institutions), $214.00 (foreign individuals), $120.00 (foreign residents), and $406.00 (foreign institutions). Foreign air speed delivery is included in all *Clinics* subscription prices. All prices are subject to change without notice. **POSTMASTER:** Send change of address to *Sleep Medicine Clinics*, Elsevier Health Sciences Division, Subscription Customer Service, 3251 Riverport Lane, Maryland Heights, MO 63043. Customer Service: **Tel: 1-800-654-2452 (U.S. and Canada); 314-447-8871 (outside U.S. and Canada). Fax: 314-447-8029. E-mail: journalscustomerservice-usa@elsevier.com (for print support); journalsonlinesupport-usa@elsevier.com (for online support).**

Reprints. For copies of 100 or more of articles in this publication, please contact the Commercial Reprints Department, Elsevier Inc., 360 Park Avenue South, New York, NY 10010-1710. Tel.: 212-633-3812; Fax: 212-462-1935; E-mail: reprints@elsevier.com.

Printed and bound by CPI Group (UK) Ltd, Croydon, CR0 4YY

Transferred to Digital Print 2012

GOAL STATEMENT

The goal of *Sleep Clinics of North America* is to keep practicing physicians up to date with current clinical practice by providing timely articles reviewing the state of the art in patient care.

ACCREDITATION

The *Sleep Clinics of North America* is planned and implemented in accordance with the Essential Areas and Policies of the Accreditation Council for Continuing Medical Education (ACCME) through the joint sponsorship of the University of Virginia School of Medicine and Elsevier. The University of Virginia School of Medicine is accredited by the ACCME to provide continuing medical education for physicians.

The University of Virginia School of Medicine designates this enduring material activity for a maximum of 15 *AMA PRA Category 1 Credit(s)*™ for each issue, 60 credits per year. Physicians should only claim credit commensurate with the extent of their participation in the activity.

The American Medical Association has determined that physicians not licensed in the US who participate in this CME enduring material activity are eligible for a maximum of 15 *AMA PRA Category 1 Credit(s)*™ for each issue, 60 credits per year.

Credit can be earned by reading the text material, taking the CME examination online at http://www.theclinics.com/home/cme, and completing the evaluation. After taking the test, you will be required to review any and all incorrect answers. Following completion of the test and evaluation, your credit will be awarded and you may print your certificate.

FACULTY DISCLOSURE/CONFLICT OF INTEREST

The University of Virginia School of Medicine, as an ACCME accredited provider, endorses and strives to comply with the Accreditation Council for Continuing Medical Education (ACCME) Standards of Commercial Support, Commonwealth of Virginia statutes, University of Virginia policies and procedures, and associated federal and private regulations and guidelines on the need for disclosure and monitoring of proprietary and financial interests that may affect the scientific integrity and balance of content delivered in continuing medical education activities under our auspices.

The University of Virginia School of Medicine requires that all CME activities accredited through this institution be developed independently and be scientifically rigorous, balanced and objective in the presentation/discussion of its content, theories and practices.

All authors/editors participating in an accredited CME activity are expected to disclose to the readers relevant financial relationships with commercial entities occurring within the past 12 months (such as grants or research support, employee, consultant, stock holder, member of speakers bureau, etc.). The University of Virginia School of Medicine will employ appropriate mechanisms to resolve potential conflicts of interest to maintain the standards of fair and balanced education to the reader. Questions about specific strategies can be directed to the Office of Continuing Medical Education, University of Virginia School of Medicine, Charlottesville, Virginia.

The faculty and staff of the University of Virginia Office of Continuing Medical Education have no financial affiliations to disclose.

The authors/editors listed below have identified no professional or financial affiliations for themselves or their spouse/ partner:

Francesca Bisulli, MD; Cynthia Brown, MD (Test Author); Oliviero Bruni, MD; Gaetano Cantalupo, MD; Al W. de Weerd, MD, PhD; Martina della Corte, MD; Christopher P. Derry, MB BS, MRCP, PhD; Elena Gardella, MD, PhD; Madeleine M. Grigg-Damberger, MD (Guest Editor); Katie Hartner, (Acquisitions Editor); Wytske A. Hofstra-van Oostveen, MD, PhD; Sanjeev V. Kothare, MD; Elina Liukkonen, MD, PhD; Tobias Loddenkemper, MD; Alice Mallucci, MD; Luana Novelli, PhD; Dinesh V. Raju, MD, PhD; Antonino Romeo, MD; Guido Rubboli, MD; Carlo Alberto Tassinari, MD; and Martina Vendrame, MD, PhD.

The authors/editors listed below identified the following professional or financial affiliations for themselves or their spouse/ partner:

Charles M. Epstein, MD is a patent holder for Neuronetics, Inc., and is an industry funded research/investigator for Baxter Pharmaceuticals and GSK.
Raffaele Ferri, MD is a consultant for Sapio Life.
Nancy Foldvary-Schaefer, DO, MS (Guest Editor) is an industry funded research/investigator for UCB Pharma, Lundbeck, Teva Pharmaceuticals, and CleveMed, and is on the Speakers' Bureau for UCB Pharma.
Teofilo Lee- Chiong, Jr., MD (Consulting Editor) is employed by Respironics, and is an industry funded research/investigator for Respironics and Embla.
Federica Provini, MD is a consultant for Sanofi-Aventis.
Rodney A. Radtke, MD is a consultant and is on the Speakers' Bureau for UCB and GSK, and is a consultant for Eisai and Supernus.
Paolo Tinuper, MD is on the Speakers' Bureau for Cyberonics, Eisai, and Sanofi-Aventis; and is on the Speakers' Bureau and Advisory Board for GSK, Janssen-Cilag, Novartis, and UCB.

Disclosure of Discussion of Non-FDA Approved Uses for Pharmaceutical Products and/or Medical Devices.

The University of Virginia School of Medicine, as an ACCME provider, requires that all faculty presenters identify and disclose any off-label uses for pharmaceutical and medical device products. The University of Virginia School of Medicine recommends that each physician fully review all the available data on new products or procedures prior to clinical use.

TO ENROLL

To enroll in the Sleep Clinics of North America Continuing Medical Education program, call customer service at 1-800-654-2452 or visit us online at www.theclinics.com/home/cme. The CME program is available to subscribers for an additional fee of $114.00.

Sleep Medicine Clinics

THE CLINICS ARE NOW AVAILABLE ONLINE!

Access your subscription at:
www.theclinics.com

Contributors

CONSULTING EDITOR

TEOFILO LEE-CHIONG Jr, MD
Professor of Medicine and Chief, Division
of Sleep Medicine, National Jewish Health;
Associate Professor of Medicine, University
of Colorado Denver School of Medicine,
Denver, Colorado

GUEST EDITORS

MADELEINE M. GRIGG-DAMBERGER, MD
Professor of Neurology, Medical Director of
Pediatric Sleep Services, Associate Director of
the Clinical Neurophysiology Laboratory,
Department of Neurology, University of New
Mexico School of Medicine, Albuquerque,
New Mexico

NANCY FOLDVARY-SCHAEFER, DO, MS
Professor of Neurology, Cleveland Clinic
Lerner College of Medicine of Case Western
Reserve University; Director, Sleep Disorders
Center and Staff, Epilepsy Center Cleveland
Clinic Neurological Institute, Cleveland, Ohio

AUTHORS

FRANCESCA BISULLI, MD
Department of Neurological Sciences, IRCCS
Istituto delle Scienze Neurologiche, University
of Bologna, Bologna, Italy

OLIVIERO BRUNI, MD
Department of Developmental Neurology and
Psychiatry, Centre for Paediatric Sleep
Disorders, Sapienza University, Rome, Italy

GAETANO CANTALUPO, MD
Child Neurologist, Child Neuropsychiatry Unit,
University of Parma, Parma, Italy

AL W. DE WEERD, MD, PhD
Department of Clinical Neurophysiology and
Sleep Centre SEIN, Zwolle, The Netherlands

MARTINA DELLA CORTE, MD
Faculty of Medicine and Psychology, S. Andrea
Hospital, Rome, Italy

**CHRISTOPHER P. DERRY, MB BS,
MRCP, PhD**
Consultant Neurologist, Edinburgh and South
East Scotland Epilepsy Service, Department of
Clinical Neurosciences, Western General
Hospital, Edinburgh, United Kingdom

CHARLES M. EPSTEIN, MD
Professor of Neurology, Department of
Neurology, Emory University School of
Medicine, Atlanta, Georgia

RAFFAELE FERRI, MD
Department of Neurology, I.C., Sleep Research
Centre, Oasi Institute for Research on Mental
Retardation and Brain Aging (IRCCS),
Troina (EN), Italy

NANCY FOLDVARY-SCHAEFER, DO, MS
Professor of Neurology, Cleveland Clinic
Lerner College of Medicine of Case Western
Reserve University; Director, Sleep Disorders
Center and Staff, Epilepsy Center Cleveland
Clinic Neurological Institute, Cleveland, Ohio

ELENA GARDELLA, MD, PhD
Epileptologist, Danish Epilepsy Center, Epilepsihospitalet, Dianalund, Denmark; Epilepsy Center, San Paolo Hospital, University of Milan, Milan, Italy

MADELEINE M. GRIGG-DAMBERGER, MD
Professor of Neurology, Medical Director of Pediatric Sleep Services, Associate Director of the Clinical Neurophysiology Laboratory, Department of Neurology, University of New Mexico School of Medicine, Albuquerque, New Mexico

WYTSKE A. HOFSTRA-VAN OOSTVEEN, MD, PhD
Department of Neurology, Medisch Spectrum Twente Hospital, Enschede; Department of Clinical Neurophysiology and Sleep Centre SEIN, Zwolle, The Netherlands

SANJEEV V. KOTHARE, MD
Division of Epilepsy and Clinical Neurophysiology, Department of Neurology, Center for Pediatric Sleep Disorders, Harvard Medical School, Children's Hospital, Boston, Massachusetts

ELINA LIUKKONEN, MD, PhD
Pediatric Neurologist, Epilepsy Unit, Department of Pediatric Neurology, Helsinki University Central Hospital, Helsinki, Finland

TOBIAS LODDENKEMPER, MD
Assistant Professor of Neurology, Division of Epilepsy and Clinical Neurophysiology, Children's Hospital Boston, Harvard Medical School, Boston, Massachusetts

ALICE MALLUCCI, MD
Faculty of Medicine and Psychology, S. Andrea Hospital, Rome, Italy

LUANA NOVELLI, PhD
Department of Developmental Neurology and Psychiatry, Centre for Paediatric Sleep Disorders, Sapienza University; Department of Neuroscience, AFaR-Fatebenefratelli Hospital, Rome, Italy

FEDERICA PROVINI, MD
Department of Neurological Sciences, IRCCS Istituto delle Scienze Neurologiche, University of Bologna, Bologna, Italy

RODNEY A. RADTKE, MD
Department of Medicine (Neurology), Duke University Medical Center, Durham, North Carolina

DINESH V. RAJU, MD, PhD
Department of Medicine (Neurology), Duke University Medical Center, Durham, North Carolina

ANTONINO ROMEO, MD
Department of Neurosciences, Epilepsy Center, Fatebenefratelli e Oftalmico Hospital, Milano, Italy

GUIDO RUBBOLI, MD
Epileptologist, Danish Epilepsy Center, Epilepsihospitalet, Dianalund, Denmark; Neurology Unit, Bellaria Hospital, IRCCS Institute of Neurological Sciences, Bologna, Italy

CARLO ALBERTO TASSINARI, MD
Professor, Neuroscience Department, University of Parma, Parma, Italy

PAOLO TINUPER, MD
Department of Neurological Sciences, IRCCS Istituto delle Scienze Neurologiche, University of Bologna, Bologna, Italy

MARTINA VENDRAME, MD, PhD
Assistant Professor of Neurology, Division of Clinical Neurophysiology and Sleep, Department of Neurology, Boston University Medical Center, Boston, Massachusetts

Contents

> Optimum use of electroencephalography (EEG) can be improved by an understanding of the underlying signals and the nature of the recording and display technology. Topics reviewed in this section include the source of EEG signals; electrical noise; behavior of the amplifiers, filters, sampling, and displays; construction of EEG montages; quantitative EEG; and electrical safety. The author discusses how these considerations impact data quality and interpretation.

> The development of organized sleep/wake states is a major feature of the neonatal period and developing infant. Although subsequent changes in the sleep/wake cycle with age are less profound, they represent predictable physiologic changes occurring as a function of age. Similarly, there are characteristic electroencephalography (EEG) patterns seen as a function of maturity in the neonate and developing child. These EEG changes continue to evolve into adulthood, offering an electrophysiologic marker of brain development.

> Too many sleep specialists and technologists lament they lack sufficient training in recognizing abnormalities in the limited electroencephalography (EEG) channels recorded in a polysomnograph (PSG). Moreover, increasing numbers of patients with epilepsy, dementias, and extrapyramidal diseases are being referred to sleep centers, many of whom require recording of their PSGs with expanded EEG montages. This article reviews the range of normal, abnormal, and benign EEG variants encountered in patients undergoing PSG with conventional and expanded EEG montages. Because comprehensive in-laboratory PSGs are rarely requested for patients with severe acute encephalopathies, coma, or status epilepticus, discussion of these is omitted.

> Videopolysomnography with expanded electroencephalography (VEEG PSG) combines expanded EEG and PSG to evaluate unexplained paroxysmal nocturnal

events. VEEG PSG can also provide a more comprehensive assessment of patients with neurologic disorders undergoing PSG. VEEG PSG has several advantages over routine PSG, including (1) improving the likelihood of recognizing interictal and ictal EEG activity; (2) allowing for more precise evaluation of EEG background; and (3) correlating clinical with other neurophysiologic parameters. This article reviews epileptic EEG abnormalities encountered when evaluating patients with unexplained nocturnal events in the sleep laboratory and discusses strategies to optimize the diagnostic yield of EEG and videorecordings.

Seizures and epilepsies present with multiple causes and multiple clinical features, and change across the lifespan. Epilepsy is not a single disease but a diverse group of disorders that have in common an abnormally increased predisposition to epileptic seizures. A systematic approach to epileptic seizures and epilepsies is a first step toward the diagnosis and treatment of these disorders. Description of findings is crucial for selection of the most helpful diagnostic and therapeutic approach, defining relationships to sleep and sleep-related interactions, and comorbidities.

Many sleep disorder symptoms and some primary sleep disorders are two to three times more common in people with epilepsy than the general population. Adults with epilepsy and sleep complaints have significantly lower quality of life than those without sleep problems. Sleep problems in children with epilepsy are associated with negative effects on daytime behavior and academic performance. Late-onset or worsening seizure control in older adults may herald obstructive sleep apnea. Identifying and treating sleep disorders in people with epilepsy improves seizure control and quality of life in some cases. This article reviews the recent evidence for this claim.

Sleep deprivation can activate seizures in people with epilepsy, and a few without it. Sleep activates Interictal epileptiform discharges (IEDs). In many patients with epilepsy, IEDs are often seen only during sleep. The presence, type, and location of IEDs on an electroencephalogram (EEG) can help characterize the type of epilepsy and location of the epileptic focus, as well as predict whether seizures are likely to recur. Recording sleep in an EEG (with or without sleep deprivation or sedation) can increase the likelihood that IEDs will be found. This review provides a summary of research related to these issues.

Interaction between circadian rhythmicity and epilepsy or seizures may have important implications in diagnostic and therapeutic options, as EEGs and treatment can be individualized. In studies in humans and animals, seizure occurrence has been shown to have a 24-hour (ie, diurnal) rhythmicity, depending on the type of seizure and lobe of origin. A pilot study in humans suggested that temporal and frontal seizures not only occur in diurnal patterns but also are time locked to the circadian phase. A study in rats showed a true endogenous-mediated circadian rhythm in seizure occurrence in a rodent model of limbic epilepsy.

Nocturnal frontal lobe epilepsy (NFLE) is an epileptic syndrome characterized by a peculiar motor pattern with ballistic movements, bimanual-bipedal activity, rocking axial and pelvic torsion, and/or sustained dystonic posturing or tremor of the limbs often associated with emotional behaviors. Distinguishing NFLE seizures from non-epileptic sleep-related events, in particular arousal disorders, is often difficult and sometimes impossible by history taking alone. Because of its limited social impact, NFLE is usually considered a benign condition, but about a third of the cases are drug resistant. This article discusses the diagnostic and therapeutic challenges of NFLE.

Distinguishing epileptic seizures from nonepileptic disorders of sleep can be challenging. This article covers 3 main areas: a brief review of epileptic and nonepileptic disorders associated with paroxysmal events from sleep; a discussion of important features to be uncovered in the history; and a review of the value and limitations of investigations in this setting.

Central pattern generators (CPGs) are genetically determined neural circuits that produce self-sustained patterns of behavior that subserve innate motor activities essential for survival. In higher primates, CPGs are largely under neocortical control. Certain motor manifestations observed in parasomnias and epileptic seizures share similar semiological features resembling motor behaviors, which can be the expression of the same CPG. Epilepsy and sleep can lead to a temporary loss of control of neocortex on lower neural structures. We suggest that this transitory neocortical dysfunction facilitates the emergence of stereotyped inborn motor patterns that depend on the activation of the same CPGs.

Rolandic and occipital benign epilepsies of childhood are strictly linked to sleep but often no specific alterations of sleep organization were found. The spike activation is mostly evident in the first sleep cycle and related to EEG sigma band. NREM 1 and 2 sleep facilitate the spreading of epileptic discharges of benign childhood epilepsies while in NREM 3-4 sleep the spreading capacity is reduced. REM sleep inhibits both phenomena. Cyclic alternating pattern (CAP) modulates epileptiform discharges and seizures in lesional epilepsies, but shows no effect in the benign childhood epilepsies. Specific alterations of CAP structure (reduction of CAP rate and A1 phases in NREM 2) may shed light on the pathophysiology of cognitive disturbances of these children.

Encephalopathy with electrical status epilepticus in sleep (ESES) syndrome is a rare form of epilepsy in childhood. Results of treatment with antiepileptic medications or immunotherapy are variable. Epilepsy surgery should be considered in patients with a symptomatic cause. Cognitive outcome is more favorable in patients with an idiopathic form. Any newly observed seizure type or behavioral or developmental/cognitive symptom in children aged younger than 10 years with focal epilepsy should alert the clinician to the possibility of ESES syndrome. The exact pathophysiological mechanisms of ESES and associated functional impairments are still unresolved.

Sudden unexpected death in epilepsy (SUDEP) is the sudden unexpected death of a seemingly healthy individual with epilepsy. SUDEP is the commonest cause of death directly attributable to epilepsy, and most often occurs at or around the time of a seizure and during sleep. Sleep, respiration, arousal responses, and caudal brainstem serotoninergic neurons probably play roles in SUDEP, but more research is needed to understand these relationships. This article reviews the medical literature on the epidemiology, risk factors, and preventive measures for SUDEP in people with epilepsy, and discusses the roles of sleep, respiration, impaired autonomic functioning, and nocturnal seizures.

Foreword

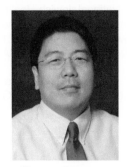

Teofilo Lee-Chiong Jr, MD
Consulting Editor

The Brain—is wider than the sky—
For—put them side by side—
The one the other will contain
With ease—and You—beside—

The Brain is deeper than the sea—
For—hold them—Blue to Blue—
The one the other will absorb—
As sponge—Buckets—do—

The Brain is just the weight of God—
For—Heft them—Pound for Pound—
And they will differ—if they do—
As Syllable from Sound—
—Emily Dickinson

The human brain, weighing about 3 lbs., is not the largest among mammals; those of the elephant (11 lbs.) and sperm whale (18 lbs.) are heavier. It does not even have the highest brain-to-body mass ratio—this distinction belongs to the shrew. Our *Homo sapien* brain is relatively small; indeed, it is smaller than those of Neanderthals, who have been extinct for over 35,000 years.

But what a brain! We *are* what our brains have made us, limited only by what our body can withstand. The human brain has created all facets of human civilization—

- Over 6500 living languages, and countless more from nameless peoples from time immemorial to both enlighten as well as confuse;
- Engineering and exploration to extend the reach of humans beyond their grasp;
- The building of governments, and the destruction of war;

- Music to excite and incite, and music to uplift the human spirit;
- Commerce and fashion to create demand for goods beyond the basic necessities of living;
- Sports to discipline the body; education to unleash thought and creativity; and
- Religions to provide answers that philosophy and science cannot.

Various analogies for the human brain have been proposed throughout the ages. The ancient Greeks considered the brain a puppeteer that is able to control our actions by strings. The word "neuron" is derived from the Greek word *neûron* meaning "a sinew, string, or wire." The French philosopher Rene Descartes suggested that the mind is like a watch that is wound and set in motion by God. The brain has been considered a complex machine during the industrial age, and a vast switchboard during the era of telecommunications. More recently, the brain is most popularly thought of as a data-processing device, ie, a computer, albeit a very fast one. This last comparison is not unreasonable, especially given the rapid increase in speed and capacity of our computers, and had led to some attempts to ascribe to both the brain and the computer comparable "disorders" (brain = computer): stroke = bad hardware sectors; dementia = failed RAM chip; attention deficit hyperactivity disorder = memory fragmentation; headache = malware; and seizures = static charge surge.

Many wonder whether computers will ever replace humans—in many instances, they already do. Computers have outperformed humans in mathematical calculations, and on February 10, 1996, "Deep Blue" became the first computer to win a chess game against a reigning world chess champion.

Sleep Med Clin 7 (2012) xi–xii
doi:10.1016/j.jsmc.2012.02.003

sleep.theclinics.com

Perhaps a time will come when computers will create languages, undergo explorations, control governments, declare war, enjoy music, worry about their looks, exercise to keep in shape, teach future generations, and believe in a god. Perhaps, a time will come when computers will even outperform humans in deceit, treachery, dishonesty, greed, and cruelty. When that time comes, if it comes, what then is the brain to do, where there is nothing at all to do?

Teofilo Lee-Chiong Jr, MD
Division of Sleep Medicine
National Jewish Health
University of Colorado Denver School of Medicine
1400 Jackson Street, Room J221
Denver, CO 60206, USA

E-mail address:
Lee-ChiongT@NJC.ORG

Preface

Sleep-Related Epilepsy and Electroencephalography

Relationships between sleep and epilepsy have been described since antiquity. In recent decades, polysomnography (PSG) and video electroencephalography (EEG) have extended early clinical observations. In turn, heightened awareness of these complex relationships has increased the role of the sleep clinician and sleep laboratory in the evaluation and treatment of patients with epilepsy and unexplained events in sleep.

In this volume of *Sleep Medicine Clinics*, experts in the fields of epileptology, sleep medicine, and EEG provide an overview of the basic concepts of EEG and seizure/epilepsy classification and highlight specific sleep-related epilepsies and aspects of the field that are relatively well established or rapidly evolving.

We begin with the nuts and bolts of EEG by Dr Epstein, who discusses the origin of the scalp EEG and illustrates common electrode artifacts, filters, sampling rates, and derivations and montages for the polysomnographer. Drs Raju and Radtke and Drs Vendrame and Kothare discuss the ontogeny of normal EEG, benign variants commonly mistaken for epileptic activity, and nonepileptiform EEG abnormalities and their significance in polysomnographic recordings. We discuss the indications for combining EEG and PSG to evaluate unexplained nocturnal events and assess patients with neurological disorders in the sleep laboratory. We illustrate various ictal and interical EEG abnormalities and EEG localization rules and offer strategies to optimize the yield of EEG and video recordings in the sleep laboratory. Recognizing seizures and epilepsies in the sleep clinic and laboratory requires knowledge of seizure semiology, its implications on epilepsy localization, and the history of epilepsy classification. In the last of these introductory articles, Drs Vendrame and Loddenkemper review the

approach to evaluating patients with seizures and provide the framework for classifying epilepsy using the clinical history, neuroimaging, and electrophysiological testing.

Sleep is an important modulator of interictal EEG abnormalities and seizures. Sleep deprivation and sleep disorders activate some types of epilepsy. Furthermore, seizures in certain epilepsies are closely linked with the sleep/wake cycle, underscoring the importance of routinely assessing sleep/wake complaints in patients with epilepsy. We then review the prevalence of sleep complaints and primary sleep disorders in people with epilepsy and the diagnostic yield of sleep and sleep deprivation on the EEG. Drs Hofstra-van Oostveen and de Weerd discuss the impact of circadian rhythms on seizure occurrence in different epilepsy syndromes.

Next, several epileptic disorders characterized by seizures appearing predominately or exclusively in sleep are highlighted. Dr Provini and colleagues discuss nocturnal frontal lobe epilepsies (NFLE) and the diagnostic challenges these syndromes pose to sleep specialists and epileptologists alike. The differentiation between NFLE and disorders of arousal and other paroxysmal nocturnal events is then reviewed by Dr Derry. Dr Rubboli and colleagues discuss the role of central pattern generators (CPGs), neural circuits producing stereotyped motor activities essential for survival, and the hypothesis that activation of CPGs produces similar motor behaviors in parasomnias and epileptic seizures. Dr Bruni and colleagues review rolandic and occipital benign epilepsies of childhood, the most common epileptic disorders in childhood and strictly linked to sleep. Drs Liukkonen and Grigg-Damberger describe electrographic status epilepticus in slow-wave sleep, an EEG pattern characterized

Sleep Med Clin 7 (2012) xiii–xiv
doi:10.1016/j.jsmc.2012.02.001

by continuous spike-wave discharges during NREM sleep, typically associated with seizures, cognitive regression, and motor impairments. Finally, Dr Grigg-Damberger discusses sudden unexpected death in epilepsy (SUDEP), the most common cause of death directly attributable to epilepsy and a research priority in the scientific community. The roles of sleep, respiration, impaired autonomic functioning, and nocturnal seizures in SUDEP are reviewed.

We hope you enjoy this volume of *Sleep Medicine Clinics* on sleep-related epilepsy and EEG and find it a useful resource when evaluating patients in your sleep clinic and laboratory. These reviews illustrate a multitude of opportunities available to sleep and epilepsy investigators for clinical and basic research in this exciting, rapidly evolving field.

Madeleine M. Grigg-Damberger, MD
Department of Neurology
University of New Mexico School of Medicine
MSC10 5620, One University of NM
Albuquerque, NM 87131-0001, USA

Nancy Foldvary-Schaefer, DO, MS
Cleveland Clinic Lerner College of Medicine of
Case Western Reserve University
Epilepsy Center
Cleveland Clinic Neurological Institute
9500 Euclid Avenue, FA 20
Cleveland, OH 44195, USA

E-mail addresses:
mgriggd@salud.unm.edu (M.M. Grigg-Damberger)
foldvan@ccf.org (N. Foldvary-Schaefer)

The Nuts and Bolts of Electroencephalography

Charles M. Epstein, MD

KEYWORDS

- Electroencephalography • Polysomnography • Epilepsy
- Technical polysomnography
- Technical electroencephalography

Electroencephalography (EEG) and polysomnography (PSG) have evolved together since their infancy. **Fig. 1** shows single-channel sleep EEG samples performed by Charles Henry in 1939, in an era when EEG and PSG were identical enterprises and every recording was an adventure. Since then, the number of channels, convenience, and flexibility of recording have grown enormously but the fundamentals of detecting and interpreting electrical signals from the human body have changed far less. This article reviews some of the basics of EEG technology and discusses how an understanding of them can help inform both recording and interpretation.

ORIGIN OF THE SCALP EEG

The electrical activity of neurons falls primarily into 2 categories: postsynaptic potentials and action potentials. Postsynaptic potentials are slow fluctuations of the voltage across neuronal cell membranes, extending over many milliseconds. These fluctuations represent excitatory and inhibitory postsynaptic potentials, caused by the arrival of various neurotransmitters at synapses on the cell body and dendrites. Such potentials may also arise by direct electrical contact in so-called gap junctions.

Action potentials are brief, explosive depolarizations that only last a millisecond or less and are triggered by postsynaptic potentials near the origin of the axon at the cell body, and then conducted rapidly along axons for distances ranging from millimeters to meters. Action potentials are too small, brief, and unsynchronized for their effects to do anything but cancel out over the great distance between the brain and the scalp. Instead, EEG recorded at the scalp seems to represent the ever-changing sum of synchronous postsynaptic potentials arising from broad cerebral cortical areas.

For EEG signals to be detected through the skull and other intervening tissues, synchronous activity must extend over cortical areas of 10 cm^2 or more, which does not mean that all of the neurons in that area are behaving synchronously; perhaps only a small fraction of them are. Ten cm^2 is the cortical expanse possessed by a medium-sized rodent.[1] Because a rodent brain is capable of doing many different things simultaneously, this consideration may place significant limitations on the level of detail in the information that can be extracted from scalp EEG.

Fig. 2 shows a sketch of large pyramidal cells oriented vertically through the layers of the human cerebral cortex. Excitatory neurotransmitter receptors tend to be clustered distally in the dendrites and inhibitory receptors closer to the cell body. Excitation of the dendritic membrane generates a net flow of negative charge into the extracellular space of the upper cortical layers. Inhibition of the proximal cell membrane produces a net positivity in the extracellular space at deeper layers. The resulting extracellular dipoles tend to be distributed vertically through the depth of the cortex. Multiplied across millions of neurons, this stratification of electrical charge produces the scalp EEG.

AMPLIFICATION AND ELECTRICAL NOISE

The resting potential across the neuronal membrane represents an astonishing voltage in a microscopic space; scaled up to familiar sizes, it would

The author has no financial or other conflicts of interest to report related to this article.
Department of Neurology, Emory University School of Medicine, 1365A Clifton Road, Northeast, Atlanta, GA 30322, USA
E-mail address: charles.epstein@emory.edu

Sleep Med Clin 7 (2012) 1–12
doi:10.1016/j.jsmc.2012.01.005

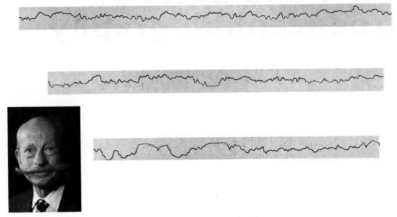

Fig. 1. Strips of single-channel sleep EEG recorded in 1939 by Chuck Henry.

throw sparks and produce serious shocks. By the time this activity reaches the scalp, their neuronal voltages are attenuated thousandfold, to the range of 20 to 50 µV. This magnitude is roughly the size of a weak radio signal and must be amplified enormously before it can be processed and displayed.

A 50 µV EEG signal at the scalp is far smaller than the many sources of noise that threaten to disrupt or obliterate it and is subject to distortion at many stages of the recording process. First, the signal must be amplified many thousands of times for proper analysis; the multiplication factor is called *gain*. But amplification of the EEG is straightforward; more bothersome is the large

range of other electrical noise (from the body and the external environment) that can swamp the EEG entirely (**Fig. 3**). Certain electrical activity (from muscle contraction, cardiac conduction, and eye movement) represents noise when it appears in the EEG channels but it is a desired PSG signal when recorded in the appropriate PSG channels.

Many artifactual potentials that corrupt the EEG signal in PSG arise from the clutter of electrical wires and equipment that surrounds us in modern buildings, producing electrical noise that permeates our bodies whenever we are inside them. The largest source of such noise is the 60-cycle field from nearby electrical equipment and power lines, which can easily be hundreds of times larger than the EEG.

Many years ago, frustrated neurophysiologists attempted to avoid environmental noise by recording inside metal enclosures (Faraday

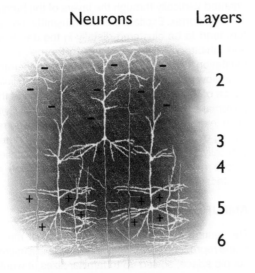

Fig. 2. The larger neurons in the layers of the cerebral cortex, with long vertically oriented dendrites. The + and − signs indicate vertical separation of charge in the extracellular space during postsynaptic potentials. Synchrony of such potentials across many square centimeters of cortex produces a detectable potential difference at the overlying scalp.

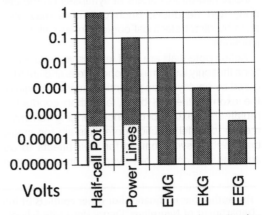

Fig. 3. The enormous range of electrical activity that can be recorded from the human body. Note that the vertical axis is a logarithmic scale in volts. EKG, electrocardiogram; EMG, electromyogram.

cages). Such enclosures remain necessary for magnetic resonance imaging and for the infinitesimal signals of magnetoencephalography but in EEG and PSG they can usually be avoided with the use of modern amplifiers.

Because electrical noise can be orders of magnitude larger than EEG and other neurophysiological signals (see **Fig. 3**), it may seem surprising that we ever see the EEG at all. The key is that enormous as the interfering signals may be, many of them are almost identical on closely adjacent portions of the body. Thus, an exact subtraction of the activity from nearby electrodes can remove the noise those electrodes have in common (common-mode signal) and record only the activity that is different at those electrodes (differential-mode signal.)

This accurate subtraction of the common-mode signal requires a precisely balanced input stage called a differential amplifier, which classically involves a 3-electrode input: a hot positive terminal, a hot negative terminal, and a neutral or ground connection. The ground lead is explicit in electromyography (EMG) and electrocardiography (EKG). In EEG and PSG, a single ground electrode serves multiple channels and is most often placed on the forehead.

The cleanup factor for a differential amplifier is called the common-mode rejection ratio and is supposed to be 10,000 or greater. In practice, problems like unequal electrode properties, poor ground connections, or noise sources in direct contact with the body can degrade amplifier performance, allowing 60-cycle artifact and other noise to appear in the EEG.

It is easy to think that the 60-Hz noise can simply be removed with the notch filters but other types of common-mode signals that accompany it cannot. Thus, the notch filters should be left off whenever humanly possible, allowing 60-Hz noise to serve as the electrical equivalent of a canary in a mine shaft.

ELECTRODES

EEG, EMG, and EKG electrodes provide the essential interface between lead wires and human tissues. Placing dry metal electrodes directly on dry skin is usually ineffective at conducting electrical potentials; skin preparation is necessary to remove cutaneous oils and reduce the insulating effect of keratin. An ionic solution, or electrolyte, provides an essential conductive layer on the scalp.

However, the interface between the electrolyte and the metal electrode produces a chemical half-cell potential, which is, essentially, half of an electric battery and can be much larger even than the 60-Hz noise (see **Fig. 3**). Avoiding possible interference requires careful design of the amplifier, use of a low-frequency filter (LF), and matching electrodes to produce minimal size and variation in the half-cell potential.

For the latter reason, gold and silver-silver chloride electrodes have been widely preferred. Disposable stick-on electrodes with a layer of conductive gel and a small amount of silver-silver chloride tend to be more uniform and are easier to use on areas that are free of hair. However, all skin connections are imperfect and manifest a certain amount of *impedance*, which is the term for all of the factors that oppose current flow.

The effectiveness of the differential amplifier depends on equal impedances at the 2 hot input terminals. Large and unequal electrode impedances can allow unpredictable amounts of common-mode noise to appear at the output. Most often, the common-mode noise is a 60-Hz artifact. Occasionally it represents other activity, including EKG and pickup from the ground electrode on the forehead. **Fig. 4** is a complex example of the latter. Poor electrode connections were obscured because the 60-Hz filter was turned on, but this artifact was detected because of its pattern across multiple derivations. With fewer

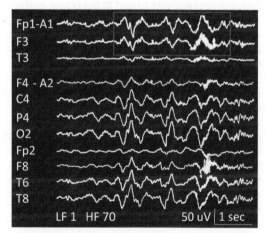

Fig. 4. Ground recording artifact in a segment of paper EEG using an ipsilateral ear reference montage. Note that only selected channels from the left and right hemisphere are shown, to give a more compact display. Outlined in red is frontal slow activity over the left hemisphere. Directly below it there seems to be a burst of posterior temporal, parietal, and occipital slowing on the right. Close inspection shows that the right-sided posterior activity is actually the inverse of the left-sided frontal activity. The latter has been picked up from the ground electrode on the forehead. All of the apparent slowing on the right is ground recording artifact. HF, high frequency filter.

channels it might have been extremely difficult to recognize. The best way to avoid unpredictable common-mode artifacts is not to apply the 60-Hz filters routinely but to use good technique and keep the electrode impedances low.

GROUND

In North America, ground has 3 different but overlapping meanings: (1) True earth ground (a physical connection to the whole planet through metal plumbing or other low-resistance conduits) is a wonderful zero-potential point—a near-infinite reservoir for storing or withdrawing electrons. Stray charges, like lightning, head for earth ground. (2) Ground in electrical circuits is a reference point that remains at a virtual zero voltage and may or may not be connected to earth. (3) In the classic 3-terminal differential amplifier, the recording ground is the neutral reference lead.

Be advised that confusing the 3 meanings of ground can be fatal, because one of the 2 wires in alternating current (AC) power lines is almost always connected to earth ground at the local power station. To operate electrical devices plugged into the AC wall jack, the current flows from the hot wire of the power line to the neutral wire at earth ground. Connecting the reference ground on patients to earth ground would, therefore, connect patients to part of the power system. If patients are connected to earth ground, any stray currents (especially those from the hot power line) will happily flow through patients on the way there.

All grounded metal surfaces and grounded electrodes are potential routes through which a stray current can electrocute patients. A third power wire, which represents a second and more direct earth ground connection, is required for all hospital equipment. This additional ground, commonly referred to as "the" ground, increases safety overall, but in rare situations also constitutes a risk if the connection fails or patients contact voltage from another source.

The core principal of modern neurophysiological safety standards is that the recording ground on patients cannot form a direct connection to the power line grounds or to other sources of earth ground. Patients should not be in contact with any other earth ground, although they may inevitably encounter it in the form of hospital plumbing fixtures. In most modern electronic equipment, every electrode jack is separated from patients and the rest of the recording system by an optical isolation system.

Traditionally, discussions of electrical safety have focused on ground loops, which may be formed when patients are connected to more than one recording ground through different pieces of medical equipment. With proper isolation of the electrodes, ground loops are no longer a safety issue but may still contribute substantially to electrical noise.

ANALOG VERSUS DIGITAL RECORDING

Over the past few decades, the transformation from analog to digital PSG has brought substantial advantages. The greatest of these is the ability to review EEG and respiratory activity independently at the optimum time scale for each. Even during the era of paper, many scorers and readers found it desirable to page through a PSG 2 or more times, concentrating separately on sleep stages, respiration, arousals, and EKG. The 30-second epoch of PSG compressed the data close to the limit of resolution for sleep spindles and well beyond it for many forms of epileptic EEG activity. At the same time, 30-second epochs are still too fast for easy recognition of some respiratory events, such as prolonged mild hypopneas. Reading the PSG at multiple display resolutions from 10 seconds to several minutes per screen page improves both speed and accuracy.

The ability to alter the display resolution, filters, sensitivity, and EEG montages can improve analysis of suboptimal data and helps greatly to refine interpretation of the recording. The ease with which scored data can be summarized into a - hypnogram assists greatly in understanding the findings and communicating them to other physicians and patients. The savings in paper, ink, and space required to store a complete PSG is enormous, and the digital storage capacity needed for a full PSG and multichannel EEG is smaller than that for the simultaneous video that now often accompanies it.

The downsides of digital PSG are subtler. Knowing that gain and filter settings can be optimized after the fact, technologists may become less conscientious in adjusting them, which is a dereliction that can easily spread to poor electrode connections, loose sensors, and other sources of artifact that are *not* subsequently correctible. Studies may be run with the 60-Hz notch filter on routinely, a maneuver that seems to clean up the record but also allows the intrusion of difficult and often irremediable artifacts, as noted later. Physicians may come to depend excessively on the graphical summary and on automatic reports rather than on their own review of the raw data, thus, overlooking errors in scoring, epileptiform activity, and potentially dangerous arrhythmias. Even at 10 seconds per screen, PSG on a computer monitor has less high-frequency resolution than paper.

FILTERS

In the analog era, the filters used to select frequencies of interest, and get rid of those we would prefer not to see, consisted of resistors and capacitors. Final filtering of data for display is now performed in software. However, hardware filtering is still desirable at the limits of recording. Before the analog-to-digital conversion that transfers the electrical signal into the computer, a LF that eliminates activity less than approximately 0.1 Hz helps to block the considerable drift that may occur in the electrode half-cell potentials. LF drift may be caused by drying out or diluting the electrolyte, sweating, movement artifacts, and galvanic skin responses.

A particular LF setting (eg, 0.3 Hz) specifies the cutoff frequency at which the amplitude of that frequency is reduced by a set percentage (classically about 30%). The amplitude of frequencies slower than the LF cutoff frequency will be reduced more drastically. Note the contradictory terminology for EEG or PSG low and high frequency filters (HF): What clinicians call the low filter is known to engineers as a high-pass filter and what clinicians call the high filter is known to engineers as a low-pass filter.

HF filters are designed to attenuate faster activity; the HF cutoff frequency is that above which the amplitude is reduced. Many digital systems have steeper roll off for HF, which reduces demand on the sampling rate of the analog-to-digital converter.

To avoid aliasing of the digital signal (see next paragraph), an HF is needed to limit excess high frequency activity (primarily EMG).[2] **Fig. 5** illustrates the properties of a simple LF and HF produced by 2 sets of resistors and capacitors. Compared with a few physical components, digital filters can produce much steeper slopes in the stopband than those shown in **Fig. 5**. Nonetheless, it is clear that the boundary between the passband and the stopband is never exact.

LIMITATIONS OF COMPUTER MONITOR SCREEN RESOLUTION

With one exception, digital PSG technology has advanced sufficiently that the technical issues of sampling rate, bit resolution, dynamic range, and storage space should no longer be a concern. The one exception is the computer monitor resolution. Even a high-definition 1080 display has less

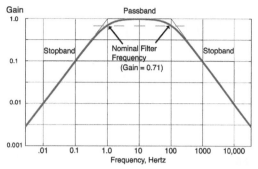

Fig. 5. Log-log plot of an LF at 1.0 Hz, high filter at 100 Hz, and the resulting passband. The dotted green line indicates the nominal filter frequencies, at which 71% of the signal still passes through, meaning that a considerable amount of activity in the adjacent stopband is not, in fact, completely blocked. Simply moving the straight descending sections of the red curve to the left or right can plot other filter frequencies. This elegant symmetry of the HF and LF is present only in a logarithmic display.

than 2000 discrete points, or pixels, across the screen. This is actually much poorer spatial resolution that was available using paper. With a portion of the screen devoted to annotations, a 30-second EEG sample will be assigned approximately 50 pixels per second. The highest-frequency activity that can be displayed accurately at 50 pixels per second is around 10 to 12 Hz. Even worse, data frequencies more than 25 Hz will be subject to *aliasing*, an irreversible alteration of the data that generates spurious activity at lower frequencies. A minimum computer monitor resolution for PSG of 1600 × 1200 pixels is recommended. Allowing for notations, a 30-second epoch over a horizontal span of 1600 pixels would result in an effective sampling rate less than 50 Hz and some frequencies will be distorted down to the alpha range. Viewing the PSG at shorter display times (eg, 10-second or even 5-second epochs) will improve the resolution of the waveforms.

SAMPLING RATES

Fig. 6 shows the effect of a decreasing sampling rate on a continuous sine wave as the sampling frequency decreases. Below about 5 samples per wave, there is increasing distortion of the original waveform. Below the critical frequency of 2 samples per wave, aliasing causes some of the original waves to be lost and generates spurious waveforms at lower frequencies. On occasion, aliasing generates activity that can be mistaken for EEG.[2] Classically, aliasing is avoided by (1) increasing the sampling rate or (2) filtering the analog signal before digitization to

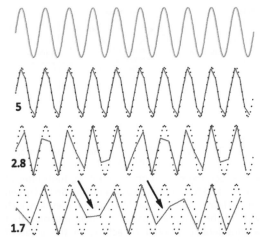

Fig. 6. Progressive distortion of a continuous sine wave as the analog-to-digital sampling rate decreases. At the top, in green, are the original continuous data. The dotted blue curves in the lower 3 graphs outline the original waveform at 20 samples per wave. The solid red lines show the waveform as seen by the computer at the indicated sampling rates. Arrows indicate the appearance of aliasing, or spurious activity at lower frequencies, at sampling rates less than twice per wave.

remove waveforms with a frequency faster than half the analog-to-digital sampling rate. However, neither of these data-processing techniques will help with the limited real estate of computer screen displays.

In an attempt to avoid aliasing, digital display manufacturers commonly use special processing techniques; these techniques in turn can behave like an extra high filter, further degrading the appearance of frequencies above the low alpha range. Muscle activity can be unexpectedly attenuated. Narrow epileptic spike discharges, in particular, can be decimated (**Fig. 7**). Conversely, benign waveforms in the background can closely resemble interictal epileptic discharges (IEDs) in displays of 30 seconds per page (**Fig. 8**C, D). The moral is that *reading for epileptic discharges must be done at display speeds faster than 30 seconds per page.*

DERIVATIONS AND MONTAGES

A derivation is the pair of electrodes in a given EEG channel. A montage is the collection of derivations in a particular screen display. A common frustration among beginning electroencephalographers is the insistence of their mentors on using multiple montages to review a given record. This practice is not an obscure hazing ritual; it derives instead from the regrettable fact that no single montage can give optimal display of all EEG abnormalities.

Montages come in 2 major families: bipolar (differential) and referential. Bipolar montages form chains along the scalp; are relatively free of artifact; and, most importantly, produce *instrumental phase reversal*, which causes surface-negative spikes and sharp waves to point toward each other and makes them intuitively easier to recognize (see **Fig. 8**A). The greatest disadvantage of bipolar montages is that they may obscure activity that covers broad areas and give an inaccurate representation of where the highest-amplitude activity actually resides.

Referential montages distribute the negative inputs for multiple channels to different locations on the scalp and then cluster the positive inputs from all those channels at a single reference point. An ideal reference would be electrically silent, completely free of EMG, EKG, and its own underlying EEG. The signal from the negative, exploring electrode would then give a perfect representation of the activity beneath it.

The perfect reference does not exist. The references that do exist have their unique advantages and disadvantages. Because of the long interelectrode distance, a vertex reference magnifies activity from the temporal lobes; conversely, references at the ears or mastoids magnify activity from the central regions. Both of these can, however, be contaminated by EEG activity near the reference electrode, which interpreters must learn to recognize.

An average reference, which electronically computes the average of most of the electrodes on the head (see **Fig. 8**B), is attractive because it seems to give all of the exploring electrodes equal weighting and is free of the EKG artifact that often bedevils ear, mastoid, and even vertex references. However, like the others, an average reference can be contaminated, in this case, by activity that is large and widespread in one scalp area.

All EEG montages should be designed to give a simple, logical mapping of electrode locations on the scalp. Montages that skip around excessively may satisfy their inventors but place a needless burden on other interpreters.

A major technical difference from the analog era is that the original recordings are commonly made in referential mode, with all channels connected to a common reference electrode. The data are then digitally reformatted to produce any combination of electrode connections that the interpreter desires. Typically, the reference electrode, which is separate from the neutral ground electrode, is placed in the midline around the central parietal region.

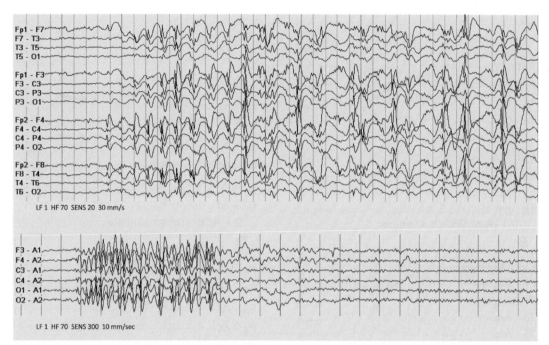

Fp1 - F7
F7 - T3
T3 - T5
T5 - O1

Fp1 - F3
F3 - C3
C3 - P3
P3 - O1

Fp2 - F4
F4 - C4
C4 - P4
P4 - O2

Fp2 - F8
F8 - T4
T4 - T6
T6 - O2

LF 1 HF 70 SENS 20 30 mm/s

F3 - A1
F4 - A2
C3 - A1
C4 - A2
O1 - A1
O2 - A2

LF 1 HF 70 SENS 300 10 mm/sec

Fig. 7. At the top, a burst of generalized spike wave in a conventional 16-channel EEG montage at 30 mm/s. A sensitivity of 20 uV/mm is needed to define this high-voltage discharge. At the bottom, the same burst in sleep derivations at 10 mm/s. Although the evolution of the burst frequency from faster to slower is clearly visible, the narrow spikes have mostly been erased by compression into an inadequate number of screen pixels. Note the sensitivity setting of 300 uV/mm required to match the long interelectrode distances of the sleep channels. HF, high frequency.

EEG ABNORMALITIES IN PSG RECORDING

Given the limited number of EEG channels in standard PSGs, any possibility of recognizing IEDs or ictal EEG activity depends on the location of the electrodes. After 5 or 6 years of age, most focal IEDs emanate from the temporal regions. Limited EEG derivations that lack either or both of the ear/mastoid electrodes are less likely to detect temporal IEDs.

Recording focal seizures on PSG is a rare event; however, when present, these are likely to be most prominent in the temporal and frontal regions. The crossed-ear references, central and frontal electrodes recommended by the American Academy of Sleep Medicine Scoring Manual,[3] are conveniently located to sample these areas, provided that both of the ears (or mastoids) are included. Purely midline derivations, such as Fz-Cz (permitted as an alternative EEG derivation in the manual) are unlikely to provide information about focal epilepsy. Thus, polysomnographers interested in looking for supportive evidence for epilepsy should be using a larger number of EEG channels than needed for sleep scoring alone (see **Fig. 8**C, D). Occasionally, when a mesial

temporal focus is reflected most strongly at the ear/mastoid electrode, interictal epileptic activity can seem to come from the wrong side. For polysomnographers, such false lateralization is probably less important than recognition of a serious abnormality.

All polysomnographers are trained in using EEG to stage wakefulness and sleep, and are thus reasonably prepared to recognize generalized slowing in the waking record. Identification of focal slowing, like that of focal spikes or sharp waves, is contingent on having enough EEG channels to assess areas of both hemispheres independently. However, an unsuspected brain lesion large enough to produce regional EEG slowing is a rare event.

Of much greater concern to polysomnographers is missing IEDs or ictal electrographic seizure activity in a PSG. Recognizing the footprints of epilepsy is not always an easy task. To make it even more challenging, the classic recording techniques for recognizing and distinguishing IEDs display 18 to 21 channels of EEG at 10 seconds per screen, with multiple montages used routinely.

The good news is that digital PSG technology provides the ability to do these things for every

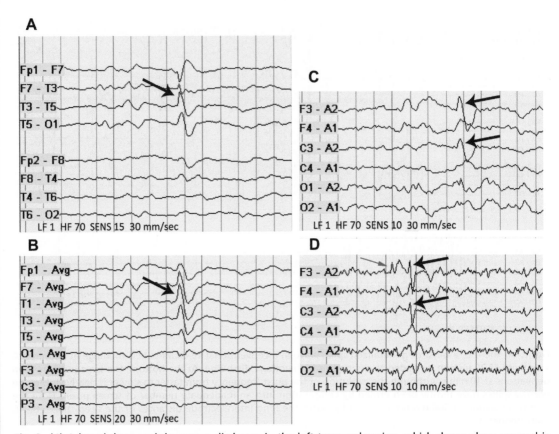

Fig. 8. (*A*) A broad sharp-and-slow wave discharge in the left temporal region, which shows phase reversal in conventional bipolar EEG derivations (*arrow*). (*B*) The same sharp-slow discharge using average reference derivations. Unlike the bipolar chain, this type of EEG display shows the actual location of the sharp wave in the electrode with highest amplitude, here T_1 (*arrow*). (*C*) The same discharge shown using sleep EEG derivations and display times of 10 seconds per page. (*D*) The same discharge in sleep derivations at 30 seconds per page (*arrow*). Note that just to the left of the sharp-slow complex, indicated by the red arrow, is a benign up-going slow wave that closely resembles it at this display speed.

patient. The bad news is that reviewing digital PSG data to identify IEDs and seizures properly takes not just extensive training and experience in EEG but also large amounts of additional review time. Even for experienced electroencephalographers, recognizing evidence of epilepsy can be challenging, especially when a limited number of EEG derivations are recorded and displayed. Interictal and ictal epileptiform discharges must not only be detected but also distinguished from a wide variety of normal variants and recording artifacts that closely resemble them. Spiky, sharply contoured, paroxysmal, and rhythmic nonepileptic activity is common in the EEG and PSG (**Fig. 9**).

Identifying IEDs in a digital PSG is not dependent on any single feature but rather on recognizing a complex pattern likely to be epileptic. Attributes that increase the likelihood a spike or sharp waveform is epileptic include the following: (1) IEDs have a sharp or spiky component; but spikiness alone is

not in any way a diagnostic finding. (2) After the neonatal period a spike or sharp wave is usually surface negative. So, in strings of bipolar derivations (see **Figs. 7** and **8**), the spike-wave discharges show a surface-negative phase reversal and point toward each other over their area of maximal scalp electronegativity. Phase reversal makes an IED much easier to recognize. (3) Spikes and sharp waves are most often followed by a slow wave. (4) IEDs are small explosions within the cortex that interrupt the ongoing background and are not ordinarily parts of rhythmic sequences of normal EEG waves. Statistically, IEDs and seizures are most likely to occur in non–rapid eye movement (NREM) sleep and are easiest to recognize in NREM 1 and NREM 2 sleep.

It is useful to remember a criterion first described by John Knott decades ago: the apparent spike-wave complex must be more than a random amalgam of various pointy shapes and

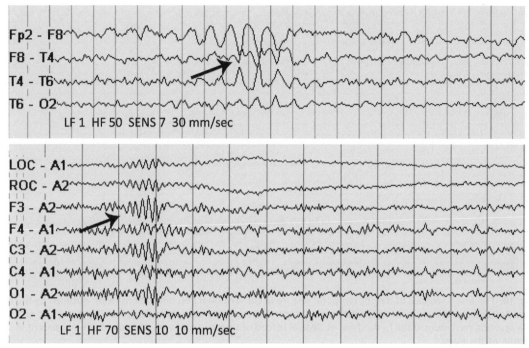

Fig. 9. At top, a train of spikey activity right temporal during drowsiness, shown in 4 bipolar EEG channels (*arrow*). At bottom, the same activity in sleep derivations, where it is maximal at the ear electrode A_2 (*arrow*). This classic rhythmic midtemporal theta of drowsiness is completely benign.

slow waves that are present elsewhere in that portion of the recording. Finally, and most important, polysomnographers should not expect to find evidence of epilepsy often when it is not suspected.

Generalized spike-wave discharges (the hallmark of genetic or primary generalized epilepsies) tend to occur at regular rates around 3 per second in wakefulness but may seem to be more fragmentary in sleep and in older patients. Bursts of generalized spike waves lasting only a few seconds are usually asymptomatic. However, bursts that last longer than 5 seconds are increasingly likely to be accompanied by changes in behavior and, thus, to represent actual seizures (see **Fig. 7**). Note that in the bottom half of **Fig. 7**, the spike components are greatly attenuated by the limited number of screen pixels at 30 seconds per page; the pattern could easily be mistaken for a less-specific burst of rhythmic delta.

Focal-onset seizures most often do NOT contain spike activity. Instead, focal electrographic seizures are characterized by rhythmic activity in the theta, alpha, or delta range, which may start gradually or suddenly, evolve, and then end abruptly (**Fig. 10**). The evolution of a focal electrographic seizure includes changes in EEG frequency (usually from faster to slower) and spatial distribution (commonly from a limited number of EEG channels to a broader area of the scalp). Rhythmic activity that does not evolve should not be interpreted as epilepsy. In a limited number of sleep derivations, evolution in frequency can often be easier to recognize than evolution in space.

COMPUTERIZED EEG

Quantitative EEG analysis (QEEG) by Fourier transform was performed in Europe and America as early as the 1930s[4] and became practical with the development of more powerful, accessible, and personal digital computers in the 1970s and 1980s. Although many different quantitative techniques have been used, the most common remains a digital version of the Fourier transform applied by Knott and others 70 years ago. The Fourier theorem states that any infinitely repeating series, including the most complicated EEG, can be represented as a collection of sine waves having different frequencies, amplitudes, and phases. The Fourier transform identifies those sine waves. **Fig. 11** shows 2 examples.

Software to graph EEG background trends, spikes, seizures, and respiratory events is now widely available. The uses of trending software to help identify seizures and other changes[5] are illustrated in **Fig. 12**. Other digital EEG computer

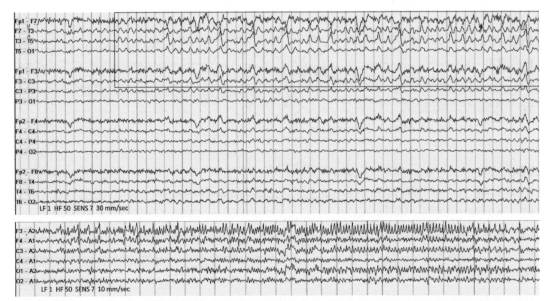

Fig. 10. The first 9 seconds of a right temporal seizure in conventional EEG derivations (*top*), outlined by the red box. Bottom, the seizure in sleep recording at 30 seconds per page. The seizure occupies all but the first and last few seconds, maximum in the F$_3$-A$_2$ channel. Spatial spread of seizure activity to other channels is apparent in the middle of the page.

software programs are intended to assist interpreters by actually identifying IEDs and seizures. Such software represents, at best, a tradeoff in sensitivity and specificity; when applied to long recordings from sleep patients, who are overall unlikely to experience epileptic seizures, the false-positive rate increases to astronomic levels.

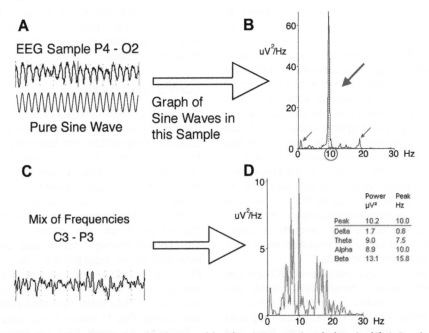

Fig. 11. (*A*) A short sample of EEG that closely resembles the sine wave just below it. (*B*) A Fourier transform confirms that the EEG sample in (*A*) can be represented by one large sine wave around 10 Hz (*red circle*) plus a couple of smaller sine waves, at 1 Hz and 19 Hz (*arrows*). (*C*) A more complex EEG sample requires (*D*) multiple sine waves on the frequency graph. However, these can easily be collected into quantitative estimates of the major EEG frequencies (*inset table*).

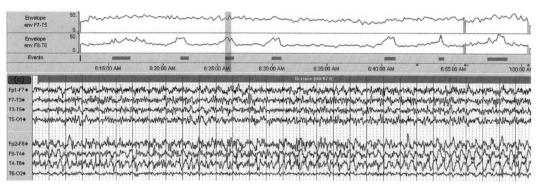

Fig. 12. At top, envelope trends from a series of right-hemisphere seizures in an intensive care patient. The bumps in the lower right hemisphere trend are produced by seizures. The red horizontal bars beneath the envelope display mark the seizures as visually identified by a human interpreter. The gray bar in the envelope display indicates the segment of the raw EEG at the bottom. Even though the raw EEG is taken from the middle of a seizure and compressed to 30 seconds per page, evolution of the seizure is difficult to recognize in this sample. Total trend duration is almost 1 hour.

Over the past several decades, hundreds of skilled mathematicians, engineers, and researchers have spent uncounted person-years pursuing what sounds like a straightforward task: to extend and improve EEG interpretation by computerized techniques. Software intended to quantify EEG background, recognize IEDs and seizures, and even make specific diagnoses has been commercially available for more than 30 years. In practice, however, the quality of the results ranges from marginally useful for skilled interpreters to dangerously inaccurate for the less adept.[6]

There are at least 3 reasons why computerized diagnostic software programs have failed to achieve what their developers had hoped for. One reason is misunderstanding the clinical problem. Moderate success has been reported in distinguishing between unmedicated, uncomplicated, classic cases of brain disorders and carefully selected, unmedicated normal controls.[7] Unfortunately, this is not a particularly useful result. The clinical need is to accurately diagnose atypical cases in the setting of multiple complications and possibly multiple disorders. Second is the lack of a gold standard. The recent "Jeopardy" game victory of the IBM Watson computer (IBM, Armonk, New York) consisted of doing, marginally better and faster, something that humans already knew how to do (while using hundreds of high-powered servers and a score of engineers). But nobody knows if it is even possible to use EEG to make specific diagnoses in complex situations. Finally, thousands of different EEG variables, computed from scores of electrodes, would have to be collated against hundreds of different brain conditions in thousands of patients. Such an enterprise would rival the cost and complexity of the Manhattan Project. In the United States, the threshold for marketing of seizure-recognition and other quantitative EEG programs is low. Their sale is allowed under the Food and Drug Administration 510(k) grandfather clause, which deems them "substantially equivalent"[8] to systems allowed before 1976 and no more than an adjunct to visual interpretation. At most, EEG and PSG readers should use quantitative techniques as supplements to human skills, and not their replacements.

SUMMARY

1. Use good technique and keep the electrode impedances low. Do not be fooled by the idea that 60-Hz filters will make everything satisfactory.
2. Take advantage of the flexibility that digital EEG and PSG afford but beware of its limitations. Freely adjust montages, gain, and filter settings. Most especially, change the display speed for better resolution. Use QEEG to summarize data trends cautiously.
3. Keep patients away from earth ground.

REFERENCES

1. Tao JX, Baldwin M, Ray A, et al. The impact of cerebral source area and synchrony on recording scalp electroencephalography ictal patterns. Epilepsia 2007;48:2167–76.
2. Epstein CM. Aliasing in the visual EEG: a potential pitfall of video display technology. Clin Neurophysiol 2003;114:1974–6.
3. Iber C, American Academy of Sleep Medicine. The AASM manual for the scoring of sleep and associated

events: rules, terminology and technical specifications. Westchester (IL): American Academy of Sleep Medicine; 2007.

4. Knott JR, Gibbs FA. A Fourier transform of the EEG from one to eighteen years. Psychol Bull 1939;36: 512–3.

5. Scheuer M. Continuous EEG monitoring in the intensive care unit. Epilepsia 2002;43(Suppl 3): 114–27.

6. American Clinical Neurophysiology Society Guidelines. Assessment of digital EEG, QEEG and EEG brain mapping: a report of the AAN and the ACNS. Available at: http://www.acns.org/. Accessed January 12, 2012.

7. John ER, Prichep LS, Fridman J, et al. Neurometrics: computer-assisted differential diagnosis of brain dysfunctions. Science 1988;239:162–9.

8. Premarket Notification (510k). Available at: http://www. fda.gov/MedicalDevices/DeviceRegulationandGuidance/ HowtoMarketYourDevice/PremarketSubmissions/ PremarketNotification510k/default.htm. Accessed January 12, 2012.

Sleep/Wake Electroencephalography Across the Lifespan

Dinesh V. Raju, MD, PhD, Rodney A. Radtke, MD*

KEYWORDS

- Electroencephalography • Sleep • Neonate • Infant

The development of organized sleep/wake states is a major feature of the neonatal period and developing infant. Although subsequent changes in the sleep/wake cycle with age are less profound, they represent predictable physiologic changes occurring as a function of age. Similarly, there are characteristic electroencephalography (EEG) patterns seen as a function of maturity in the neonate and developing child. These EEG changes continue to evolve into adulthood, offering an electrophysiologic marker of brain development.

PATTERNS OF SLEEP ACROSS THE LIFESPAN
Young Adult

Sleep patterns in the young adult are the most studied and best defined, and commonly serve as the basis with which the sleep patterns of other age groups are compared. Normal healthy young adults exhibit a predictable and well-characterized pattern of alternating cycles of rapid eye movement (REM) and non-REM (NREM) sleep across a typical night of sleep. Each cycle lasts 90 to 120 minutes, with 4 to 6 cycles expected across a night of sleep. The initial cycle is usually slightly shorter and they become longer as the night progresses. With the initial descent into sleep, a few minutes of light sleep (N1) is initially seen, followed by deeper stages of sleep (N2, N3). Usually there are 10 to 25 minutes of N2 sleep followed by increasing delta activity leading into N3, the deepest stage of sleep. After approximately 90 minutes of sleep, there usually are a few minutes of lighter sleep (stage N2 or N1) followed by the development of REM sleep. The first period of REM sleep is usually the shortest (<5 minutes) and often has only subtle rapid eye movements that make it more difficult to identify.

Deeper sleep (N3) is primarily seen in the first 2 sleep cycles, and often is the dominant sleep stage early in the night. With each sleep cycle, the REM duration usually increases and the later portion of the night is spent alternating between stage N2 and REM. During a typical night sleep, a young adult spends 75% to 80% in NREM and 20% to 25% in REM sleep. NREM sleep is usually divided into stage N1 (2%–5% of total sleep time [TST]), N2 (45%–55% of TST), and N3 (18%–23% of TST).[1–4]

Infant

Development of organized sleep/wake states and subsequent evolution to a circadian sleep/wake cycle is a major developmental accomplishment of a neonate. Age-appropriate sleep ontogeny is a sensitive marker of central nervous system development in this age group. As opposed to the well-defined sleep pattern of the young adult, infants have cycles composed of quiet sleep, active sleep (the physiologic precursor of REM sleep), and wakefulness. Cycle duration is variable, in the range 50 to 300 minutes, and the initial descent into sleep is most commonly into active sleep. The EEG/polygraphic characteristics of these sleep stages are discussed later. By age 3 months, infants start to develop a circadian rhythm and, by age 4 months, sleep is usually concentrated during the nighttime hours.[1,4,5]

Child

There are more limited studies of sleep/wake changes in this age group. During the first 2 to

Department of Medicine (Neurology), Duke University Medical Center, Durham, NC 27719, USA
* Corresponding author.
E-mail address: rod.radtke@duke.edu

Sleep Med Clin 7 (2012) 13–22
doi:10.1016/j.jsmc.2012.01.001
1556-407X/12/$ – see front matter © 2012 Elsevier Inc. All rights reserved.

3 years, sleep becomes consolidated in a long nocturnal sleep period, usually about 10 to 12 hours in duration. Typically, the child initially has two naps, a short one in the morning and a longer one in the afternoon. Gradually the morning nap is abandoned and then, usually by age 4 to 5 years, sleep is consolidated into a single nocturnal sleep period. At age 1 year, REM sleep occupies approximately 33% of TST. This proportion decreases to the adult value (20%–25%) by about age 4 to 5 years. Initially, the sleep cycle duration is about 60 minutes, but lengthens to the adult value (90 minutes) by about age 5 years. Between the ages of 5 and 10 years, less prominent changes are noted. During these years, the single nocturnal sleep period shortens to 9.5 to 11 hours, the percentage of N3 sleep decreases modestly, and naps are unusual.[6]

Older Adult

Several changes occur in sleep in older adults. These changes include increased nocturnal arousals and awakenings, decreased sleep efficiency, a mild increase in stage N1, marked decrease in stage N3, and relative preservation of REM sleep. As a result of these factors, the elderly typically require more time in bed to obtain their usual 7 to 8 hours of sleep. The latency to the first appearance of REM sleep decreases and the amount of REM sleep is distributed more uniformly across the night; both patterns are also seen in depression. The amplitude, duration, and occurrence of sleep spindle activity decrease, and there is a loss of the consolidation of sleep in the nocturnal period with more wakefulness during the night and more frequent naps during the day.

As noted earlier, one of the biggest changes in sleep in the elderly is the decrease in stage N3 sleep. Healthy elderly without primary sleep problems spend less than 10% of their TST in N3, compared with 25% to 35% in young adults. Older adults had an average of 27 arousals per hour of sleep compared with young adults who averaged 10 per hour of sleep. Sleep efficiency (TST/time in bed) in older adults is typically around 80% compared with young adults who average greater than 90%. Older healthy adults average 18% of REM sleep time compared with 20% to 25% in younger adults.[1–3,5] Sleep among elders is characterized by increased number and duration of awakenings, decreased sleep efficiency, with an increase in wake time after sleep onset.

A recently published meta-analysis studied age-related changes in sleep architecture among 65 studies of all-night polysomnography (PSG) or actigraphy done on 3577 healthy subjects, aged 5 years to 102 years.[5] The results of this study, summarized here, reinforce many of the observations outlined earlier. With increasing age, there is a gradual reduction in the TST. However, this trend in school-aged children was present only with recordings during school nights, suggesting that the reduction in TST during school-age years reflects externally imposed sleep restrictions. There is a small but significant increase in sleep latency (the time an individual takes to fall asleep) of about 10 minutes from age 20 to 80 years. The percentage of stage N1 sleep increases during adulthood, likely reflecting greater sleep disruption. From ages 5 to 60 years, there is a significant increase in the percentage of stage N2 sleep, which is likely caused by the marked decrease of stage N3 sleep. Infants may spend 50% of TST in REM sleep and, by age 4 to 5 years, the percentage of TST spent in REM approaches the adult values of 20% to 25%. The latency of REM sleep increases with age. Neonates preferentially enter active sleep (the precursor of REM sleep). By the age of 6 months, an infant immediately enters REM sleep approximately 20% of the time. By age 2 years, sleep-onset REM sleep is rare and the usual latency to REM sleep is 60 minutes. The percentage of TST spent in stage N3 or slow wave sleep decreases with increasing age. In young children, stage N3 sleep can account for 40% of TST and usually reduces to 15% to 25% by the teenage years.[5]

EEG PATTERNS ACROSS THE LIFESPAN
Term Neonate to Age 3 Months

During this early stage of life, the EEG can be divided into wakefulness, active sleep, and quiet sleep.

Wakefulness and active sleep

In the term neonate, similar EEG patterns are seen in both wakefulness and active sleep. Active sleep is usually characterized by a low-voltage irregular pattern, with continuous 25 to 50 μV theta and less than 25 μV lower-amplitude delta activity. A second pattern is sometimes seen in the initial descent into sleep and is termed a mixed pattern, which is similar to the low-voltage pattern described earlier but has higher-amplitude delta activity (**Fig. 1**). Differentiating wakefulness from active sleep in a neonate is not possible from EEG patterns alone. Active sleep, considered to be the precursor of adult REM sleep, characteristically has irregular respiration, increased heart rate variability, and frequent body and eye movements.[7,8] The loss of muscle tone is less consistently identified than in adult REM sleep and

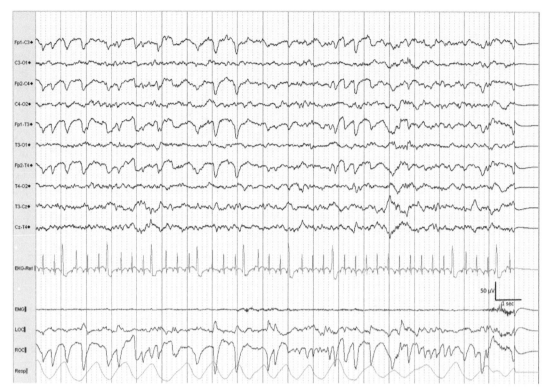

Fig. 1. Active sleep is seen in this term infant with low-voltage theta and delta activity and rapid eye movements seen in the eye leads (FP1, FP2, ROC, and LOC). The EMG shows reduced activity. (*Courtesy of* Aatif Husain, MD.)

often the technologist's report of the patient's eyes being closed is the strongest confirmation of sleep state.

Quiet sleep

Two patterns are seen during quiet sleep in the term infant: trace alternant and high-voltage slow. The trace alternant pattern can be seen from birth up to 46 weeks' gestational age and is characterized by symmetric bursts of delta activity (50–300 μV) lasting a few seconds with a similar duration of lower-amplitude mixed frequencies (25–50 μV). By 44 weeks' gestational age, the EEG of quiet sleep predominantly shows the high-voltage slow pattern with high-voltage (50–200 μV) theta and delta activity (**Fig. 2**).[7,8]

Age 3 Months to 2 Years

Wakefulness

As the infant enters toddlerhood, wakefulness is manifested with increasingly rhythmic and developed delta activity, which is seen initially centrally and occipitally. As the child approaches age 2 years, the central and occipital delta activity is gradually replaced with theta activity, which is still predominantly seen posteriorly. This occipital dominant rhythm increases with age (**Table 1**)

and is an important part of the assessment of the waking EEG.[9]

Drowsiness

Drowsiness is manifested as high-amplitude delta that reduces in amplitude with age. A common pattern seen with drowsiness is hypnagogic hypersynchrony, which is a high-amplitude discharge of 3 to 5 Hz that appears suddenly and is usually diffuse but can have an anterior, posterior, or temporal predominance and can be continuous or intermittent (**Fig. 3**). This pattern is seen in nearly all children by age 2 years and is usually absent by adolescence.[9,10]

Sleep

Sleep spindles (distinctive EEG markers of stage N2) may be seen as early as 3 weeks and are normally present by 2 to 3 months of age. Until 1 to 2 years of age, often more than half of the sleep spindles in a given PSG are asynchronous (**Fig. 4**).[8,11] By age 1 year, sleep spindles are synchronous 30% of the time and fully synchronous by age 2 years. Well-developed K-complexes are usually present by 6 months of age.[7,8,12] Recognizable stage N1, N2, and N3 can be identified as early as 4 to 4.5 months term, and are usually present by 5 to 6 months of age. Mature forms of

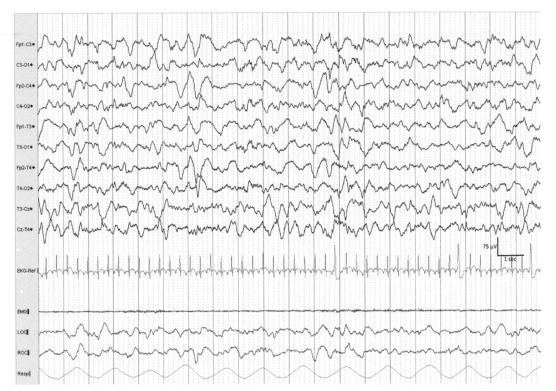

Fig. 2. Quiet sleep is seen in this term infant with high-voltage theta and delta activity. (*Courtesy of* Aatif Husain, MD.)

vertex sharp waves are usually seen by 6 months of age. New rules for scoring sleep in infants and children 2 months term or older have been published as part of the new scoring manual. A position paper supporting the development of these rules and citing the evidence (or consensus) on which they were based accompany the rules.[9]

After about 6 months of age, children's EEG sleep patterns more consistently resemble the well-recognized adult patterns. Children normally enter NREM sleep from the drowsy state. According to Grigg-Damberger and colleagues,[9] the

onset of NREM sleep is identified if the dominant background rhythm "occupies less than 50% of a 30-second epoch, and one or more of the following EEG patterns appear: (1) a diffuse lower voltage mixed frequency activity; (2) hypnagogic hypersynchrony; (3) rhythmic anterior theta of drowsiness; (4) diffuse high voltage occipital delta slowing; (5) runs or bursts of diffuse, frontal, frontocentral, or occipital maximal rhythmic 3–5 Hz slowing; (6) vertex sharp waves; and/or (7) postarousal hypersynchrony."

Stage N1 sleep is frequently manifested by vertex waves, which are sharp waves of high amplitude (250 μV), duration of less than 200 milliseconds, with a central and paracentral predominance (Cz, C3, C4) (**Fig. 5**). Vertex waves are usually seen by age 16 months. Stage N2 sleep is characterized by sleep spindles and K-complexes. Sleep spindles become increasingly synchronous between the hemispheres by age 2 years. The K-complex, seen best in the frontal region (Fz, F3, and F4), begins with a high-amplitude (200 μV) negative deflection and subsequent lower-amplitude positive wave, and overall duration of at least 0.5 seconds. K-complexes are usually present by age 6 months. Sleep spindles may follow or precede K-complexes.[12] Stage N3 or slow wave sleep is characterized by

Table 1	
Normative values of the mean occipital dominant rhythm during development	
Age	**Occipital Dominant Rhythm (Hz)**
3–4 mo	3.5–4.5
5–6 mo	5–6
3 y	8
9 y	9
15 y	10

Data from Grigg-Damberger M, Gozal D, Marcus CL, et al. The visual scoring of sleep and arousal in infants and children. J Clin Sleep Med 2007;3(2):201–40.

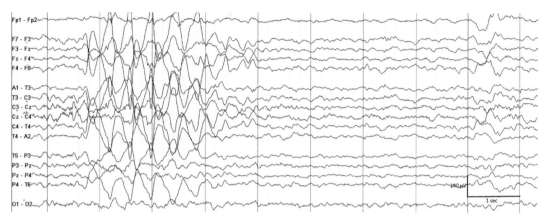

Fig. 3. Hypnagogic hypersynchrony, with high-voltage discharge at 3 to 5 Hz, is seen in this 14-year-old patient illustrated on a transverse montage.

high-amplitude, slow activity (0.5–2 Hz).[2,9,10] The adult pattern of REM sleep replaces active sleep, with mixed delta and theta activity becoming low-amplitude synchronous activity.

Age 2 to Early Adulthood

Wakefulness
Wakefulness is manifested by a sinusoidal posterior dominant rhythm that reaches the lower limit of the adult normal value of 8 Hz by age 3 years in most children. This activity is seen best in occipital regions but can also be seen in central regions. This alpha activity gradually increases in frequency up to young adulthood. A key characteristic of the alpha activity is attenuation of amplitude with eye closure. The amplitude of the alpha activity increases with age and can be greater than 100 μV by age 10 years, but then begins to reduce in amplitude. Rhythmic theta activity can be seen over the temporal and occipital regions and, less frequently, in the frontocentral region during wakefulness, especially during the teenage years.[1,7]

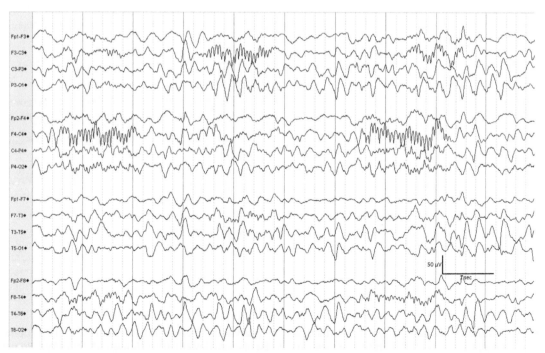

Fig. 4. Asynchronous sleep spindles are seen in this recording of a 1-year-old child. (*Courtesy of* Aatif Husain, MD.)

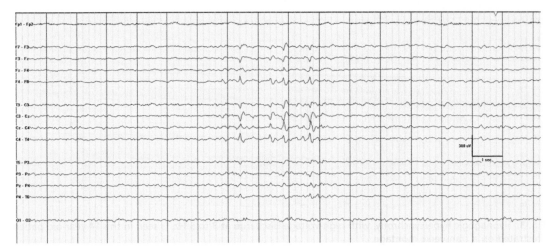

Fig. 5. Vertex waves seen in the central leads in this 13-year-old patient shown on a transverse montage.

Posterior slow activity is common in children between the ages of 6 and 14 years (**Fig. 6**). Posterior slow waves of youth are delta frequency waveforms that occur sporadically over the occipital region. Waking alpha activity is usually superimposed on this delta activity. The slow waves may be asymmetric and asynchronous but block with eye opening and are considered a normal variant. They are frequently seen in children aged 8 to 14 years.[1,7] Slow alpha variants may also be seen over the occipital region during wakefulness. This activity is manifested by trains of occipital activity of 4 to 5 Hz that block with eye opening and are thought to represent a subharmonic of the normal alpha frequency activity.

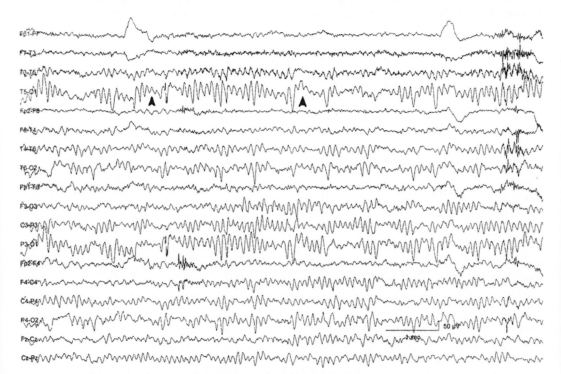

Fig. 6. Posterior slow waves of youth, the delta activity (marked by the *arrowheads*) underlying the occipital dominant alpha activity on the left side, are seen in this EEG of an adolescent. (*From* Rowan AJ, Tolunsky E. Primer of EEG with a mini-atlas. Philadelphia: Butterworth Heinemann (Elsevier); 2003. p. 121; with permission.)

Drowsiness and sleep

Slow, roving eye movements manifested as deflections of 0.5 to 1 Hz with opposite polarities in the left and right frontal eye leads heralds the transition to sleep (**Fig. 7**). Drowsiness is also manifested with a reduction of the occipital dominant rhythm by 1 Hz or greater. The EEG of NREM and REM sleep during this age group is similar to that described earlier for children aged 3 months to 2 years but with less ambiguous transitions from one stage of sleep to another. Vertex waves in this age group tend to be sharper, more repetitive, and of higher amplitude, which can sometimes raise concern for possible epileptiform features.[1,9,10,13]

Early and Middle Adulthood

Wakefulness

In the adult, the EEG shows an occipital dominant alpha activity usually in the range of 10 Hz with the eyes closed. Brazier and Finesinger,[14] using 500 young adult controls, identified a mean alpha frequency of 10.2 ($\pm$ 0.9) Hz. Based on this and similar studies, the low end of the normative range is usually considered to be 8 or 8.5 Hz. With eyes open and visual fixation, the alpha activity is replaced by low-amplitude fast activity. About 10% of normal adults do not have discernable occipital dominant activity and another 10% of normal adults have an occipital dominant activity of low-amplitude alpha activity with mixed beta activity.

This pattern is usually described as a low-voltage fast background, and is considered a variant of normal.[1,15]

Drowsiness and NREM sleep

The transition to sleep begins with slowing of the dominant occipital rhythm by at least 1 Hz. Roving eye movements, seen as slow undulating deflections of the electrooculogram (EOG) with opposite polarities in the right and left eyes, are physical manifestations of drowsiness and may be the only sign of transition to sleep in patients without a well-formed occipital dominant rhythm. Brief periods of theta at the vertex can also be seen in drowsiness. The beginning of stage N1 sleep is traditionally characterized by the presence of vertex waves, mostly background activity of 2 to 7 Hz, dropout of background alpha activity, and roving eye movements. Increased beta activity, usually 18 to 25 Hz and predominantly in the central regions, is also seen during stage N1 sleep. Stage N2 sleep contains low-amplitude activity of 2 to 7 Hz with superimposed sleep spindles and K-complexes. Sleep spindles are sinusoidal waves with a frequency range of 11 to 16 Hz, lasting for 0.5 seconds or more, predominantly in the central regions (**Fig. 8**). Sleep spindles often initially increase and then decrease in amplitude (giving them a spindlelike appearance) and most often have a frequency of 12 to 14 Hz.[16] With increasing age, there is a progressive reduction in the number of sleep spindles during sleep and an increase in

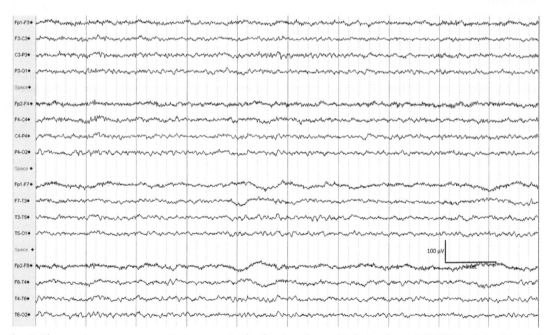

Fig. 7. Slow roving eye movements are seen in the frontopolar and inferior frontal (F7/F8) leads in this adult patient. (*Courtesy of* Aatif Husain, MD.)

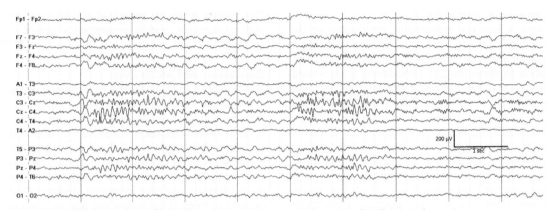

Fig. 8. Stage N2 sleep is identified in this adult with symmetric sleep spindles illustrated on a transverse montage.

the intervals between sleep spindles.[11] K-complexes are biphasic or triphasic sharp waves that usually begin with an initial negative deflection and subsequent positive deflection with a duration of 0.5 seconds or more. K-complexes are best seen over the frontal regions (**Fig. 9**).[12,16] They can recur every 60 to 100 seconds and can have high amplitudes. K-complexes can be followed by sleep spindles and, in some cases, brief periods of alpha activity.[12] Stage N3 or slow wave sleep is identified by activity of 0.5 to 2 Hz that occupies more than 20% of an epoch; this activity has peak-to-peak amplitude of more than 75 μV when measured in the frontal regions.[2,13,15,17–19]

REM sleep
The EEG of REM sleep is characterized by diffuse (but predominantly in the posterior regions) low-amplitude activity composed of mixed frequencies that resemble wakefulness (**Fig. 10**). The electromyogram (EMG) shows significantly reduced or absent activity at the chin lead. Rapid eye movements, for which this stage of sleep is named,

may not be seen in all epochs of REM sleep. Rapid eye movements are characterized by rapid deflections of opposite polarity between the right and left frontal leads, with a frequency of 1 to 2 Hz. Sawtooth waves, sharply contoured activity of 2 to 5 Hz predominantly over the central regions, can be seen before the onset of rapid eye movements.[10,15,18]

Late Adulthood

Wakefulness
In elderly adults, the occipital dominant rhythm slows to the lower end of the alpha range. After the age of 60 years, the occipital dominant rhythm is often 8 to 9 Hz. The voltage and reactivity of the alpha rhythm decrease with increasing age. With eye closure, the alpha rhythm can be seen in more frontal and central regions.[1,7]

Drowsiness and sleep
In addition to the EEG characteristic described earlier for young and middle-aged adults, elderly adults can have bilateral synchronous delta

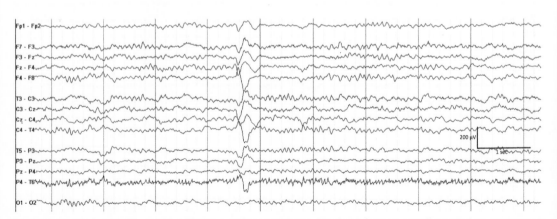

Fig. 9. Stage N2 sleep is characterized by K-complexes, high-amplitude biphasic waves illustrated on a transverse montage.

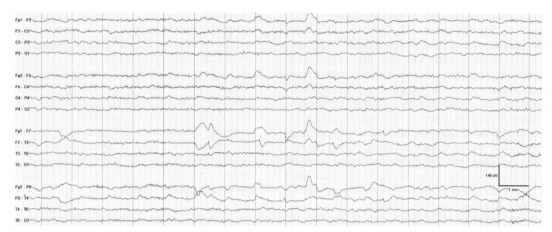

Fig. 10. REM sleep is seen in this sample with low-voltage activity and rapid eye movements recorded in the fronto-topolar and inferior frontal leads in this 19-year-old patient.

activity at sleep onset, sometimes termed delta-onset sleep. Also, instead of the common transition from drowsiness to N1 and then N2 sleep, elderly adults more often transition from drowsiness directly into N2 sleep. The EEG characteristics of the sleep stages are otherwise similar to those described earlier for younger adults.[13]

NORMAL EEG VARIANTS DURING SLEEP

Posterior occipital sharp transients of sleep (POSTS) are commonly seen during stages N1 and N2 (**Fig. 11**). They are sharply contoured, positive waves, 100 to 200 milliseconds in duration and 50 to 100 μV in amplitude. These waveforms are seen predominantly over the occipital region and are usually bisynchronous. POSTS are initially seen in light sleep between the ages of 3 and 5 years, but are present into adulthood. There are several other EEG patterns that occur during drowsiness or sleep that have an epileptiform appearance but are not associated with an increased risk for seizures. These patterns are considered benign or normal variants and include

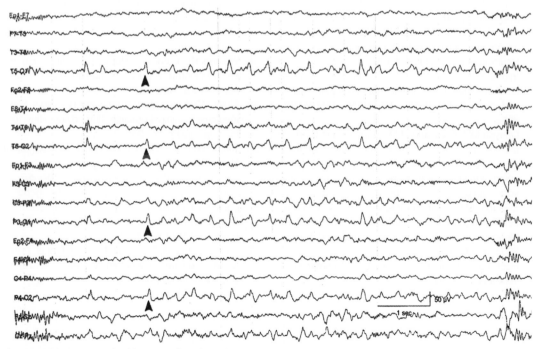

Fig. 11. POSTS are marked by *arrowheads* in this EEG. (*From* Rowan AJ, Tolunsky E. Primer of EEG with a mini-atlas. Philadelphia: Butterworth Heinemann (Elsevier); 2003. p. 129; with permission.)

small sharp spikes (SSS), wicket spikes, 14-Hz and 6-Hz positive bursts, and rhythmic midtemporal theta bursts of drowsiness (RMTD). SSS are low-amplitude, usually biphasic discharges with durations less than 75 milliseconds that occur predominantly over the temporal regions bisynchronously or independently. Unlike pathologic sharps or spikes, there is minimal disruption of the background baseline and no accompanying slow wave. Wicket spikes can occur during drowsiness or sleep and are characterized by runs of high-amplitude (200 μV or more) arch-shaped discharges occurring predominantly in the temporal regions. Positive bursts of 14 Hz and 6 Hz are brief (<1 second) trains of moderate-amplitude (<75 μV) positive spikes that occur at frequencies of 14 or 6 Hz predominantly in the posterior temporal regions in adolescents during sleep. RMTD is manifested by 4-Hz to 7-Hz rhythmic sharp discharges with waxing and waning amplitude that are seen independently or bisynchronously in the midtemporal regions during the early stages of sleep.[20–22] The last 2 patterns, 14-Hz and 6-Hz positive bursts and RMTD, are more commonly seen in adolescents.

REFERENCES

1. Lee-Chiong T, editor. Sleep: a comprehensive handbook. New York: John Wiley; 2006.
2. Gaudrea H, Carrier J, Montplaisir J. Age-related modifications of NREM sleep EEG: from childhood to middle age. J Sleep Res 2001;10(3):165–72.
3. Brezinová V. The number and duration of the episodes of the various EEG stages of sleep in young and older people. Electroencephalogr Clin Neurophysiol 1975;39(3):273–8.
4. Iglowstein I, Jenni OG, Molinari L, et al. Sleep duration from infancy to adolescence: reference values and generational trends. Pediatrics 2003;111(2): 302–7.
5. Ohayon MM, Carskadon MA, Guilleminault C, et al. Meta-analysis of quantitative sleep parameters from childhood to old age in healthy individuals: developing normative sleep values across the human lifespan. Sleep 2004;27(7):1255–73.
6. Sheldon SH. Sleep in infants and children. In: Lee-Chiong TL, Sateia MJ, Carskadon MR, editors. Sleep medicine. Philadelphia: Hanley and Belfus; 2002. p. 99–103.
7. Fisch BJ. Fisch and Spehlmann's EEG primer. New York: Elsevier; 1999.
8. Jenni OG, Borbély AA, Achermann P. Development of the nocturnal sleep electroencephalogram in human infants. Am J Physiol Regul Integr Comp Physiol 2004;286(3):R528–38.
9. Grigg-Damberger M, Gozal D, Marcus CL, et al. The visual scoring of sleep and arousal in infants and children. J Clin Sleep Med 2007;3(2):201–40.
10. Iber C, Ancoli-Isreal S, Chesson A, et al, for the American Academy of Sleep Medicine. The AASM manual for the scoring of sleep and associated events: rules, terminology and technical specifications. 1st edition. Westchester (IL): American Academy of Sleep Medicine; 2007.
11. Nicolas A, Petit D, Rompré S, et al. Sleep spindle characteristics in healthy subjects of different age groups. Clin Neurophysiol 2001;112(3):521–7.
12. Halász P. K-complex, a reactive EEG graphoelement of NREM sleep: an old chap in a new garment. Sleep Med Rev 2005;9(5):391–412.
13. Santamaria J, Chiappa KH. The EEG of drowsiness in normal adults. J Clin Neurophysiol 1987;4(4): 327–82.
14. Brazier MA, Finesinger JE. Characteristics of the normal EEG: a study of the occipital cortical potentials in 500 normal adults. J Clin Invest 1944;23: 303–11.
15. Sibler MH, Ancoli-Israel S, Bonnet MH, et al. The visual scoring of sleep in adults. J Clin Sleep Med 2007;3(2):121–31.
16. McCormick L, Nielsen T, Nicolas A, et al. Topographical distribution of spindles and K-complexes in normal subjects. Sleep 1997;20(11):939–41.
17. Smith JR, Karacan I, Yang M. Ontogeny of delta activity during human sleep. Electroencephalogr Clin Neurophysiol 1977;43(2):229–37.
18. Williams RL, Karacan I, Hursch CJ, editors. Electroencephalography (EEG) of human sleep: clinical applications. New York: John Wiley; 1974.
19. Sibler MG, Krahn LE, Morgenthaler TI, editors. Sleep medicine in clinical practice. 2nd edition. New York: Informa Healthcare; 2010.
20. Tatum WO 4th, Husain AM, Benbadis SR, et al. Normal adult EEG and patterns of uncertain significance. J Clin Neurophysiol 2006;23(3):194–207.
21. Radhakrishnan K, Santoshkumar B, Venugopal A. Prevalence of benign epileptiform variants observed in an EEG laboratory from south India. Clin Neurophysiol 1999;110(2):280–5.
22. Santoshkumar B, Chong JJ, Blume WT, et al. Prevalence of benign epileptiform variants. Clin Neurophysiol 2009;120(5):856–61.

Recognizing Normal, Abnormal, and Benign Nonepileptiform Electroencephalographic Activity and Patterns in Polysomnographic Recordings

Martina Vendrame, MD, PhD[a], Sanjeev V. Kothare, MD[b],*

KEYWORDS

- Electroencephalogram • Variants • Nonepileptiform
- Epileptiform

Electroencephalography (EEG) is a clinical electro-physiologic test, which provides a continuous measure of cerebral function of changing voltage fields at the scalp surface that result from ongoing synaptic activities in the underlying cerebral cortex. EEG reflects spontaneous intrinsic inhibitory and excitatory postsynaptic activity in the underlying cerebral cortex generated by cortical neurons with afferent inputs from subcortical thalamic and brainstem reticular formation. Thalamic afferents are largely responsible for entraining cortical neurons to produce the dominant alpha rhythm and sleep spindles.

An EEG is abnormal if it contains: (1) epileptiform activity or electrographic seizure patterns; (2) slow waves inappropriate to the state of wake/sleep; (3) amplitude abnormalities; or (4) certain patterns resembling normal activity but deviating from it in frequency, reactivity, distribution, or other features.[1] Abnormalities in EEG need to be distinguished from normal patterns, benign variants, and artifacts.

Too many sleep specialists and technologists lament they lack sufficient training in recognizing abnormalities in the limited EEG channels recorded on a polysomnograph (PSG). Moreover, increasing numbers of patients with epilepsy, dementias, and extrapyramidal diseases are being referred to sleep centers, many of whom require recording of their PSGs with expanded EEG montages. Given this, the authors review the range of normal, abnormal, and benign EEG variants encountered in patients undergoing PSG with conventional and expanded EEG montages. Because comprehensive in-laboratory PSGs are rarely requested for patients with severe acute encephalopathies, coma, or status epilepticus, discussion of these is omitted.

DEVIATIONS FROM NORMAL EEG PATTERNS

Deviations from normal EEG patterns that may be encountered in a PSG include: (1) abnormal slowing of the dominant posterior rhythm (DPR); (2)

Financial disclosure and conflict of interest statement: There are no disclosures and no conflict of interest.
[a] Division of Clinical Neurophysiology and Sleep, Department of Neurology, Boston University Medical Center, Neurology C-3, 72 East Concord Street, Boston, MA 02118, USA
[b] Division of Epilepsy and Clinical Neurophysiology, Department of Neurology, Center for Pediatric Sleep Disorders, Harvard Medical School, Children's Hospital, Boston, MA 02115, USA
* Corresponding author.
E-mail address: sanjeev.kothare@childrens.harvard.edu

Sleep Med Clin 7 (2012) 23–38
doi:10.1016/j.jsmc.2011.12.008
1556-407X/12/$ – see front matter © 2012 Elsevier Inc. All rights reserved.

abnormal reactivity of the DPR; (3) excessive beta activity; (4) abnormalities in sleep spindles, vertex activity, and other PSG markers of sleep; and (5) indeterminate or undifferentiated sleep. On rare occasions, triphasic waves or periodic lateralized epileptiform discharges may be observed in a PSG, most often recorded in a hospitalized patient.

The Dominant Posterior Alpha Rhythm

Interpretation of an EEG (or scoring an epoch of sleep in a PSG) begins by analyzing whether a DPR is present, bilateral, symmetric, and within the expected normal frequency range for age and state. The DPR (also called the dominant alpha rhythm or the alpha rhythm) is probably the most important EEG pattern and rhythm. The alpha rhythm is often of highest amplitude over the occipital, posterior temporal, and parietal scalp regions. In one-third of healthy adults, the alpha rhythm extends into the temporal and central regions, which results in the DPR equally seen in the frontal, central, and occipital channels linked to the mastoid references when recording EEG during a routine PSG (**Fig. 1**).

The alpha rhythm is usually best seen with eyes closed during periods of physical relaxation and relative mental inactivity; it attenuates or is blocked by eye opening and attention, especially visual and mental effort (**Fig. 2**). This attribute is called reactivity of the alpha rhythm, and can vary from complete suppression of the activity to varying degrees of attenuation with voltage reduction. Reactivity of the DPR may be transient, or appear and then fade with continued eye closure. Some have a DPR that is nonreactive; absent reactivity of an alpha rhythm is only abnormal if it is distinctly asymmetric.

The frequency of the DPR in normal adults ranges from 8 Hz to 13 Hz or more. Most normal adults and adolescents have an alpha rhythm between 9 and 11 Hz, and only 5% have a DPR of 11.5 Hz or more.[2] The mean DPR in 500 normal adult subjects was 10.2 ± 0.9 Hz, 10.5 Hz in those adults younger than age 24 years, and 10.4 Hz in those 24 to 47 years old.[3] The DPR remains greater than 8.5 Hz even in healthy octogenarians.

In approximately 25% of normal adults, the alpha rhythm is poorly visualized, with 6% to 7% of normal adults demonstrating voltages of less than 15 Hz.[4] Because of this, the bilateral absence of a DPR is not considered abnormal. The frequency of alpha rhythm is only measured when the patient is awake and not drowsy because it decreases by 1 to 2 Hz with drowsiness. In the baseline calibration period of a PSG, the DPR is best measured and assessed during periods of eye opening and closure.

DPRs first appear in infants 3 to 4 months' term as irregular, relatively high-amplitude (50–100 μV

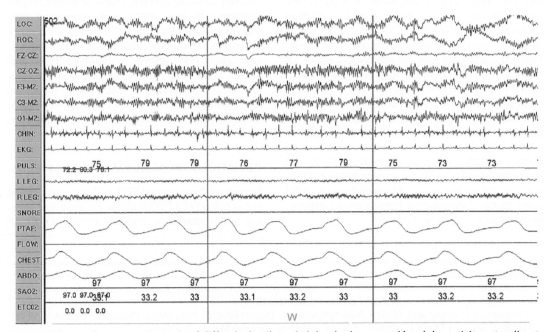

Fig. 1. Diffuse alpha activity. Example of diffusely distributed alpha rhythm caused by alpha activity extending to the temporal and central regions. A 30-second PSG epoch shows an example of diffusely distributed alpha rhythm caused by alpha activity extending to the temporal and central regions in a 41-year-old awake man. (*Courtesy of* M. Grigg-Damberger.)

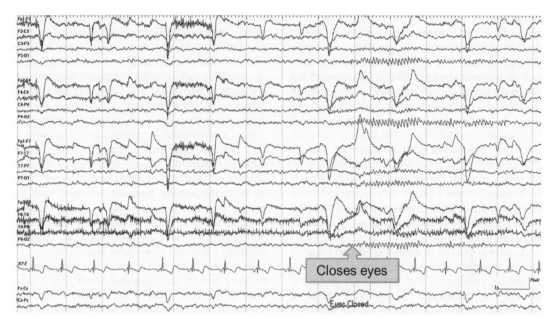

Fig. 2. Dominant posterior alpha rhythm. Normal symmetric reactivity of the DPR to eye opening. Note how the 10- to 10.5-Hz dominant posterior alpha rhythm over the posterior regions (P3-O1, P4-O2, P7-O1, and P8-O2) appears with eye closure in this 12-year-old child. The alpha rhythm is usually best seen with eyes closed during periods of physical relaxation and relative mental inactivity; it attenuates or is blocked by eye opening and attention (especially visual and mental effort). (*Courtesy of* M. Grigg-Damberger.)

or greater), reactive 3.5- to 4.5-Hz activity over the occipital regions. Many infants achieve 5 to 6 Hz by 5 to 6 months of age, 70% have 5- to 6-Hz alpha-like activity by 12 months' term, and 82% have a mean occipital frequency of 8 Hz (range 7.5–9.5 Hz) by 36 months of age.[5] Most children have a 9- to 11-Hz posterior alpha rhythm by 8 years of age, and normal adult occipital alpha frequencies are typically reached by 13 years. The mean posterior alpha frequency is 9 Hz in 65% of the 9-year-olds and 10 Hz in 65% of normal children by age 15.

Be advised that a young child does not close the eyes until drowsy, so the frequency of the posterior rhythm when a young child's eyes spontaneously close often represents drowsiness. As seen in adults, during drowsiness the DPR is often 1 to 2 Hz slower than the child's actual DPR. Reactivity of the DPR to passive eye closure can be first seen as early as 3 months of age, and is usually first present by 5 to 6 months.[6,7]

Abnormalities of the DPR

Electroencephalographers use the term slowed background for a waking posterior alpha rhythm that is too slow for age and state. A DPR that never exceeds 8 Hz in an awake adult is abnormal because a DPR of less than 8 Hz is seen in less than 1% of normal adult subjects at any age.[1,8] The absolute lower limits of abnormal for the frequency of the

DPR are: less than 5 Hz at age 1, less than 6 Hz at age 3, less than 7 Hz at age 5, and less than 8 Hz at age 8 years.[9]

A unilateral decrease in the frequency of the DPR is considered abnormal if there is a consistent left-right difference of greater than 0.5 Hz, but differences of less than 1 Hz are difficult to appreciate without signal analysis methods such as spectral analysis.[1] The DPR is usually of higher amplitude on the right. A DPR with an amplitude that is 50% or more lower on the left compared with the right, or 35% or more on the right compared with the left, may be abnormal. Voltage asymmetries are best measured using referential EEG derivations (eg, O1-M2 and O2-M1). Asymmetries in the DPR amplitude when not accompanied by other EEG abnormalities should be interpreted with caution because they can occur in healthy individuals. Asymmetries in the DPR voltage need to recognized by the technologist while recording, and should prompt confirmation that the interelectrode distances are equal for the locations of homologous electrodes. If the distance between O1-M2 is less than O2-M1, the amplitude of O1-M2 may appear falsely lower.

Clinical Significance of Abnormalities in the DPR

In general, bilateral slowing of the DPR is most often caused by conditions that slow brain metabolism. Some are transient (associated with acute toxic or metabolic encephalopathies) whereas others are chronic (including dementias, cerebral atrophy, or bilateral cerebral lesions such as bilateral strokes). Bilateral slowing of the DPR is a sign of encephalopathy, and its degree often reflects the severity of the cerebral dysfunction, that is, the more the slowing, the more severe the cerebral dysfunction. The most common conditions associated with a bilaterally slowed DPR are metabolic disorders and dementias or, less often, bilateral cortical lesions (such as bilateral strokes). Bilateral absence of an alpha rhythm with bilateral occipital needle-like spikes can be seen in patients with congenital or early-acquired binocular blindness.

A unilateral slowed or absent DPR can be seen with: (1) ipsilateral damage to the occipital cortex (ie, stroke, contusion, and tumor); (2) ipsilateral damage to thalamus; (3) transient ischemic attacks; (4) milder head injuries; and (5) following a seizure or migraine. **Fig. 3** shows a significantly slower and poorly sustained DPR on the left. Unilateral failure of the DPR to attenuate (react) with eye opening or mental concentration is called the Bancaud phenomenon, and is seen with ipsilateral temporal or parietal cortical lesions such as tumors or infarcts.[10] However, asymmetries in frequencies of the posterior rhythm occasionally are falsely lateralizing when the dominant generator of the posterior rhythm involves the medial surface of one cerebral hemisphere and projects contralaterally.

Normal and Abnormal Beta Activity

Beta activity are EEG frequencies greater than 13 Hz. Beta activity is most often seen over the frontal and central scalp regions, usually at a frequency of 18 to 25 Hz, less often at 14 to 16 Hz, and rarely at 35 Hz. Beta activity may become more prominent or accentuated by mental, lingual, or cognitive efforts. Beta activity typically has a voltage of 5 to 20 µV. The voltage of beta activity in 98% of adults is less than 20 µV, and beta voltages greater than 25 µV are considered abnormal.[8]

Beta activity often increases with drowsiness. In very young children, prominent beta activity appears in NREM 1 sleep, which may be maximal posteriorly. The abrupt onset of prominent 20- to 25-Hz beta activity typically maximal over the central and postcentral regions heralds drowsiness in some children and sometimes persists during NREM 1 and 2 sleep, first seen at 5 to 6 months of age and rarely after age 7 years.

Excessive prominent augmentation of 15- to 25-Hz beta activity during wakefulness and drowsiness in an older child or an adult is most often the result of a medication effect, particularly seen with benzodiazepines and barbiturates.[11] Benzodiazepines, barbiturates, and chloral hydrate are potent activators of beta activity, often increasing beta activity in the 14- to 16-Hz bandwidth. Increased theta activity may accompany excessive beta activity in some cases.

Central nervous system stimulants such as methylphenidate, amphetamines, cocaine, tricyclic antidepressants, and levothyroxine also increase beta activity, but such activity is often low in voltage.[12] Withdrawal from alcohol or barbiturates may produce a similar low-voltage EEG with beta activity.[12,13] The beta-inducing effects of medications on the EEG are more pronounced in children compared with adults, and in acute rather than chronic use.[12] **Fig. 4** shows increased beta activity on a PSG, caused by clonazepam.

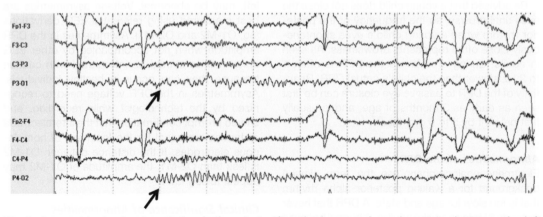

Fig. 3. Asymmetric dominant posterior rhythm. A significantly slower and poorly sustained DPR on the left (*arrow*). Note the asymmetric dominant posterior rhythm in this 10-second EEG fragment recorded in a 36-year-old man who had a left occipital ischemic stroke in the past. The dominant posterior rhythm is 10 Hz over P4-O2 (*arrow*); 7 to 8 Hz intermixed with 3 to 5 Hz over P3-O1. (*Courtesy of* M. Grigg-Damberger.)

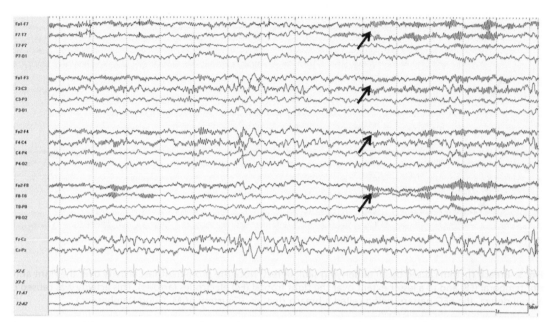

Fig. 4. Increased beta activity in a PSG, due to clonazepam. A 15-second fragment of EEG recorded in a 12-year-old boy in NREM 2 sleep shows excessive medium to high beta activity maximal bianteriorly (*arrows*). (*Courtesy of* M. Grigg-Damberger.)

Beta activity is usually symmetric. Persistently reduced voltages of beta activity greater than 50% suggest a cortical gray abnormality within the lower amplitude hemisphere. Lesser intermittent voltage asymmetries may simply reflect normal physiologic skull asymmetries.[8] A persistent focal suppression or attenuation of beta activity over a scalp region or hemisphere is a reliable localizing sign, and a hallmark of a structural lesion involving the underlying cerebral cortex or from an extradural fluid collection (such as a subdural hematoma). Focal attenuation of faster activities on the side of the lesion is most commonly associated with occlusive vascular disease.[14]

A marked focal increase in beta activity is most often caused by an underlying skull defect (most often a craniotomy or burr hole). Known as a breach rhythm, this pattern is characterized by sharply contoured waveforms with beta activity that is often threefold higher than that seen over other scalp regions (**Fig. 5**).[15] Misidentifying the sharply contoured waveforms evident in the region of the breach rhythm because of interictal epileptiform discharges (IEDs) is a common perilous pitfall in EEG interpretation.[16] The defect in the skull (most often a craniotomy, burr hole, or fracture) creates a low-resistance pathway for EEG currents, resulting in a localized increase in beta activity that is maximal near the margins of the skull defect. The amplitude of underlying theta and alpha activity is similarly enhanced through the defect, and this

leads to the sharply contoured waveforms being misidentified as discharges.[17] Of note, focal delta slowing over a skull defect is not caused by the skull defect, but reflects the acute or chronic underlying focal structural lesion. Asymmetric eye movements can be seen in patients with frontal skull defects. On rare occasions, beta activity is increased on the scalp region overlying a brain tumor or a focal cortical dysplastic lesion.[14]

Abnormalities in the Polysomnographic Markers of Sleep

Abnormalities of the distinctive PSG markers of sleep, such as sleep spindles and vertex waves, may be seen in PSG recording using standard and expanded EEG montages. Sleep spindles first appear in NREM 2, and may persist in early NREM 3 sleep. Sleep spindles most often occur at a frequency of 12 to 14 Hz (but range from 10 to 16 Hz), and recur at a frequency of 3 to 6 bursts per minute in stable undisturbed NREM 2 sleep. Sleep spindles first appear 3 to 4 weeks' term (43–44 weeks conceptional age) over the midline central (vertex, Cz) region. The absence of sleep spindles by 3 months' term is considered abnormal. At 3 and 6 months' term, 50% of sleep spindles are synchronous, shifting at times from side to side. Sleep spindles are synchronous by 12 months in 70% of cases. By age 2 years, sleep spindles appear synchronously over both hemispheres and are approximately symmetric.[18]

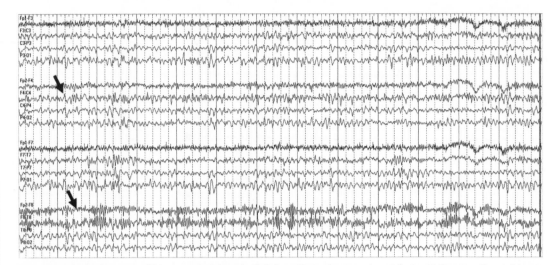

Fig. 5. Breach rhythm caused by an underlying skull defect. Note the prominent fast activity over the right anterior temporal (F8) and to a lesser extent over the right frontal (F4) electrodes (*arrows*). This activity was caused by a skull defect, the EEG pattern being called a breach rhythm. (*Courtesy of* M. Grigg-Damberger.)

The unilateral absence, decreased amplitude, or decreased frequency of sleep spindles is associated with an underlying ipsilateral pathologic condition, which can be found within the cortex or along the thalamocortical axis.[19] **Fig. 6** shows an example of asymmetric sleep spindles caused by a unilateral thalamic stroke. Sleep-spindle activity may be influenced by various hypnotic-sedative drugs.[20] Benzodiazepines and barbiturates also increase sleep-spindle activity. Bilateral prolonged spindles have been seen in recordings of patients with chronic and/or excessive benzodiazepines and barbiturate use.[20] An uncommon pattern of

almost continuous sleep spindles during NREM 2 (called extreme spindles) has been observed in individuals with severe intellectual disability.[21,22]

Sharp transients of sleep that can be mistaken as epileptic discharges

Vertex waves in adults are biphasic sharp transients with maximal negativity over the midline central region (Cz) typically lasting 200 milliseconds. Vertex waves in children often have large amplitudes (50–150 μV, rarely >250 μV in Cz-M1).[23] Vertex waves are usually symmetric and maximal over the midline, often extending to

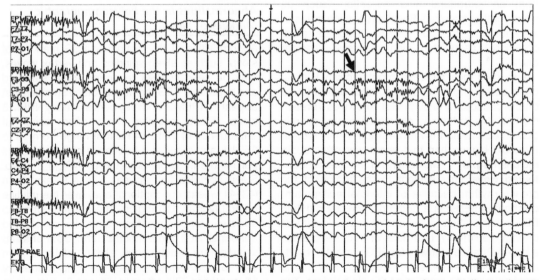

Fig. 6. Asymmetric sleep spindles caused by a thalamic stroke. Note the asymmetric sleep spindles in this 10-second EEG fragment. Sleep spindles were present on the left (*arrow*) (maximal C3, Cz) and absent on the right. The loss of sleep spindles on the right was caused by a thalamic stroke.

adjacent areas, especially in children. Vertex waves in children aged 2 to 4 years can appear of high voltage and sharply contoured, and may be asymmetric lateralizing to the right or left central (C3 or C4), but typically maximal over the midline.[23,24] When these occur in brief runs and are particularly spiky, they may be mistaken for IEDs (**Fig. 7**).

SLOW ACTIVITY INAPPROPRIATE FOR STATE/AGE

Inappropriate or excessive slowing in an EEG includes activities that are abnormally slow for the age and state of the patient. Slow activity can be subdivided according to whether it is localized or generalized, bilaterally synchronous or asynchronous, and continuous or intermittent. Generalized slowing is bilateral and relatively diffuse (although sometimes maximal over the anterior, central, or posterior regions). Lateralized slow activity is restricted to one hemisphere, whereas regional slow activity is limited to one lobe or part of a lobe. Basic patterns of slow-wave activity in EEG include: (1) focal (localized or regional) slow waves; (2) generalized synchronous slow waves; and (3) generalized asynchronous slow waves. **Table 1** summarizes the patterns of abnormal slow-wave activity as well as their clinicopathologic associations and significance.

Abnormal focal slow waves are typically in the theta (<8 Hz) or delta (<4 Hz) frequency range and usually are restricted to a few nearby

electrodes, less often lateralized to a hemisphere. Focal slowing is usually secondary to a superficial and/or deep focal disturbance of cerebral function in that hemisphere, and reflects interruption in corticocortical and corticosubcortical fiber connections. Focal arrhythmic delta (FAD) activity is often called focal polymorphic delta activity, although focal arrhythmic delta slow activity is the now preferred EEG terminology.

FAD activity consists of arrhythmic delta slow waves with variable frequency, amplitude, and morphology, which can be seen persistently in a specific site throughout the recording. FAD activity is the hallmark of an underlying structural lesion in the white matter. About two-thirds of patients with FAD have a subcortical structural lesion.[25,26] The specificity of the etiology of FAD in an EEG is poor. Ischemic stroke, hemorrhagic stroke, and tumors all can cause FAD. FAD usually lateralizes to the side of the lesion. FAD produced by parasagittal lesions can project the same abnormal slowing to the contralateral hemisphere, and anterior structural lesions can produce bilateral abnormalities. A unilateral frontal lesion can cause bilateral FAD, although usually of higher amplitude and with a wider field of slowing on the side of the lesion. Furthermore, both frontal and parietal lesions can cause delta slowing that is of highest amplitude over the temporal areas.

Transient or short-lived FAD can also be seen following seizures, migraine, and transient ischemic attacks. FAD in these clinical settings would be expected to: (1) resolve over time during

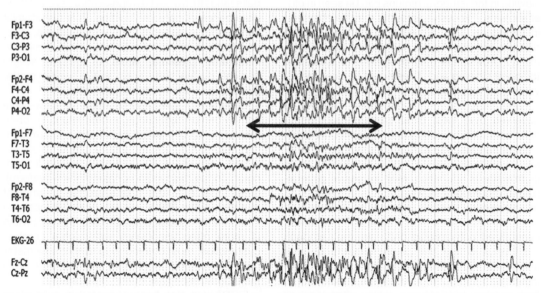

Fig. 7. Run of sharply contoured vertex activity in a 9-year-old child. High-voltage vertex waves in a young child. Note the run of high voltage, sharply contoured vertex waves that are maximal over the midline central (Cz) region in this child in NREM 2 sleep (*arrow*). (*Courtesy of* M. Grigg-Damberger.)

Table1
Patterns of slow-wave abnormality in the electroencephalogram

Slow-Wave Activity	Clinicopathologic Correlations
Localized (focal or regional) slow waves	Focal structural damage to subcortical white matter and/or thalamus (stroke, hemorrhage, contusion, tumor, and brain abscess) Focal, often transient, disorders of cerebral blood flow or metabolism (migraine, postictal state, and transient ischemic attack)
Generalized asynchronous slow waves	Generalized disturbance of cerebral function (cerebral anoxia, postictal state, and coma) Widespread degenerative or cerebrovascular disease that involves subcortical white matter; Mild or moderate amounts are seen in 10%–15% of normal adults with no detectable abnormality
Bilaterally synchronous slow waves	Deep midline gray matter involvement by: Metabolic, toxic, or endocrine encephalopathies (hepatic encephalopathy) or Local structural lesions that compress, distort, or involve deep midline structures of midbrain, diencephalon, or mesial/orbital frontal lobes (tumors/strokes) Diffuse degenerative diseases that damage subcortical and cortical gray matter more than white matter (Alzheimer, dementia, and progressive supranuclear palsy)

continuous EEG monitoring or subsequent EEGs, or to be intermittent; (2) involve substantial theta activity rather than slower delta activity; (3) disappear with eye opening or external stimuli; and/or (4) be reactive to sleep/wake changes.

Brief intermittent runs of low-amplitude FAD slowing in the temporal regions can be seen in older subjects. Excessive amounts may be observed in individuals with dementia or cerebrovascular disease, but represent a nonspecific EEG abnormality. Drowsiness may contribute to excessive temporal slowing and, if restricted to sleep deprivation and drowsiness, is often normal.

Generalized asynchronous slow activity is observed over most or all parts of both hemispheres. It can be continuous or semicontinuous, or recur as intermittent bursts of slowing. Generalized asynchronous theta or delta slowing is normal in drowsiness and sleep. Mild excessive generalized asynchronous slowing occurs in 5% to 10% of otherwise normal individuals. Generalized asynchronous delta slow activity: (1) is called generalized polymorphic delta slowing, although the former is now the preferred term; (2) may lessen with eye opening or alerting; and (3) is associated with structural or functional impairment of both cerebral hemispheres, which often involves subcortical white matter, including diffuse metabolic encephalopathies.

Generalized asynchronous arrhythmic slow activity with the predominant EEG frequencies in the theta range (4 to <8 Hz) are seen in patients with mild to moderate encephalopathies, dementias, and systemic infections. A diffusely slowed EEG in which the dominant frequencies are in the delta range (0.5 to <4 Hz) represents a severe diffuse disturbance of cerebral function. This disturbance can be seen in the setting of severe metabolic, toxic, or infectious encephalopathies, severe increased intracranial pressure, acute or chronic severe cortical dysfunction, gray and/or white matter disease, and/or brainstem dysfunction.

Generalized synchronous rhythmic slow-wave activity can be continuous or intermittent. Discrete runs or bursts of bilateral synchronous intermittent rhythmic delta activity (IRDA), most often at a frequency of 2.5 Hz (and often having a slight notch on the descending phase of the waveform), often localize to the frontal (frontal intermittent rhythmic delta; FIRDA) or the occipital (occipital intermittent rhythmic delta; OIRDA) regions. FIRDA is more often associated with global cerebral dysfunction, most commonly in relation to a metabolic encephalopathy. FIRDA can also be seen in the elderly, especially during drowsiness.

FIRDA has also been observed in subcortical lesions (especially tumors), alteration of midline structures, dementia, or elevated intracranial pressure.[27,28] Asymmetric FIRDA has been associated with an underlying brain lesion,[29] and should prompt investigations for structural lesions.[29] Intermittent rhythmic delta slowing in children is more often maximal over the occipital regions (OIRDA). OIRDA can be transiently seen in children following a seizure, trauma, or migraine.[30] However, when observed in children with absence epilepsy, OIRDA carries a favorable prognosis for their epilepsy.[31]

Temporal intermittent rhythmic delta activity (TIRDA) can be seen in up to 40% of patients with temporal lobe epilepsy and, when present, lateralizes to the side of the epileptic focus.[32,33] One study reported TIRDA in 13% of patients with juvenile absence epilepsy in whom focal IEDs also occurred, despite it being classified as a generalized epilepsy.[34] TIRDA, although a nonspecific EEG abnormality, can be seen in patients with either temporal or extratemporal epilepsies.[35]

NORMAL SLOW ACTIVITY MISTAKEN FOR ABNORMAL ACTIVITY

Adult sleep specialists need to know that the waking DPR in children between ages 1 and 15 years contains intermittent theta and delta slowing, the quantity of which decreases and the frequency of which increases with age.[36] The intermixed slowing is often arrhythmic or semirhythmic, of moderate voltage (<100 μV), and of range 2.5 to 4.5 Hz (**Fig. 8**).[37] Intermixed slowing is particularly prominent between ages 5 and 7 years. Fifteen percent to 20% of normal children aged 8 to 16 years have independent runs of 5 to 8 Hz activity over the frontal and central regions.[38–40]

Posterior slow waves of youth (PSWs) may be misinterpreted as abnormal occipital slowing (**Fig. 9**). PSWs are a normal EEG pattern seen during wakefulness in children and characterized by intermittent runs of delta waveforms that have individual alpha waveforms superimposed or fused on the delta waveform. These waves are typically of moderate voltage (≤120% of the DPR voltage) and bilateral, but often asymmetric over the occipital regions. PSWs, like the DPR, attenuate with eye opening and disappear with drowsiness; they typically occur in rapid succession or are separated from each other by 1 to a few seconds. Pathologic (abnormal) PSWs are often larger in amplitude (>150% of the amplitude of the DPR), disrupt the underlying DPR, are not associated with overriding alpha activity, and are less reactive to eye opening.[4] PSWs are most prominent in children aged 8 to 14 years, and uncommon in those younger than age 2 or after age 21. However, 2 studies reported PSWs in 7% to 10% of adults aged 18 to 30 years.[23,41]

Hypnagogic Hypersynchrony

Hypnagogic hypersynchrony (HH) is a well-recognized normal pattern seen during NREM 1 sleep in children from age 3 months to 13 years. HH consists of paroxysmal bursts or runs of diffuse bisynchronous sinusoidal high voltage (often 200–350 μV) and 3- to 5-Hz bursts that tend to begin abruptly and occur intermittently or continuously for several minutes during sleep onset, maximal over the frontocentral regions.

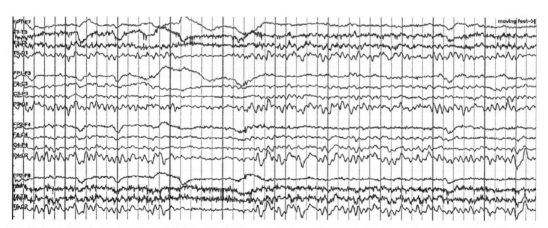

Fig. 8. Intermixed slowing in a child's wake background. Appropriate for age intermixed theta-delta slowing activity in the waking posterior background of a child. The waking dominant posterior rhythm in children between ages 1 and 15 years often contains intermixed theta and delta slowing, which is typically bilateral, less than 150% of the amplitude of the dominant alpha rhythm. Note the intermixed arrhythmic 2- to 4-Hz activity in the T5-O1, P3-O1, T6-O2, and P4-O2 channels in this 10-second EEG fragment recorded during wakefulness in an 8-year-old.

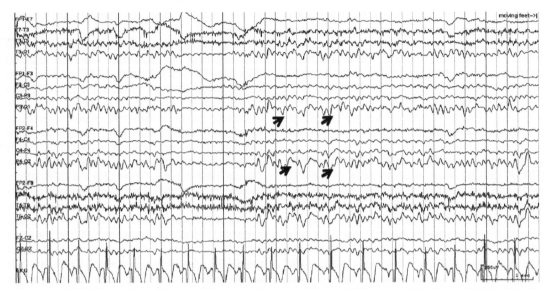

Fig. 9. Posterior waves of youth. The dominant posterior rhythm in this 7-year-old consists of 8-Hz intermixed with 2- to 2.5-Hz posterior slow waves of youth (*arrows*). Note how the dominant posterior rhythm is fused on the slow waves. Posterior slow waves of youth are accentuated by hyperventilation, always bilateral but often asymmetric, reactive to eye opening, and disappear with drowsiness and sleep.

Because HH tends to occur in runs or bursts and is often high-voltage and paroxysmal, it is sometimes mistaken for generalized IEDs (**Fig. 10**).

Normal Sharp Transients that can be Mistaken as Epileptiform or Seizures

Positive occipital sharp transients
Positive occipital sharp transients of sleep (POSTS) are surface positive, bisynchronous, occipital sharp waves lasting 200 to 300 milliseconds. POSTS have a voltage of 20 to 50 mV and usually occur in brief runs of 4 to 5 Hz during NREM 1 and 2 sleep. They can be seen in children as young as 4 years and usually are not seen in adulthood. POSTS that are particularly sharp, asymmetric, and/or occur in runs can fool the unwary who mistake them at first glance for IEDs (**Fig. 11**).

Lambda waves
Lambda waves are high-amplitude biphasic or triphasic waveforms that appear in the occipital derivations when a patient scans a textured or complex picture with fast saccadic eye

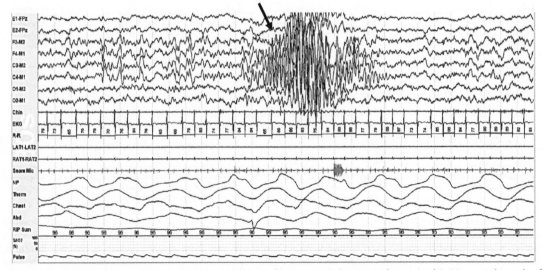

Fig. 10. Hypnagogic hypersynchrony. Paroxysmal burst of hypnagogic hypersynchrony in this 30-second epoch of PSG recorded in NREM 1 sleep in a 5-year-old child (*arrow*). (*Courtesy of* M. Grigg-Damberger.)

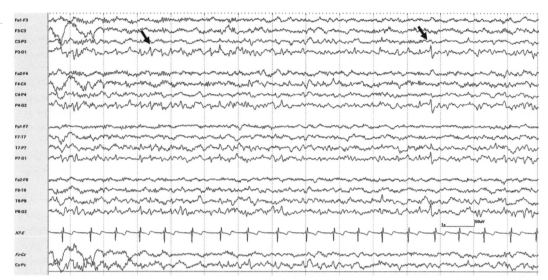

Fig. 11. Positive occipital sharp transients of sleep (POSTS) seen as surface-positive waves in the occipital regions. Note the sharply contoured surface-positive POSTS in this 15-second EEG fragment recorded during NREM 2 sleep in a 12-year-old child (*arrows*). (*Courtesy of* M. Grigg-Damberger.)

movements (**Fig. 12**). The International Glossary of EEG defines lambda waves as "diphasic sharp transients over the occipital regions of the head of waking subjects during visual exploration," further detailing that: (1) the main component is surface positive relative to other areas; (2) they are time-locked to saccadic eye movements; and (3) they are generally less than 50 µV in amplitude.[42] Lambda waves are often sharply contoured, asymmetric, and sometimes of higher amplitude than the DPR, and occasionally mistaken for IEDs. Lambda waves are most

common in children, but may be seen in young adults. Observing prominent lambda waves and uncertain of their nature, the technologist can, by placing a plain white sheet of paper in front of the patient, eliminate the visual input necessary for their generation.[8]

Rhythmic midtemporal theta bursts of drowsiness

Rhythmic midtemporal theta bursts of drowsiness (RMTD; psychomotor variant) refer to temporal intermittent rhythmic theta activity, not

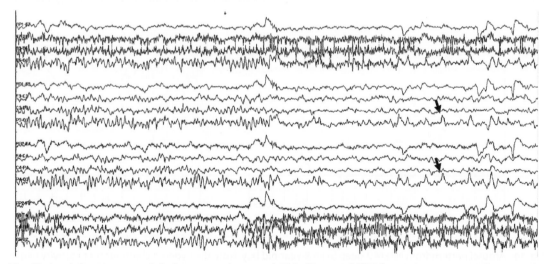

Fig. 12. Lambda waves noted during an awake record. This 10-second EEG fragment on an anterior-posterior bipolar montage shows prominent lambda waves (*arrows*) in the occipital derivations when a 9-year-old child is awake and scanning a picture.

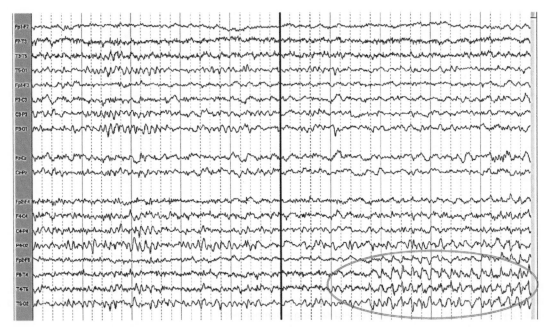

Fig. 13. Rhythmic midtemporal theta bursts of drowsiness (RMTD). Note the run of unilateral rhythmic midtemporal theta activity over the right temporal region in this 10-second EEG fragment recorded in a 50-year-old in NREM 1 sleep (*circle*).

accompanied by polymorphic slowing. RMTD is typically seen in drowsiness, and waves typically phase-reverse over the midtemporal regions (**Fig. 13**).[43] RMTD can occur bilaterally or unilaterally, and may shift from side to side. When RMTD has a notched appearance, it can be mistaken for spike-and-wave discharges. The specific occurrence of RMTD only during drowsiness and NREM 1 sleep should help confirm its benign nature.[43]

Arousal patterns from sleep

Arousal patterns also need to be distinguished from epileptiform abnormalities. In children and adults, arousals from sleep represent a quick phenomenon with a change from sleep into a waking stage, usually with a very well developed posterior alpha rhythm. This transition may be marked by a sequence of K-complexes, which may appear as a run of high-amplitude sustained activity maximal in the frontal and central regions.[44] In

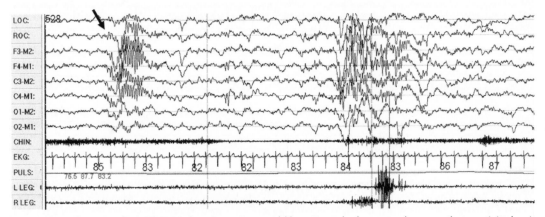

Fig. 14. Arousal pattern from NREM 2 sleep in an 8-year-old boy. Note the hypersynchronous theta activity beginning in the fifth second of this 30-second epoch of PSG in an 8-year-old boy during NREM 2 sleep. The child arouses, and paroxysmal sharply contoured 3-Hz frequencies intermixed with faster frequencies are seen (*arrow*). These EEG patterns are normal for age. (*Courtesy of* M. Grigg-Damberger.)

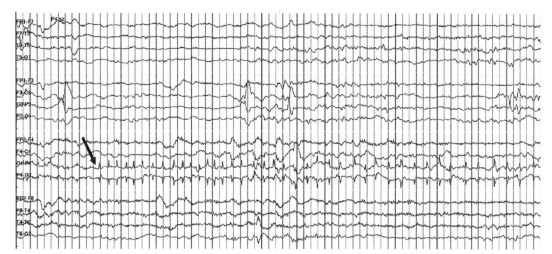

Fig. 15. Electrode popping artifact noted at electrode P4 (*arrow*). An electrode pop involving the right parietal (P4) electrode is shown in this 10-second EEG fragment, and is most likely caused by a poorly applied electrode. The electrode pop causes repetitive sharp transients that involve only one electrode, and are caused by abrupt changes in the impedance of the electrode.

children, sustained rhythmic theta and delta activity can be seen, and may mimic IEDs. **Fig. 14** shows an example of a rhythmic paroxysmal arousal from NREM 2 sleep in a child.

In infancy (3–4 months), 3- to 4-Hz rhythmic occipital activity is often noted on arousal.[45] The main feature that distinguishes these arousal patterns from epileptic activity is the fact that this occipital pattern can be blocked with eye closure. At later ages, these patterns can have higher frequencies, namely 5 Hz at age 5 months and 6 to 8 Hz at 12 months, with amplitudes of 50 to 100 μV.[45] Arousal patterns in children aged 1 to 3 years often consist of diffuse high-voltage 4- to 6-Hz activity intermixed with slower frequencies.[46] Another normal EEG pattern sometimes mistaken as epileptiform is the frontal arousal rhythm (FAR). FAR is characterized by intermittent rhythmic, often sharply contoured theta activity, most prominent over the frontal regions, and

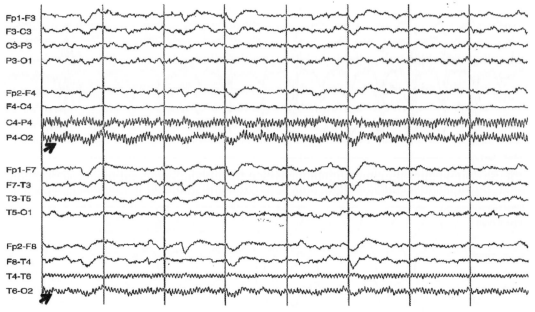

Fig. 16. Artifact in P4 and T6. Alternating current (60 Hz) artifact noted at electrode C4. Note the 60-Hz artifact in this 10-second EEG fragment over P4 and T6 (*arrows*).

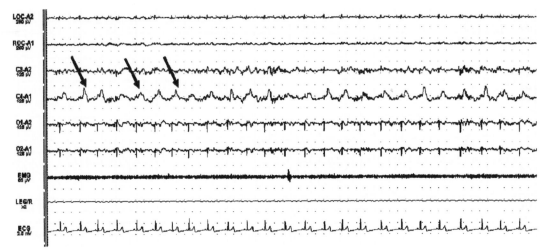

Fig. 17. Pulse artifact in C4. Pulse artifact is noted in this 10-second EEG fragment in the midline region, as sinusoidal waves with frequency corresponding to pulse rate (note matching frequency of the pulse artifact and heart rate) (*arrows*). (*Courtesy of* Timothy Hoban.)

especially common in children between age 2 and 12 years.[47] Some report that this pattern may be associated with epilepsy, and caution should be used in interpreting it as benign.[47]

ARTIFACTS THAT CAN RESEMBLE INTERICTAL EPILEPTIC DISCHARGES OR SEIZURES

Artifacts produced by electrode malfunction may also resemble IEDs. Some can be easily recognized and confirmed by troubleshooting the EEG equipment by the technologist (voltage and impedances, electrode box connections, and integrity of EEG electrodes on the scalp). Examples of common artifacts that can mimic IEDs or seizures include electrode popping, alternating current (60 Hz) artifact, and sweat, pulse, and respiratory artifacts. Movement artifacts can often be easily identified by reviewing the time-locked video when the event is observed on the PSG.

Electrode pops appear as single or multiple sharp waveforms with abrupt vertical transients that do not modify the background activity, due to abrupt impedance change in an electrode

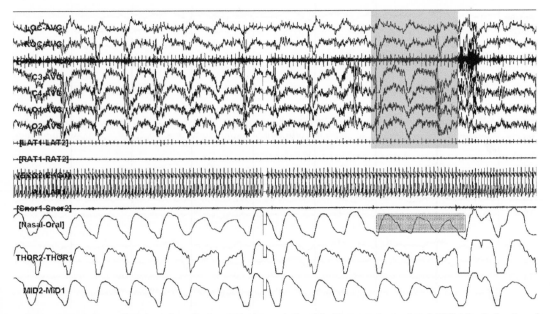

Fig. 18. Respiration artifact invades all the EEG channels in this 30-second epoch of PSG (*shaded column*). (*Courtesy of* Timothy Hoban.)

(**Fig. 15**). Pops are identified easily by their characteristic appearance and distribution limited to a single electrode. Sharp transients that occur at a single electrode should be considered artifacts until proved otherwise (although this is sometimes challenging when recording so few EEG derivations on a routine PSG). Rhythmic electrode popping can resemble a seizure but can be recognized when it occurs in a single electrode. Alternating current (60 Hz) artifact presents at exact frequency (60 Hz) (**Fig. 16**). It can involve one or more electrodes. To identify this artifact, the paper speed can be increased to 60 mm per second so that the individual waveforms can be counted (1 cycle/mm). This problem occurs when the impedance of one of the electrodes becomes significantly large between the electrodes and the amplifier ground, leading to the ground becoming active.

A pulse artifact can be seen when an EEG electrode is placed over a pulsating scalp vessel. The vessel pulsation can cause rhythmic movements of the electrode, which appear as slow waves (**Fig. 17**). This activity may simulate a seizure or rhythmic slow activity. One easy way to identify this artifact is to recognize that there is a direct relationship between the electrocardiogram and the pulse waves: the pulse waves occur slightly after the QRS complex (200–300 milliseconds). Respiration artifact can present as slow or sharp waves that occur synchronously with inhalation or exhalation. This activity usually involves only a few electrodes, typically those on which the patient is lying (**Fig. 18**).

SUMMARY

Recognizing EEG abnormalities and distinguishing epileptic from nonepileptic patterns and artifacts are important for polysomnographers. The most common pitfall is misidentifying normal variants and artifacts as epileptic patterns. Although the ability to recognize these patterns comes with experience, less experienced polysomnographers should be aware of the range of normal rhythms seen on EEG.

REFERENCES

1. Fisch BJ. Fisch and Spehlmann's EEG primer: basic principles of digital and analog EEG. 3rd edition. New York: Elsevier; 2006.
2. Aminoff MJ. Autonomic dysfunction in central nervous system disorders. Curr Opin Neurol Neurosurg 1992;5(4):482–6.
3. Brazier MA, Finesinger JE. Characteristics of the normal electroencephalogram. I. A study of the occipital cortical potentials in 500 normal adults. J Clin Invest 1944;23(3):303–11.
4. Kellaway P. Orderly approach to visual analysis: elements of the normal EEG, and their characteristics in children and adults. In: Ebersole JS, Pedley TA, editors. Current practice of clinical electroencephalography. 3rd edition. Philadelphia: Lippincott Williams & Wilkins; 2003. p. 100–59.
5. Gibbs EL, Lorimer FM, Gibbs FA. Clinical correlates of exceedingly fast activity in the electroencephalogram. Dis Nerv Syst 1950;11(11):323–6.
6. Werner SS, Stockard JE, Bickford RG. The ontogenesis of the electroencephalogram of prematures. Atlas of Neonatal Electroencephalography. 1st edition. New York City: Raven Press; 1977. p. 47–91.
7. Niedermeyer E. Maturation of the EEG: development of wake and sleep patterns. In: Niedermeyer E, Lopes da Silva F, editors. Electroencephalography: basic principles, clinical applications and related fields. 4th edition. Philadelpha: Lippincott, Williams and Wilkins; 1999. p. 189–214.
8. Tatum WO, Husain AM, Benbadis SR, et al. Normal adult EEG and patterns of uncertain significance. J Clin Neurophysiol 2006;23(3):194–207.
9. Luders H, Noachtar S. Atlas of epileptic seizures and syndromes. Philadelphia: Saunders; 2001.
10. Westmoreland BF, Klass DW. Defective alpha reactivity with mental concentration. J Clin Neurophysiol 1998;15(5):424–8.
11. Michail E, Chouvarda I, Maglaveras N. Benzodiazepine administration effect on EEG fractal dimension: results and causalities. Conf Proc IEEE Eng Med Biol Soc 2010;2010:2350–3.
12. Blume WT. Drug effects on EEG. J Clin Neurophysiol 2006;23(4):306–11.
13. Courtney KE, Polich J. Binge drinking effects on EEG in young adult humans. Int J Environ Res Public Health 2010;7(5):2325–36.
14. Green RL, Wilson WP. Asymmetries of beta activity in epilepsy, brain tumor, and cerebrovascular disease. Electroencephalogr Clin Neurophysiol 1961;13:75–8.
15. Westmoreland BF, Klass DW. Unusual EEG patterns. J Clin Neurophysiol 1990;7(2):209–28.
16. Markand ON. Pearls, perils, and pitfalls in the use of the electroencephalogram. Semin Neurol 2003; 23(1):7–46.
17. Cobb WA, Guiloff RJ, Cast J. Breach rhythm: the EEG related to skull defects. Electroencephalogr Clin Neurophysiol 1979;47(3):251–71.
18. Dehghani N, Cash SS, Rossetti AO, et al. Magnetoencephalography demonstrates multiple asynchronous generators during human sleep spindles. J Neurophysiol 2010;104(1):179–88.
19. Dehghani N, Cash SS, Halgren E. Emergence of synchronous EEG spindles from asynchronous MEG spindles. Hum Brain Mapp 2011;32(12): 2217–27.

20. Jankel WR, Niedermeyer E. Sleep spindles. J Clin Neurophysiol 1985;2(1):1–35.

21. Shibagaki M, Kiyono S, Watanabe K. Spindle evolution in normal and mentally retarded children: a review. Sleep 1982;5(1):47–57.

22. Husain AM. Electroencephalographic assessment of coma. J Clin Neurophysiol 2006;23(3):208–20.

23. Fisch BJ. Fisch and Spehlmann's EEG primer. 3rd printing revised and enlarged ed. New York: Elsevier; 2002.

24. Mizrahi EM. Avoiding the pitfalls of EEG interpretation in childhood epilepsy. Epilepsia 1996; 37(Suppl 1):S41–51.

25. Gilmore PC, Brenner RP. Correlation of EEG, computerized tomography, and clinical findings. Study of 100 patients with focal delta activity. Arch Neurol 1981;38(6):371–2.

26. Marshall DW, Brey RL, Morse MW. Focal and/or lateralized polymorphic delta activity. Association with either 'normal' or 'nonfocal' computed tomographic scans. Arch Neurol 1988;45(1):33–5.

27. Scollo-Lavizzari G, Matthis H. Frontal intermittent rhythmic delta activity. A comparative study of EEG and CT scan findings. Eur Neurol 1981; 20(1):1–3.

28. Calzetti S, Bortone E, Negrotti A, et al. Frontal intermittent rhythmic delta activity (FIRDA) in patients with dementia with Lewy bodies: a diagnostic tool? Neurol Sci 2002;23(Suppl 2):S65–6.

29. Accolla EA, Kaplan PW, Maeder-Ingvar M, et al. Clinical correlates of frontal intermittent rhythmic delta activity (FIRDA). Clin Neurophysiol 2011; 122(1):27–31.

30. Gullapalli D, Fountain NB. Clinical correlation of occipital intermittent rhythmic delta activity. J Clin Neurophysiol 2003;20(1):35–41.

31. Riviello JJ Jr, Foley CM. The epileptiform significance of intermittent rhythmic delta activity in childhood. J Child Neurol 1992;7(2):156–60.

32. Brigo F. Intermittent rhythmic delta activity patterns. Epilepsy Behav 2011;20(2):254–6.

33. Di Gennaro G, Quarato PP, Onorati P, et al. Localizing significance of temporal intermittent rhythmic delta activity (TIRDA) in drug-resistant focal epilepsy. Clin Neurophysiol 2003;114(1):70–8.

34. Gelisse P, Serafini A, Velizarova R, et al. Temporal intermittent delta activity: a marker of juvenile absence epilepsy? Seizure 2011;20(1):38–41.

35. Haim S, Friedman-Birnbaum R. Pyoderma gangrenosum in immunosuppressed patients. Dermatologica 1976;153(1):44–8.

36. Henry C. Electroencephalograms of normal children. Monogr Soc Res Child Dev 1943;9:39.

37. Eeg-Olofsson O. Longitudinal developmental course of electrical activity of brain. Brain Dev 1980;2(1):33–44.

38. Aird RB, Gastaut Y. Occipital and posterior electroencephalographic rhythms. Electroencephalogr Clin Neurophysiol 1959;11:637–56.

39. Petersen I, Sorbye R. Slow posterior rhythm in adults. Electroencephalogr Clin Neurophysiol 1962;14:161–70.

40. Kuhlo W. Posterior slow rhythms. In: Redmond A, editor. Handbook of Electroencephalography and Clinical Neurophysiology, vol. 6A. Amsterdam: Elsevier; 1976. p. 89–104.

41. Niedermeyer E. The normal EEG of the waking adult. In: Niedermeyer E, Lopes da Silva F, editors. Basic principles, clinical applications and related fields. Philadelphia: Lippincott Williams and Wilkins; 2005. p. 167–87.

42. IFSECN. A glossary of terms commonly used by clinical electroencephalographers. Electroencephalogr Clin Neurophysiol 1974;37:538–48.

43. Lipman IJ, Hughes JR. Rhythmic mid-temporal discharges (RMTD): an electro-clinical study. Epilepsia 1969;10(3):416–7.

44. Grigg-Damberger M, Gozal D, Marcus CL, et al. The visual scoring of sleep and arousal in infants and children. J Clin Sleep Med 2007;3(2):201–40.

45. Andre M, Lamblin MD, d'Allest AM, et al. Electroencephalography in premature and full-term infants. Developmental features and glossary. Neurophysiol Clin 2010;40(2):59–124.

46. Hess R. The Electroencephalogram in sleep. Electroencephalogr Clin Neurophysiol 1964;16:44–55.

47. Hughes JR, Daaboul Y. The frontal arousal rhythm. Clin Electroencephalogr 1999;30(1):16–20.

Identifying Interictal and Ictal Epileptic Activity in Polysomnograms

Nancy Foldvary-Schaefer, DO, MS[a],*,
Madeleine M. Grigg-Damberger, MD[b]

KEYWORDS

- Electroencephalography (EEG) • Polysomnography (PSG)
- Video EEG PSG • Nocturnal seizures
- Sleep-related epilepsy

Recognizing epileptic electroencephalography (EEG) abnormalities and epileptic seizures in routine polysomnography (PSG) is challenging, even for those with training in EEG and epilepsy. Videopolysomnography (VPSG) with expanded EEG (VEEG PSG) combines expanded EEG and PSG to evaluate paroxysmal motor activity and behaviors in sleep, making it possible to better differentiate epileptic from nonepileptic events. VEEG PSG has several advantages over routine PSG, including (1) improving the likelihood of recognizing interictal and ictal EEG activity, (2) allowing for more precise evaluation of EEG background, and (3) correlating clinical with other neurophysiologic parameters.

VEEG PSG is usually performed to evaluate parasomnias that are (1) atypical or unusual in frequency, duration, age of onset, or too stereotyped, repetitive or focal, (2) potentially injurious or have caused injury to the patient or others, or (3) paroxysmal arousals or other sleep disruptions believed to be seizure related when the initial clinical evaluation and routine EEG are inconclusive.[1] Despite advances in neuroimaging, EEG continues to play a pivotal role in the diagnosis and management of patients with epilepsy. This article reviews interictal epileptic discharges (IEDs) and ictal electrographic seizures that sleep specialists and technologists may encounter in PSGs of patients with unexplained nocturnal events. Strategies to optimize the diagnostic yield of EEG and videorecordings in such cases are discussed.

VEEG PSG METHODOLOGY
Basic Concepts of EEG

Although EEG is discussed in more detail by Epstein elsewhere in this issue, we review some crucial concepts of EEG that are important to understand when reviewing VEEG PSG. Scalp EEG reflects fluctuating electrical voltage fields that result from continuous changing or oscillating extracellular current flow in the underlying cerebral cortex. Most of the EEG activity recorded represents a constantly changing summation and integration of excitatory and inhibitory postsynaptic potentials developed by the cell bodies and large dendrites from thousands of neighboring groups of neurons cross-talking in the underlying cerebral cortex. A single action potential does not contribute to the EEG because it is too brief, small, and distant from the recording electrode(s).

Financial Disclosure and Conflict of Interest Obligations: We have no conflicts of interest to declare regarding this paper.

[a] Cleveland Clinic Lerner College of Medicine of Case Western Reserve University, Epilepsy Center, Cleveland Clinic Neurological Institute, 9500 Euclid Avenue, FA 20, Cleveland, OH 44195, USA

[b] Department of Neurology, University of New Mexico School of Medicine, MSC10 5620, One University of NM, Albuquerque, NM 87131-0001, USA

* Corresponding author.

E-mail address: foldvan@ccf.org

Sleep Med Clin 7 (2012) 39–58

doi:10.1016/j.jsmc.2012.01.002

The pyramidal neurons in layers III and V of the cerebral cortex are believed to contribute most of the scalp EEG signal because they are aligned perpendicular to the surface of the cerebral cortex and tend to fire together. When a group of radially oriented pyramidal cortical neurons depolarize, a tangential net negativity is seen on the cortical surface, with a relative positivity in the deeper neocortical layers forming a vertical dipole for current flow.

One of the most striking features of EEG recorded from intracranial electrodes in animals and humans is the difference in electrical activity from electrode to electrode, even when the electrodes are only 1 to 2 mm apart.[2] The similarity of electrical activity from 2 scalp electrodes separated by more than a few millimeters is probably because the neurons in the vicinity of the electrode are driven by a common source. Neurons of at least 6 to 10 cm^2 of cortical surface area must fire synchronously for an IED to be detected on scalp EEG.[3,4] Neuronal generators that are deep-seated or dipoles that are horizontal to the cortical surface may not produce recognizable scalp EEG potentials.

Electrode Placement

EEG electrodes are applied to the scalp for routine EEG recordings using the International 10–20 System of electrode placement (**Fig. 1**).[5,6] In 1991, the American Clinical Neurophysiology Society (ACNS) recommended modifying the naming of the midtemporal and posterior temporal electrode placements: the left and right midtemporal electrodes (T3 and T4) were to be called T7 and T8, respectively, and the posterior temporal electrodes (T5 and T6), P7 and P8 (**Fig. 2**).[7] This recommendation was made to be in concordance with the International 10-10 System of electrode placement, which provides names and locations for additional electrodes by further dividing the distances between standard 10-20 placements. The additional electrodes of the 10-10 system are most often used for epilepsy surgery evaluations in patients with medically resistant epilepsy, detailed topographic mapping of EEG, and research. They are particularly useful when recording EEG in patients with suspected temporal lobe epilepsy (TLE) because the T7 and T8 electrodes also record activity from the lower part of the frontal lobe, and the location of the maximal electronegativity of a discharge can be helpful in differentiating mesial from neocortical TLE.

The International 10-20 System ensures that the EEG electrode placement is standardized across laboratories. Properly placed electrodes ensure the electrode placements are symmetric and evenly spaced over the correct anatomic location. When reading an EEG, electrical activity over 1 area is compared with that on the same (homologous) area on the contralateral side. Meaningful asymmetries or absence of electrical activity expected to be seen over a region (eg, sleep spindles or the alpha rhythm) can be confirmed only knowing that electrode placement is the same over time. Unequal interelectrode distances for homologous pairs of electrodes cause a false

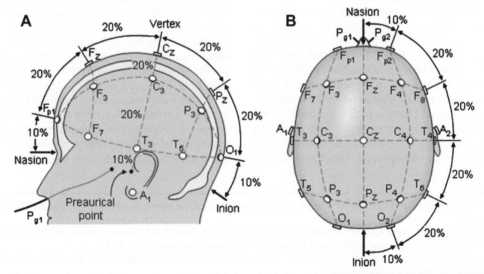

Fig. 1. The International 10-20 System seen from (*A*) left and (*B*) above the head. A, ear lobe; C, central; F, frontal; FP, frontal polar; O, occipital; P, parietal; Pg, nasopharyngeal. (*Adapted from* Sharbrough F, Chatrian GE, Lesser RP, et al. American Electroencephalographic Society guidelines for standard electrode position nomenclature. J Clin Neurophysiol 1991;8:200–2; with permission.)

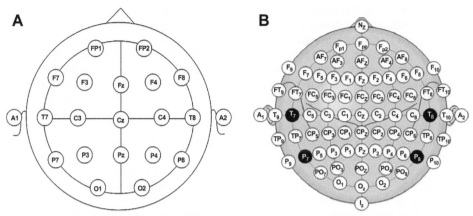

Fig. 2. The International 10-20 System with modified combinatorial nomenclature for the names and locations of electrodes (*A*). Note how the right and left midtemporal and posterior-temporal electrodes are named T7, T8, P7, and P8. This modification was first recommended by the ACNS to be in concordance with the names and locations of electrodes in the expansion of the 10-20 System, the International 10-10 System shown in (*B*). The modified combinatorial nomenclature is used to detail topographic mapping of EEG activity. ([*B*] *Adapted from* Sharbrough F, Chatrian GE, Lesser RP, et al. American Electroencephalographic Society guidelines for standard electrode position nomenclature. J Clin Neurophysiol 1991;8:201; with permission.)

amplitude asymmetry: the shorter the interelectrode distance, the lower the amplitude. Proper electrode placement becomes even more critical in routine PSG given the limited number of EEG derivations recommended by the American Academy of Sleep Medicine (AASM) scoring and recording guidelines.[8]

Basic EEG Montage Design Methods: Bipolar, Common Reference, and Average Reference

Montages are systematic and logical combinations of multiple pairs of electrodes that allow for simultaneous recording of EEG activity over the scalp.[9] Most digital EEG systems have 18 to 21 amplifiers that permit simultaneous recording of 18 to 21 channels of EEG. Each electrode is connected to an EEG amplifier. The digital EEG or PSG system connects different pairs of electrodes in any number of configurations to best show EEG activity based on the clinical question.

Montages are designed to compare EEG activity from homologous electrodes between 2 hemispheres. There are 3 basic montage designs: common reference, average reference, and bipolar. In a common reference (referential) montage, multiple scalp electrodes (lead or grid 1) are connected to a common reference (lead or grid 2). Each amplifier records the difference in electrical activity between a scalp electrode and the reference electrode. Electrodes most frequently chosen as the reference electrode(s) are the left and right mastoid (M1, M2) or the left and right auricular (A1, A2). All of the electrodes on the left scalp are typically referenced to the

ipsilateral left auricular or mastoid; those on the right to the right auricular or mastoid. Alternatively, each electrode can be referenced to the linked auricular or mastoid (ie, A1 + A2, M1 + M2) placements.

A common reference montage displays electric potential differences between each active recording electrode and the relatively biologically indifferent or neutral common reference electrode(s). If the common reference is biologically inactive, then each active scalp electrode can display the true amplitude, frequency, and phase of EEG activity over it.[9] In reality, common reference electrodes are rarely bioelectrically silent. Common reference montages are often used to confirm hemispheric asymmetries suspected on a bipolar montage and assist in the localization of epileptic abnormalities.

In routine EEG recording, the mastoid (M1 or M2) or auricular (A1 or A2) electrode placements are the most often selected common reference(s). However, a common reference should be chosen that is least likely to be involved in the electrical field of the scalp region of interest. For example, the use of the left mastoid (M1) as a reference is not advised when mapping the distribution of a left temporal spike discharge because M1 is likely to be within the field of the waveform of interest and contaminate the electrodes connected to M1. If the left temporal spike is unilateral, the contralateral mastoid (M2) could be chosen as a reference, although an electrode placement outside the temporal region is preferred.

Selecting the midline central (CZ, vertex) or parietal (PZ) as the common reference can display the wake EEG well. Reformatting and reviewing the wake EEG using a referential montage can help identify the dominant posterior rhythm, its posterior-anterior gradient, and voltage asymmetries and confirm and localize artifacts, malfunctioning electrodes, and obvious asymmetries. **Fig. 3**A shows the dominant alpha rhythm during wakefulness maximal over the parietal and occipital regions and eye movements over the frontopolar regions on a referential montage using CZ as the common reference. As shown in **Fig. 3**B, CZ is an active reference, and therefore a poor choice for common references during sleep because sleep spindles, vertex waves, K-complexes, and saw tooth waves are particularly prominent over the vertex and appear falsely distributed across all the EEG channels. The AASM Scoring Manual recommended EEG montage is an example of a common reference montage, linking right frontal, central, and occipital electrode placements to the left mastoid electrode (F4-M1, C4-M1, O2-M1), but recording the contralateral homologous EEG derivations (F3-M2, C3-M2, O1-M2) as backup.

An average reference montage may also be used to confirm the localization of EEG activity. An average reference is created by measuring, summing, and averaging electrical activity from all (or most) of the active scalp electrodes before being passed through a high-value resistor. The resulting signal in lead 2 is then used as the average reference electrode and connected to input 1 of each amplifier. Contemporary digital EEG systems perform these calculations seamlessly, providing instantaneous moment-to-moment averaged values of EEG activity from all recording electrodes. The average reference compares EEG activity over each scalp electrode with the average value of all the electrodes in use. The average reference is particularly useful in determining the maximal negativity of a focal discharge and whether bilateral discharges can be lateralized to a particular hemisphere and region.

A bipolar montage consists of serial pairs of electrodes connected together in straight lines from the front to the back of the head (longitudinal anterior to posterior), transversely (left to right) or circumferentially. Each pair of electrodes enters lead 1 and lead 2, with the lead 2 sharing lead 1 of the next channel. When an electrode is common to 2 channels (eg, F4-C4, C4-P4), it is connected to input lead 2 of the first and to input lead 1 of the next. Each EEG electrode (and the amplifier connected to it) measures and displays fluctuating voltage differences between 2 adjacent biologically active scalp electrodes.

Bipolar EEG montages are particularly useful for localizing IEDs and focal background abnormalities by identification of a phase reversal.[9] An inward or negative phase reversal is one in which the deflections point toward each other on a bipolar montage. A surface-negative phase reversal identifies which electrode is the site of maximum electronegativity (the estimated source of the IED). Most IEDs on scalp EEG are surface-negative. **Fig. 4** shows frequent spike-wave discharges that show maximal electronegativity over the left frontal (F3) region confirmed by the surface-positive downward deflection in F3-C3 and surface-negative upward deflection in F3-C3. Positive phase reversals are less common, seen in patients with skull defects, head trauma, malformations of cortical development, neonatal, and invasive EEG recordings. A positive phase reversal occurs when the summed EEG activity generates a horizontally oriented dipole of current flow. The alternative EEG montage of the AASM Scoring Manual is primarily a bipolar montage. For example, the 2-channel bipolar montage, FZ-CZ, CZ-OZ, is well suited to confirm that sleep spindles are typically maximal over CZ. When K-complexes are of equal amplitude over FZ and CZ, the FZ-CZ linkage may result in cancellation effects.[10]

Creating and Selecting Montages to Identify Normal and Abnormal Activity in an EEG

The AASM Scoring Manual requires that manufacturers of digital PSG systems permit reformatting of EEG into different montages. However, many sleep specialists and technologists are unaware of this requirement, or rarely take advantage of it. Reformatting even limited EEG montages recorded in routine PSG can be useful. When IEDs are observed in an expanded EEG tracing, it is best to make sure that the reference does not involve the electrical field of the discharge.

Review of an EEG commonly begins with a longitudinal (anterior-posterior direction) bipolar montage that connects electrodes from anterior to posterior, creating a temporal and a parasagittal chain of electrodes over each cerebral hemisphere (**Fig. 5**). This montage is often referred to as a double-banana montage. This electrode configuration allows comparison of the left and right parasagittal and temporal chains for symmetry.

The EEG can be reformatted into a longitudinal transverse (left-right direction) bipolar montage to evaluate (1) the symmetry of sleep spindles and EEG activity over the midline regions; (2) whether EEG activity is dominant over the temporal or parasagittal region in a particular hemisphere;

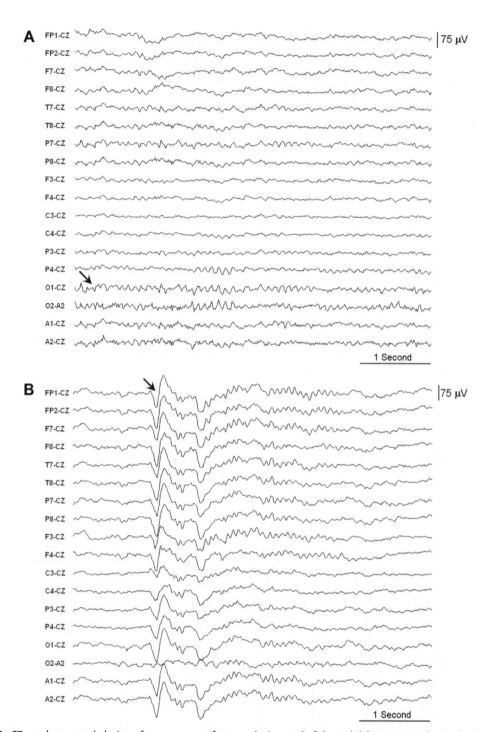

Fig. 3. CZ can be a good choice of a common reference during wakefulness (*A*) but a poor choice during non-rapid eye movement (NREM) 2 sleep, when sleep spindles are falsely projected in all the EEG channels (*B*). Note the distribution of the alpha rhythm in this 14-year-old girl, maximal in the occipital leads (*arrow, A*) and the widespread distribution of the K-complex (*arrow, B*) surface-negative at CZ.

and (3) IEDs or seizures that arise from midline or deep interhemispheric regions. **Fig. 6** shows how PSG signatures of nonrapid eye movement (NREM) sleep are displayed on a transverse bipolar montage: vertex waves typically show phase reversals over the midline central (CZ, vertex) and K-complexes over the midline frontal (FZ).

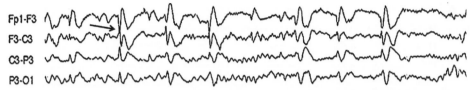

Fig. 4. Note the frequent spike-wave discharges that phase reverse over the left frontal (F3) area (*arrow*). The phase reversal is confirmed by the surface-positive downward deflection in F3-C3, and the simultaneous surface-negative upward deflection in F3-C3. A surface-negative phase reversal identifies which electrode is the site of maximum electronegativity (the estimated source of the IED). Most IEDs on scalp EEG are surface-negative.

A third commonly selected bipolar montage is a circumferential bipolar montage, also called a coronal or hatband montage. Adjacent electrodes are connected in a coronal fashion from left to right, highlighting the midline and anterior to posterior differences. This electrode configuration is particularly helpful for identifying whether IEDs or focal slowing in the posterior regions lateralize to 1 side or are maximal over the posterior temporal or occipital region. A reverse hatband montage can be used to evaluate frontopolar or anterior temporal activity. **Box 1** details the common bipolar EEG montages recommended by the ACNS when recording routine EEGs.[11]

Asymmetries suspected on a bipolar montage are best confirmed using a referential montage. Reformatting and reviewing the wake EEG using a referential montage can help identify the dominant posterior rhythm, its posterior-anterior gradient, and voltage asymmetries and confirm and localize artifacts, malfunctioning electrodes, and obvious asymmetries (**Fig. 7**).

INDICATIONS FOR VEEG PSG

The 2005 update of the AASM practice parameter for indications for PSG recommends as a guideline that in-laboratory VEEG PSG be used to evaluate parasomnias that are unusual or atypical because of the patient's age at onset; the time, duration, or frequency of occurrence of the behavior; or the specifics of the particular motor patterns in question (eg, stereotypical, repetitive, or focal).[1] The parameter further states that VEEG PSG be considered as an option when paroxysmal arousals or other sleep disruptions are suspected to be seizure related, yet the initial clinical evaluation and routine EEG are inconclusive.[1] In this

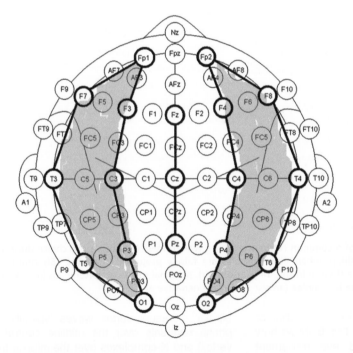

Channel Number	Longitudinal bipolar double banana
1	FP1-F3
2	F3-C3
3	C3-P3
4	P3-O1
5	FP2-F4
6	F4-C4
7	C4-P4
8	P4-O2
9	FP1-F7
10	F7-T7
11	T7-P7
12	P7-O1
13	FP2-F8
14	F8-T8
15	T8-P8
16	P8-O2
17	FZ-CZ
18	CZ-PZ
19	EKG

Fig. 5. The longitudinal anterior-posterior bipolar montage is the most common montage used in routine EEG.

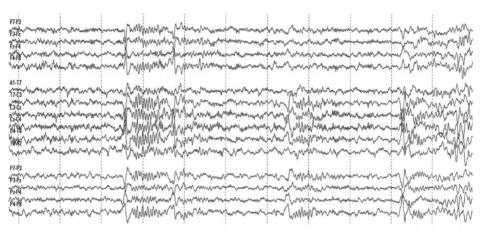

Fig. 6. Note how the polysomnographic signatures of NREM sleep (vertex activity, sleep spindles, and K-complexes) are well displayed using a transverse bipolar EEG montage.

setting, VEEG PSG requires: (1) additional derivations in an expanded bilateral montage; (2) recording surface electromyographic (EMG) activity from the left and right anterior tibialis and extensor digitorum muscles; (3) good audiovisual recording; (4) a sleep technologist present throughout the study to observe and document events; and (5) polysomnographers and electroencephalographers who are not experienced or trained in recognizing and interpreting both PSG and EEG abnormalities to seek appropriate consultation or refer patients to a center where this expertise is available.[1]

Box 1
Common bipolar EEG montages

Channel Number	Longitudinal Bipolar Double-banana	Tranverse Bipolar	Coronal Bipolar Hatband
1	FP1-F3	FP1-FP2	FP2-FP1
2	F3-C3	F7-F3	FP1-F7
3	C3-P3	F3-FZ	F7-T5
4	P3-O1	FZ-F4	T5-P7
5	FP2-F4	F4-F8	P7-O1
6	F4-C4	M1-T7	O1-O2
7	C4-P4	T7-C3	O2-P8
8	P4-O2	C3-CZ	P8-T6
9	FP1-F7	CZ-C4	T6-F8
10	F7-T7	C4-T8	F8-Fp2
11	T7-P7	T8-M2	Fp2-F4
12	P7-O1	P7-P3	F4-C4
13	FP2-F8	P3-PZ	C4-P4
14	F8-T8	PZ-P4	P4-O2
15	T8-P8	P4-P8	FP1-F4
16	P8-O2	P7-O1	F4-C4
17	FZ-CZ	O1-O2	C4-P4
18	CZ-PZ	O2-P8	P4-O2
19	EKG	EKG	EKG

Advantages of VEEG PSG Over Routine PSG

VEEG PSG has several advantages over routine PSG, including the ability to analyze behavior, correlate behavior with EEG, and more accurately detect seizure activity caused by additional recording electrodes. Aldrich and Jahnke[12] reviewed their experience with 122 patients with suspected parasomnias who underwent VPSG with 12 to 16 channels of EEG. VEEG PSG provided a definite diagnosis of epilepsy or a sleep disorder in 35% of cases, supportive evidence of either in another 30%, but was inconclusive in the rest. These investigators further found that VEEG PSG confirmed the diagnosis in 78% of 36 patients with known epilepsy, 69% of 41 patients whose paroxysmal motor nocturnal behaviors were prominent, but only 41% of 11 patients who were referred for minor motor activity in sleep.

Oldani and colleagues[13] evaluated the reliability of routine VEEG, daytime VEEG after sleep deprivation, and nocturnal VPSG to diagnose nocturnal frontal lobe epilepsy (NFLE) in 23 patients with normal awake VEEG recordings. Nocturnal VPSG confirmed the diagnosis in 87% of patients, daytime VEEG with sleep deprivation in 52%. A study of 100 consecutive adults with a history of sleep-related injury found VEEG PSG was diagnostic in 65% and helpful in another 26%, but often more than 1 night of recording was needed to confirm the diagnosis.[14]

Semiology of Epileptic Seizures for the Polysomnographer

High-quality video recordings are a necessary component of VEEG PSG because recognizing and documenting unambiguous epileptic semiology such as tonic-clonic motor activity, automatisms, and versive head movements provides

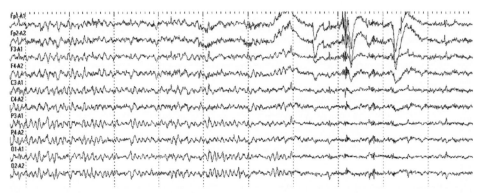

Fig. 7. Note how a common reference montage using the ipsilateral auricular electrode as reference shows the symmetry of the dominant posterior rhythm seen in the parietal and occipital regions, and eye movements noted over the frontopolar regions.

important clues to seizure localization and lateralization.[15] Minor motor manifestations characteristic of some focal epilepsies, including brief bilateral or focal tonic posturing and myoclonus, are more difficult to characterize using the clinical history alone. Staring, a sudden arrest of behavior, negative motor activity, or subtle loss of postural tone may not be recognized even by experienced observers without video recordings and patient-technologist interaction. Seizure semiology is reviewed by Vendrame and Loddenkemper elsewhere in this issue.

Vital Role of the Sleep Technologist in Confirming the Nature of Nocturnal Events

Technologists performing VEEG PSG should be trained to identify behaviors and motor activity likely to be epileptic in nature and interact with the patient to determine level of consciousness. The degree of unresponsiveness, recollection of dream content, and presence of lateralizing signs, including postictal language deficits and hemiparesis (Todd paralysis/paresis), during and immediately after the event should be ascertained. Technologists should be capable of administrating first aid to patients with generalized motor seizures, managing postictal violent or aggressive behavior, and recognizing potentially injurious situations (eg, prolonged seizures and complications such as aspiration, postictal hypoventilation, or life-threatening cardiac arrhythmias).

How Many Channels of EEG Should Be Recorded to Identify Seizures in VEEG PSG?

The 2005 AASM practice parameters for the indications for PSG do not specify how few additional derivations should be recorded because insufficient evidence had been published then to do so.[1] Only 2 studies have been published

evaluating this question, both performed by one of the authors (NFS).[16,17] In the first study, the ability of sleep medicine-trained and EEG-trained polysomnographers to correctly identify epileptic seizures using 4, 7, and 18 channels of simultaneous EEG recording at conventional PSG (30 mm/s) and EEG (10 mm/s) epoch lengths was evaluated.[16] Six polysomnographers reviewed 960 5-minute digital files of 32 sleep-related events (13 frontal lobe seizures, 11 temporal lobe seizures, and 8 arousals from sleep). The 4-channel montage included left and right central and occipital electrodes referenced to TP9 (a recognized 10/10 placement close to the auricular and mastoid reference). The 7-channel montage included FZ, CZ, PZ, F7, F8, O1, and O2 referenced to TP9.

The midline frontal, central, and parietal electrode placements were chosen to increase the yield of detecting frontal lobe seizures because these tend to propagate rapidly to the contralateral hemisphere and midline region and can be obscured by muscle artifact caused by tonic, clonic, and hypermotor activity. Furthermore, muscle artifact is often least present over CZ. The anterior temporal electrodes (F7, F8) were chosen to best identify temporal lobe seizures because most temporal lobe seizures arise from the mesial temporal regions and propagate anteriorly, appearing maximal at the F7/F8 or the mid-temporal (T7/T8) electrodes. The frontopolar (FP1, FP2) and supraorbital (SO1, SO2) electrode placements were excluded because they are so prone to ocular movements and muscle artifact.

Using pair-wise comparisons and general estimating equations, these investigators found that 6 readers identified 77% of 958 events correctly (including 74% of seizures [77% temporal, 71% frontal] and 88% of the arousals). Polysomnographers correctly identified 70% of events using the 4-channel montage; accuracy increased to only 74% reviewing 7 channels of EEG displayed in 30-second epochs and to 80% to 81% when reviewing PSG using conventional EEG epoch length, independent of the number of EEG channels available. **Fig. 8** shows the appearance of a temporal lobe seizure depending on the number of EEG channels recorded and the paper speed. **Fig. 9** shows the same for a frontal lobe seizure.

A second study in 2006 from the same center further evaluated the accuracy of electroencephalographers to distinguish seizures from nonepileptic events viewing 8-channel and 18-channel montages.[17] Three electroencephalographers reviewed 56 epileptic seizures and 60 nonepileptic events displayed using 8-channel or 18-channel EEG montages, assigning a probability of seizure score (from 0% to 100%) reflecting their

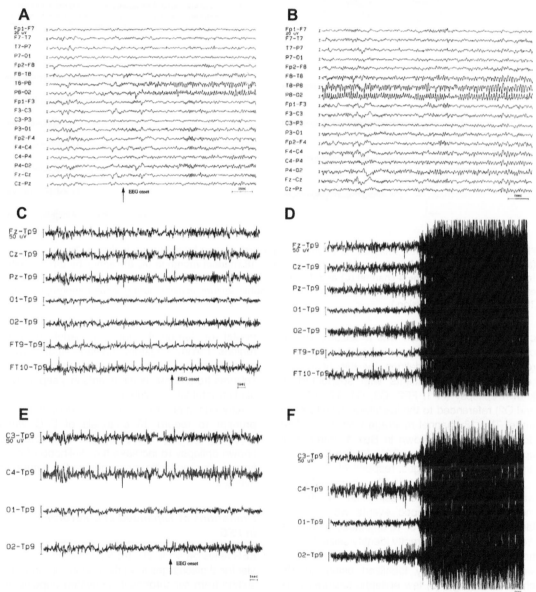

Fig. 8. The EEG onset (*arrow*) consisted of rhythmic alpha activity in the right temporal region preceding the clinical onset by 26 seconds as shown in consecutive 10-second epochs on the 18-channel anterior-posterior bipolar montage (*A, B*). The evolution of rhythmic electrographic seizure activity in the right temporal region can be appreciated on the 7-channel montage at 10 and 30 mm/s paper speed (*C, D*). However, the ictal seizure pattern is not clearly evident on the 4-channel montage even when viewed on an epoch length of 10 seconds (*E, F*). (*From* Foldvary N, Caruso AC, Mascha E, et al. Identifying montages that best detect electrographic seizure activity during polysomnography. Sleep 2000;23(2):6; with permission.)

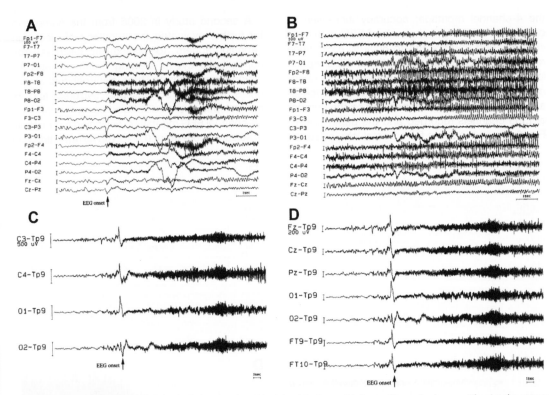

Fig. 9. A generalized motor seizure in a 13-year-old girl with frontal lobe epilepsy is shown. The ictal pattern (*arrow*) seen on consecutive 10-second epochs using the 18-channel montage (*A, B*) cannot be differentiated from muscle artifact in the 4-channel (*C*) and 7-channel (*D*) montages. (*From* Foldvary N, Caruso AC, Mascha E, et al. Identifying montages that best detect electrographic seizure activity during polysomnography. Sleep 2000;23(2):7; with permission.)

confidence that an event was a seizure. The 8-channel montage included electrode placements recommended in guidelines by the ACNS for recording PSG in patients with suspected or known epilepsy (FP1, FP2, C3, C4, T7, T8, O1, and O2) referenced to the ipsilateral TP9/10 electrode. The 18-channel montage was a standard double-banana, as shown in **Box 1**. Interreader agreement was 78% and 84% for the 8-channel and 18-channel montages, respectively.

The investigators found: (1) seizure detection was significantly better using an 18-channel montage; (2) nonepileptic events were reliably identified using either 8 or 18 channels; (3) readers were better able to correctly identify seizures from nonepileptic events using 18 channels; (4) seizures were more accurately localized using an 18-channel montage; (5) few epileptic seizures were misclassified as nonepileptic using 18 channels, but 25% were misidentified using 8 channels; (6) 56% of frontal lobe seizures were misidentified as nonepileptic events viewing 8 channels of EEG, 33% using 18 channels; and (7) using 18-channel montages, readers were more likely to accurately localize seizures emanating from the

frontal or temporal, but not parieto-occipital regions. The investigators concluded that abbreviated EEG montages are inadequate to differentiate seizures from nonepileptic events in sleep, particularly frontal lobe seizures.

Although more research is needed, it seems prudent to record 18 channels of EEG when recording PSG in patients with suspected or known epilepsy to increase the likelihood of confirming the epileptic or nonepileptic nature of event(s).

Limitations of Expanded EEG Recordings in PSG

EEG relies on scalp electrodes to record coherent electrical discharges from the underlying brain, resulting from synchronously activated populations of neurons.[18,19] One fundamental limitation is that sources must originate from relatively large cortical areas to be detected on the scalp. Scalp electrodes are relatively insensitive to activity arising within sulci (which comprise nearly 70% of the cortical surface).[20] Other deep structures are too distant for reliable scalp EEG detection, including the mesial and basal surfaces of the cerebral cortex. Electrical propagation through multiple other layers (cerebrospinal fluid, dura, skull, and scalp) further reduces source localization.[21,22] High-frequency (fast) patterns are often observed during the onset and evolution of seizures. These fast frequencies are more easily dampened than slower frequencies on scalp EEG recordings. Overall, the ictal EEG is not adequately localized in one-quarter to one-third of focal epilepsies, varying by the location, size, and pathologic substrate of the generator.[23,24]

In the case of a nondiagnostic VEEG PSG recording, long-term VEEG in a specialized unit for the care of patients with epilepsy should be considered: (1) to diagnose epileptic paroxysmal electrographic or behavioral abnormalities; (2) to classify clinical seizure type(s) in patients with documented epilepsy; (3) to characterize (lateralization, localization, distribution) EEG abnormalities associated with seizure disorders; (4) to quantify the number or frequency of seizures or IEDs; (5) to distinguish epileptic from nonepileptic events (including other parasomnias and psychogenic nonepileptic seizures); and (6) to document the response of the EEG to therapeutic interventions or modifications.

Long-term VEEG is preferred in patients with unexplained nocturnal events: (1) that do not occur nightly or every other night; (2) when a primary sleep disorder is unlikely; (3) when a history of postictal agitation, wandering, or injury is present; or (4) when the ability of the patient to cooperate is questionable. Long-term VEEG monitoring is usually performed for 3 to 7 days depending on its purpose. Antiepileptic drugs (AEDs) are typically reduced or tapered to precipitate seizures, a practice not recommended in the outpatient sleep laboratory setting.

INTERPRETATION OF VEEG PSG RECORDINGS

Interpretation of VEEG PSG requires knowledge of the clinical and manifestations of epileptic seizures, nonepileptic sleep-related movements, and parasomnias.[25] Epileptic seizures are classified as focal or generalized based on their clinical and electrographic features. Epilepsy syndromes are constellations of specific signs and symptoms that can be used to predict the natural history of a disorder. The clinical evaluation and classification of seizures, epilepsies, and epilepsy syndromes are discussed in greater detail by Vendrame and Loddenkemper elsewhere in this issue .

The time of night when nocturnal events emerge relative to sleep onset coupled with salient clinical features and the particular stage of sleep can help identify their nature. Sleep-related seizures usually arise from NREM sleep at any time of night, including just after falling asleep or before the final morning awakening. In contrast, disorders of arousal usually emerge from NREM 3 in the first third of the sleep period. The motor movements and dream enactment of rapid eye movement (REM) sleep behavior disorder (RBD) are often most prominent in the last third of the sleep period, when REM sleep predominates. Rhythmic movements associated with rhythmic movement disorder usually occur during sleep-wake transitions. Sleep-dissociative episodes emerge from wakefulness. Nocturnal panic attacks occur from NREM sleep, usually at the transition of stages NREM 2 and NREM 3.

Sleep seems to activate frontal seizures more often than temporal seizures.[26–28] Seizures in patients with frontal lobe epilepsy (FLE) typically arise from sleep, almost exclusively NREM sleep,[26–28] most often NREM 2, less often NREM 1.[29] Secondary generalization of focal seizures tends to occur more often during sleep (28%) compared with wakefulness (18%), but frontal lobe seizures tend not to secondarily generalize during sleep.[26–28,30] Epilepsies that occur only or preferentially during sleep include: (1) NFLE; (2) benign partial epilepsies of childhood (rolandic, occipital); (3) nocturnal TLE with hypermotor seizures (often mistaken at first for NFLE); (5) sleep-related idiopathic generalized tonic-clonic seizures (GTCSs); and (6) tonic seizures of the childhood-onset medically refractory epileptic encephalopathy of Lennox-Gastaut syndrome.

Definitions and Characteristic Features of IEDs

IEDs are believed to represent the macroscopic field created by the summation of electrical potentials from a population of pathologically synchronized bursting neurons.[31] The most common IEDs seen in people with epilepsy are spikes and sharp waves. Spike or sharp wave discharges have 4 fundamental characteristics: (1) the waveform disrupts the background in frequency, amplitude, or field; (2) the waveform has a sharply contoured component (the ascent of which is often steeper than the descent); (3) the waveform has an electrical field that involves more than 1 electrode; and (4) the waveform is mostly electronegative on the cerebral surface (surface-negative).[32]

A spike discharge by definition lasts 20 to 70 milliseconds and is usually biphasic (ie, composed of a surface-negative then surface-positive deflection). Sharp waves differ from spikes only in their duration, lasting 70 to 200 milliseconds. Other types of IEDs include spike or sharp wave complexes (a single spike or sharp wave followed by a slow wave of the same polarity), polyspikes (3 or more successive spikes with a frequency of more than 10 Hz), which can be followed by a slow wave (polyspike and wave), and paroxysmal fast activity (high-frequency oscillations in the β or γ frequency bands (≥14 Hz).[33]

Diagnostic Significance of the Presence or Absence of IEDs

The likelihood of detecting IEDs in EEG, PSG, or VEEG PSG depends on the seizure type, age, seizure frequency, whether the patient's epilepsy is controlled or not, and how many channels of EEG are recorded. IEDs may not be detected if the epileptic activity emanates from a small area of the cortex. As noted earlier, at least 6 to 10 cm² of cortical neurons must fire synchronously for an IED to be detected on a scalp EEG,[3,4] and IEDs that emanate from deep or medial parts of the cerebral cortex (eg, orbitofrontal or interhemispheric medial cortex) are apt to escape detection. In general, more frequent seizures tend to be associated with higher-yield IEDs.[34] Children with epilepsy are more likely to have IEDs in routine EEGs than adults.

Routine EEGs are normal in about 50% of patients with a clinical diagnosis of seizures, although the yield improves with multiple or prolonged recordings. One study showed that IEDs were never recorded in 4.4% of 919 patients who underwent long-term VEEG monitoring but in whom at least 1 epileptic seizure was recorded.[35] The absence of IEDs despite having medically resistant epilepsy was more likely to occur in patients with extratemporal (including nocturnal frontal lobe) epilepsies than patients with TLE.[35] The absence of IEDs in unmedicated patients with generalized onset seizures is exceptional in children and unusual in adults, but sufficient doses of AEDs appropriate for the seizure type may rid the EEG of IEDs and seizures. IEDs are found in the first routine EEG of 30% to 50% of adults and 80% of children with epilepsy. Repeating the EEG increases the yield by an additional 20% to 30%. The presence of IEDs after a first epileptic seizure increases the likelihood of seizure recurrence 2-fold. The absence of IEDs in a routine EEG does not prove that a paroxysmal event was not a seizure or that a patient does not have epilepsy.

Moreover, IEDs are observed in individuals with no history of seizures or epilepsy. IEDs are observed in 1.9% to 6.5% of healthy children without a history of seizures or epilepsy.[36-39] These IEDs are most often centrotemporal spikes seen in benign childhood epilepsy (BECTS) **(Fig. 10)**. Only 40% of children with BECTS ever have a seizure.

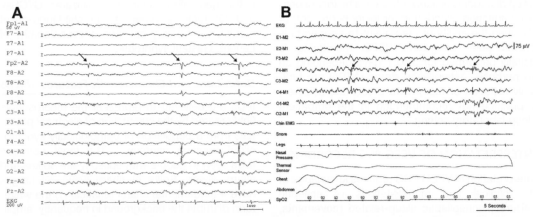

Fig. 10. Benign focal discharges of childhood. Right centrotemporal sharp waves in a child with benign focal epilepsy displayed on an 18-channel referential EEG (A) and routine PSG (B) recording. Sharp waves have a stereotyped morphology consisting of a small positivity followed by a prominent negativity and a lower amplitude slow wave maximal in the centrotemporal regions. On the referential EEG montage (A), the stereotyped dipole field has a negative polarity in the centrotemporal region and positive polarity in the frontal region (arrows) because of the tangential orientation of the generator to the cortical surface in the lower rolandic region. On the PSG recording (B), right centrotemporal sharp waves maximal at electrode placements used in routine PSG (arrows) are easily overlooked. This syndrome accounts for 15% to 25% of childhood epilepsy and features seizures characterized by unilateral focal sensorimotor seizures typically involving the face and arm that frequently evolve into generalized motor seizures restricted to sleep. In contrast to benign EEG variants described elsewhere, the term benign in this epileptic disorder refers to the spontaneous remission that occurs by 18 years of age in most cases. (*Data from* Beaussart M. Benign epilepsy of children with Rolandic (centro-temporal) paroxysmal foci. A clinical entity. Study of 221 cases. Epilepsia 1972;13(6):795–811.)

A recent study found IEDs in 14 (1.5%) of 970 healthy schoolchildren who had an overnight PSG as part of a community cohort population study. IEDs were centrotemporal spikes in 11. Generalized IEDs characteristic of primary generalized/idiopathic/genetic epilepsies can be seen in people without epilepsy, and centromidtemporal spikes are observed in 1% to 2% of EEGs of children, only 60% of whom ever have a seizure.[39,40] Generalized spike-wave discharges are also encountered in PSGs of children who (on closer questioning) often have a family history of epilepsy, and the discharges are age dependent, often remitting spontaneously in a few years in the absence of clinical seizures. Unexpected IEDs in PSGs of adults without a history of seizures or epilepsy is far less common. Finding IEDs in

a PSG requires a follow-up visit to the sleep center, a careful review of the child's personal, developmental, and family history, and often a lengthy discussion with the parents as to the significance of the finding. A more detailed discussion on IEDs in people without seizures can be found in a recent review by So.[41] The article by Bruni and colleagues elsewhere in this issue discusses the benign focal epilepsies of childhood in detail.

Normal paroxysmal EEG rhythms, normal EEG variants, and artifacts are sometimes misinterpreted as epileptic, leading to a misdiagnosis of epilepsy.[42] Most common waveforms misdiagnosed as epileptic include (1) sharply contoured waveforms in the temporal region (eg, wicket spikes or temporal theta of older adults); (2) repetitive K-complexes or vertex waves in children; and

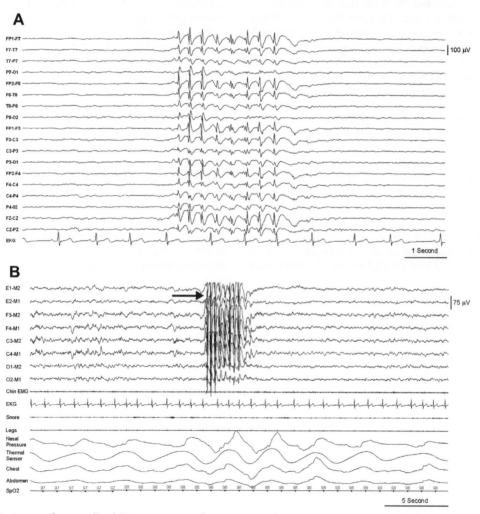

Fig. 11. A run of generalized 3-Hz to 4-Hz spike-wave complexes in a teenage with idiopathic generalized epilepsy on an 18-channel anterior-posterior longitudinal bipolar montage (*A*) and routine PSG (*B, arrow*). Note the spike-wave morphology occurring repetitively, maximal in the frontal regions with anterior to posterior amplitude decay. In contrast to focal IEDs, generalized spike-wave complexes are more readily identifiable on routine PSG because of their distribution, amplitude, and stereotyped appearance.

(3) electrode artifacts. Consultation with an experienced electroencephalographer is often required to differentiate these waveforms from epileptic activity.[43]

Generalized Seizures and Epilepsies

Generalized epileptic seizures are those conceptualized as originating at some point within, and rapidly engaging, bilaterally distributed neuronal networks.[44] Such bilateral networks can include cortical and subcortical structures, but do not necessarily imply the entire cortex is seizing. Although classically defined as lacking localizing features, it is now accepted that some generalized seizures appear asymmetric both clinically and electrographically. Most generalized epilepsies are characterized by IEDs that are generalized spike-wave or polyspike-wave discharges. These discharges are most often maximal over the mid-frontal regions (F3, FZ, and F4) with progressive amplitude decay posteriorly. However, sometimes generalized IEDs are maximal over the frontopolar or posterior regions. Although usually bilaterally synchronous and symmetric, the maximal amplitude of these IEDs may shift from side to side within the same record or in serial recordings in the same patient.

Generalized IEDs can be detected when recording the limited EEG derivations used in routine PSG (**Fig. 11**). Generalized spike-wave discharges often show phase reversals at F3 and F4 of both the spike and slow wave components. The frequency of the spike-wave bursts can be approximately 3 Hz (classic or typical), 4 to 6 Hz (atypical),[13] or less than 2.5 Hz (slow). Both typical and atypical discharges occur in idiopathic/genetic syndromes, whereas slow spike-wave complexes are usually seen in symptomatic or cryptogenic epilepsies (in which the epilepsy results from a widespread insult to the central nervous system). Those interpreting the results should recognize that, during sleep, even classic or atypical spike-wave complexes usually become slower (often <2 Hz), occur in isolation rather than in bursts, and can include polyspikes.

During generalized seizures, the EEG typically shows diffuse rhythmic activity or repetitive epileptic discharges reflecting initial involvement of both cerebral hemispheres. A primary GTCS is often preceded by a series of myoclonic jerks accompanied by recurrent high-voltage polyspike-wave bursts. Generalized voltage attenuation with superimposed 20-Hz to 40-Hz low-voltage paroxysmal fast activity lasting a few seconds at the onset of the generalized convulsion is seen in some cases. Rhythmic generalized 10-Hz to 12-Hz activity that progressively increases in amplitude is typically observed during the tonic phase of convulsion and is followed by generalized slower activity that increases in amplitude but slows in frequency from 7 to 8 Hz to 1 to 2 Hz. As the seizure continues, polyspikes interrupted by slow waves characterize the clonic phase, producing a characteristic pattern of myogenic artifact that is easy to identify even at an epoch length of 30 seconds (see later example of a secondarily generalized frontal lobe seizure). After the last burst of polyspike-wave activity, the EEG shows generalized voltage attenuation that is gradually replaced by irregular low-voltage delta activity lasting seconds to minutes until the normal background rhythms return.

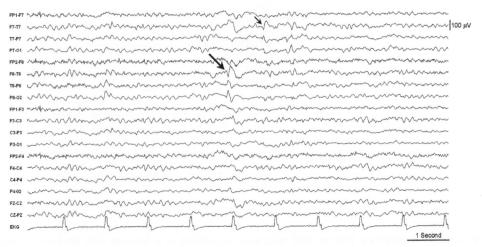

Fig. 12. A 15-second interictal EEG showing right (*larger arrow*) and left (*smaller arrow*) temporal sharp waves on an 18-channel longitudinal bipolar. Negative phase reversals are seen at T8 and T7; the midtemporal electrode placements, indicating the sources of the discharges are maximal in the cortical regions underlying these electrodes.

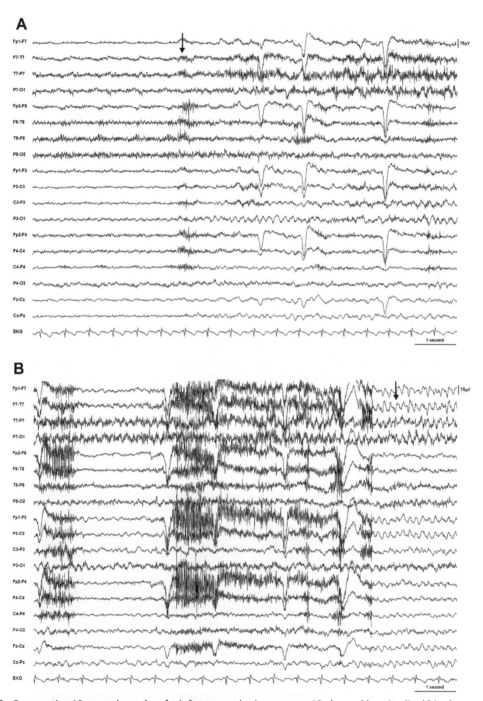

Fig. 13. Consecutive 10-second epochs of a left temporal seizure on an 18-channel longitudinal bipolar montage. seizure onset (*A, arrow*) is characterized by a change in background frequencies that is initially arrhythmic, later (*B, arrow*) evolving to rhythmic 5-Hz to 8-Hz activity with propagation to the left parasagittal region. Note that the interictal EEG immediately before seizure onset is characterized by left temporal rhythmic delta activity that was nearly continuous and not associated with clinical manifestations. The seizure was preceded by an arousal from stage N2 followed by a sudden sense of fear and anxiety 10 seconds before EEG onset. This seizure evolved to an arrest of activity with intermittent eye blinking and subtle oral automatisms (chewing and swallowing). The ictal EEG and seizure semiology are highly suggestive of TLE. An estimated 9% of patients with TLE have seizures restricted to sleep. (*Data from* Billiard MB. Epilepsies and the sleep-wake cycle. In: Sterman MB, Shouse MN, Passouant P, editors. Sleep and epilepsy. New York: Academic Press; 1982. p. 269–86.)

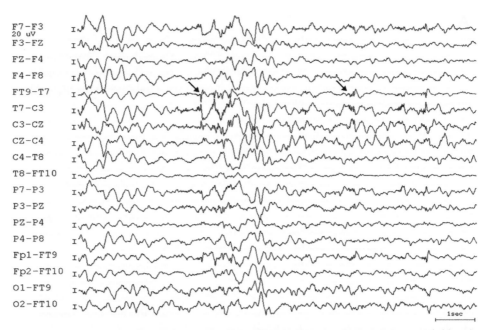

Fig. 14. A series of left hemispheric spikes shown on an 18-channel transverse montage in a child with supplementary sensorimotor area (SSMA) epilepsy. Note the negative phase reversal of the spikes at T7 followed by C3 and low-voltage fast activity in the same distribution (*arrows*). The patient had seizures characterized by an arousal from sleep with asymmetric tonic activity lasting less than 10 seconds with preserved awareness suggestive of activation of the SSMA, located in the mesial aspect of the superior frontal gyrus. Seizures arising from the SSMA have a tendency to occur predominately or exclusively in sleep. (*Data from* Morris 3rd HH, Dinner DS, Luders H, et al. Supplementary motor seizures: clinical and electroencephalographic findings. Neurology 1988;38(7):1075–82.)

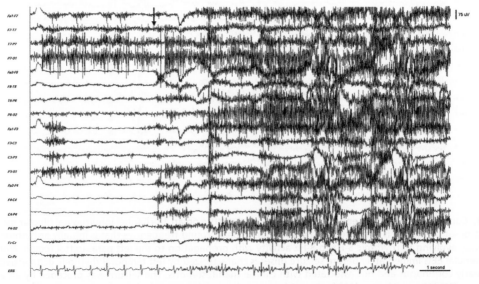

Fig. 15. A hypermotor seizure shown on an 18-channel anterior-posterior bipolar montage. EEG seizure onset (*arrow*) and the entire seizure evolution are obscured by movement artifact. Seizures were characterized by violent, thrashing movements in sleep lasting 10 to 20 seconds with preserved consciousness not responsive to medical therapy. The lack of EEG localization necessitated implantation of intracranial electrodes, which led to a resection of the left superior mesial frontal lobe. The patient has been seizure free for 5 years since surgery. Pathology revealed a malformation of cortical development.

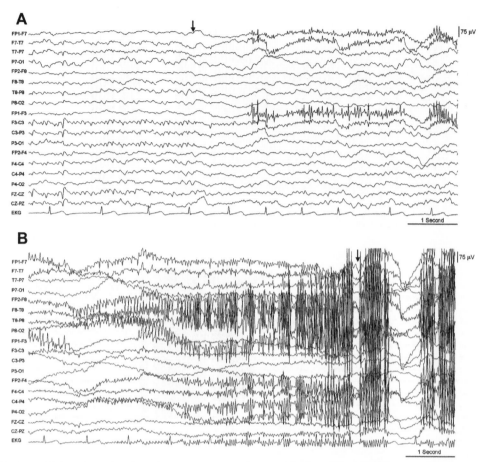

Fig. 16. Frontal lobe seizure in NFLE. Three consecutive 15-second EEG tracings displayed on an 18-channel ante-roposterior bipolar montage (*A–C*) and a 60-second PSG (*D*) of a frontal lobe seizure consisting of a behavioral arrest followed by vocation, facial distortion, and evolution to a tonic-clonic seizure. EEG seizure onset is charac-terized by fast activity (*A*) arising from the left frontal lobe maximal in the frontal polar region and evolving to the right frontal region (*B*) when clinical onset is observed. The ictal pattern becomes obscured by EMG artifact of clonic (*B, arrow*) followed by tonic (*C, arrow*) activity (in both cases, the *arrow* at the top of the screen immedi-ately precedes the motor activity described). Although the ictal EEG pattern is not readily identified on the PSG tracing (*D; solid arrow* denotes EEG seizure onset and *dotted arrow* denotes clinical seizure onset), the artifact from the tonic-clonic phase is suspicious and should prompt further review. Note the central apnea and oxygen desaturation that occurs in association with the generalized tonic-clonic phase. NFLE is a heterogeneous disorder; the familial form, known as autosomal-dominant NFLE, constitutes as much as 25% of cases. (*Data from* Marini C, Guerrini R. The role of the nicotinic acetylcholine receptors in sleep-related epilepsy. Biochem Pharmacol 2007;74(8):1308–14.)

Focal Seizures and Epilepsies

Focal epileptic seizures are those conceptualized as originating within networks limited to 1 hemi-sphere.[44] They may be discretely localized or more widely distributed. Focal seizures may origi-nate in subcortical structures. The electrographic manifestations of focal epilepsy depend on a variety of factors, including the size and location of the ictal generator, location and number of recording electrodes, and the attenuating charac-teristics of the skull and other intervening tissues.[45]

In many cases, the EEG shows IEDs from the region harboring the epileptogenic lesion. This finding is particularly true in TLE, in which a unilateral focal preponderance of IEDs predicts the area of seizure origin with a probability of more than 95% (**Fig. 12**).[46] Similarly, regional ictal EEG patterns are more common in TLE (90%), specifically those arising from the mesial temporal structures (93%), compared with so-called extratemporal epilepsies arising from outside the temporal lobe (50%), in particular from the mesial frontal lobe (24%; **Fig. 13**).[23]

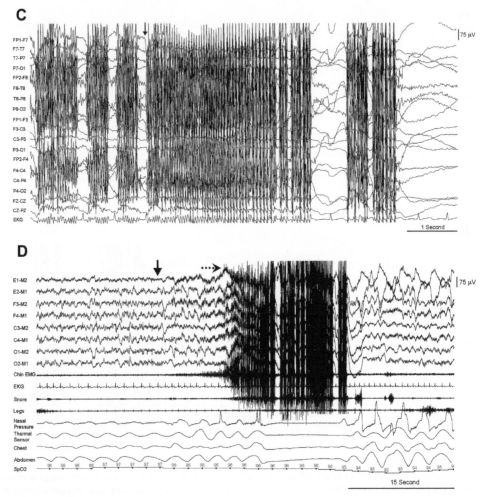

Fig. 16. (*continued*)

The EEG may be normal in patients with epileptogenic lesions arising from deep or midline regions or show generalized epileptic activity caused by rapid propagation to the contralateral hemisphere. The involvement of basal and mesial cortical areas not directly accessible to scalp EEG, rapid spreading of electric activity within and outside these areas, and tangential orientation of the spike source are responsible for the lower yield of scalp EEG in these cases.[35] Some focal epilepsies arising from the interhemispheric region are associated with IEDs and ictal patterns best observed on a coronal bipolar montage, showing the importance of tailoring the recording to the clinical history and seizure semiology (**Fig. 14**). Lateralized, generalized, or nonlateralized ictal EEG patterns are characteristic of most extratemporal focal epilepsies.[23]

Most focal seizures are characterized by rhythmic activity that evolves in frequency, field (distribution), or amplitude.[47] Repetitive spikes or

sharp waves and sudden attenuation of activity over 1 region or cerebral hemisphere are also observed. Seizures characterized by excessive motor activity may be obscured by muscle and movement artifact, rendering the EEG uninterpretable. This finding is most commonly observed in patients with FLE in whom parasomnias or nonepileptic psychogenic seizures may be erroneously diagnosed because of the apparent lack of an EEG correlate (**Fig. 15**). EEG may be normal even during a seizure if the event is brief and the epileptogenic focus is distant from the recording electrodes, another feature of FLE. Whereas TLE is the most common of the focal epilepsies in adolescents and adults, FLE more often presents with seizures during sleep that can be difficult to differentiate from other types of nocturnal events. Similarly, ictal EEG changes may not be apparent when a seizure remains confined to a limited area. The absence of EEG abnormalities does not definitively exclude the diagnosis of epilepsy.

Recognizing Artifacts in VEEG PSG Recordings

Artifacts are commonly seen in recordings of patients with unexplained nocturnal events and must be distinguished from epileptic activity and the EEG changes associated with parasomnias. Although artifacts can obscure the EEG, their stereotyped presentation may be supportive of the diagnosis in question. Examples of these artifacts include the EMG artifact of tonic and clonic seizure components (**Fig. 16**), head or body rocking artifact in rhythmic movement disorder, and the rhythmic bitemporal myogenic artifact of bruxism. Other types of artifact that mimic epileptic activity include that produced by head tremor, eye movements, and tongue movements (glossokinetic artifact). Normal patterns that are occasionally misinterpreted as epileptic include positive occipital sharp transients of sleep, repetitive vertex waves of young patients, small sharp spikes, wicket spikes, and rhythmic temporal theta of drowsiness reviewed elsewhere in this issue by Vendrame and Kothare. Physiologic artifacts in PSG at times mistaken for epileptic seizures or IEDs are further reviewed by Vendrame and Kothare elsewhere in this issue.

SUMMARY

VEEG PSG combines expanded EEG and PSG to evaluate nocturnal behaviors and motor activity when epileptic seizures are suspected and to provide a more comprehensive assessment of patients with neurologic disorders undergoing PSG. This technique has several advantages over routine PSG, including the improved ability to identify interictal and ictal EEG abnormalities and correlate clinical with neurophysiologic parameters. Additional time is required for electrode placement and data analysis and more space needed on storage media. The yield of VEEG PSG is optimized when the study is tailored and data reviewed with knowledge of the clinical history and event semiology. When VEEG PSG fails to clarify the diagnosis, long-term VEEG monitoring should be considered.

REFERENCES

1. Kushida CA, Littner MR, Morgenthaler T, et al. Practice parameters for the indications for polysomnography and related procedures: an update for 2005. Sleep 2005;28(4):499–521.
2. Cooper R, Osselton JW, Shaw JC. EEG technology. 3d edition. London; Boston: Butterworths; 1980.
3. Cooper R, Winter AL, Crow HJ, et al. Comparison of subcortical, cortical and scalp activity using chronically indwelling electrodes in man. Electroencephalogr Clin Neurophysiol 1965;18:217–28.
4. Tao JX, Ray A, Hawes-Ebersole S, et al. Intracranial EEG substrates of scalp EEG interictal spikes. Epilepsia 2005;46(5):669–76.
5. Klem GH, Luders HO, Jasper HH, et al. The ten-twenty electrode system of the International Federation. The International Federation of Clinical Neurophysiology. Electroencephalogr Clin Neurophysiol Suppl 1999; 52:3–6.
6. Jasper HH. Report on the committee on methods of clinical examination in electroencephalography. Electroencephalogr Clin Neurophysiol 1958;10: 370–5.
7. American Electroencephalographic Society guidelines for standard electrode position nomenclature. J Clin Neurophysiol 1991;8(2):200–2.
8. Iber C, American Academy of Sleep Medicine. The AASM manual for the scoring of sleep and associated events: rules, terminology and technical specifications. Westchester (IL): American Academy of Sleep Medicine; 2007.
9. Yamada T, Meng E. Practical guide for clinical neurophysiologic testing: EEG. Philadelphia: Wolters Kluwer Health/Lippincott Williams & Wilkins; 2010. p. 5–39.
10. Grigg-Damberger MM. The AASM scoring manual: a critical appraisal. Curr Opin Pulm Med 2009; 15(6):540–9.
11. Guideline 1: Minimum technical requirements for performing clinical electroencephalography. J Clin Neurophysiol 2006;23(2):86–91.
12. Aldrich MS, Jahnke B. Diagnostic value of video-EEG polysomnography. Neurology 1991;41(7):1060–6.
13. Oldani A, Zucconi M, Smirne S, et al. The neurophysiological evaluation of nocturnal frontal lobe epilepsy. Seizure 1998;7(4):317–20.
14. Schenck CH, Milner DM, Hurwitz TD, et al. A polysomnographic and clinical report on sleep-related injury in 100 adult patients. Am J Psychiatry 1989;146(9):1166–73.
15. Unnwongse K, Wehner T, Foldvary-Schaefer N. Selecting patients for epilepsy surgery. Curr Neurol Neurosci Rep 2010;10(4):299–307.
16. Foldvary N, Caruso AC, Mascha E, et al. Identifying montages that best detect electrographic seizure activity during polysomnography. Sleep 2000;23(2): 221–9.
17. Foldvary-Schaefer N, De Ocampo J, Mascha E, et al. Accuracy of seizure detection using abbreviated EEG during polysomnography. J Clin Neurophysiol 2006;23(1):68–71.
18. Creutzfeldt OD, Watanabe S, Lux HD. Relations between EEG phenomena and potentials of single cortical cells. II. Spontaneous and convulsoid activity. Electroencephalogr Clin Neurophysiol 1966;20(1): 19–37.
19. Elul R. The genesis of the EEG. Int Rev Neurobiol 1971;15:227–72.

20. Carpenter MB. Core text of neuroanatomy. Baltimore (MD): Williams & Wilkins; 1991.

21. Neshige R, Luders H, Shibasaki H. Recording of movement-related potentials from scalp and cortex in man. Brain 1988;111(Pt 3):719–36.

22. Nunez PL. Electric fields of the brain: the neurophysics of EEG. New York: Oxford University Press; 1981.

23. Foldvary N, Klem G, Hammel J, et al. The localizing value of ictal EEG in focal epilepsy. Neurology 2001; 57(11):2022–8.

24. Spencer SS, Guimaraes P, Shewmon A. Intracranial electrodes. In: Engel J, Pedley TA, editors. Epilepsy: a comprehensive textbook. New York: Lippincott Williams & Wilkins; 1998. p. 1717–48.

25. Grigg-Damberger M, Ralls F. Primary sleep disorders and paroxysmal nocturnal nonepileptic events in adults with epilepsy from the perspective of sleep specialists. J Clin Neurophysiol 2011;28(2):120–40.

26. Bazil CW, Walczak TS. Effects of sleep and sleep stage on epileptic and nonepileptic seizures. Epilepsia 1997;38(1):56–62.

27. Crespel A, Coubes P, Baldy-Moulinier M. Sleep influence on seizures and epilepsy effects on sleep in partial frontal and temporal lobe epilepsies. Clin Neurophysiol 2000;111(Suppl 2):S54–9.

28. Herman ST, Walczak TS, Bazil CW. Distribution of partial seizures during the sleep-wake cycle: differences by seizure onset site. Neurology 2001; 56(11):1453–9.

29. Minecan D, Natarajan A, Marzec M, et al. Relationship of epileptic seizures to sleep stage and sleep depth. Sleep 2002;25(8):899–904.

30. Jobst BC, Williamson PD, Neuschwander TB, et al. Secondarily generalized seizures in mesial temporal epilepsy: clinical characteristics, lateralizing signs, and association with sleep-wake cycle. Epilepsia 2001;42(10):1279–87.

31. Worrell GA, Lagerlund TD, Buchhalter JR. Role and limitations of routine and ambulatory scalp electroencephalography in diagnosing and managing seizures. Mayo Clin Proc 2002;77(9):991–8.

32. Stern JM, Engel J Jr. An atlas of EEG patterns. Philadelphia: Lippincott Williams & Wilkins; 2005.

33. Lüders HO, Noachtar S. Atlas and classification of electroencephalography. Philadelphia: Saunders; 2001.

34. Gotman J, Marciani MG. Electroencephalographic spiking activity, drug levels, and seizure occurrence in epileptic patients. Ann Neurol 1985;17(6): 597–603.

35. Stuve O, Dodrill CB, Holmes MD, et al. The absence of interictal spikes with documented seizures suggests extratemporal epilepsy. Epilepsia 2001; 42(6):778–81.

36. Eeg-Olofsson O, Petersen I, Sellden U. The development of the electroencephalogram in normal children from the age of 1 through 15 years. Paroxysmal activity. Neuropadiatrie 1971;2(4):375–404.

37. Borusiak P, Zilbauer M, Jenke AC. Prevalence of epileptiform discharges in healthy children–new data from a prospective study using digital EEG. Epilepsia 2010;51(7):1185–8.

38. Cavazzuti GB, Cappella L, Nalin A. Longitudinal study of epileptiform EEG patterns in normal children. Epilepsia 1980;21(1):43–55.

39. Sam MC, So EL. Significance of epileptiform discharges in patients without epilepsy in the community. Epilepsia 2001;42(10):1273–8.

40. Bennett DR. Control electroencephalographic study of flying personnel. Int Psychiatry Clin 1967; 4(1):23–35.

41. So EL. Interictal epileptiform discharges in persons without a history of seizures: what do they mean? J Clin Neurophysiol 2010;27(4):229–38.

42. Benbadis SR, Lin K. Errors in EEG interpretation and misdiagnosis of epilepsy. Which EEG patterns are overread? Eur Neurol 2008;59(5):267–71.

43. Berg AT, Shinnar S. The risk of seizure recurrence following a first unprovoked seizure: a quantitative review. Neurology 1991;41(7):965–72.

44. Berg AT, Berkovic SF, Brodie MJ, et al. Revised terminology and concepts for organization of seizures and epilepsies: report of the ILAE Commission on Classification and Terminology, 2005-2009. Epilepsia 2010;51(4):676–85.

45. Jayakar P, Duchowny M, Resnick TJ, et al. Localization of seizure foci: pitfalls and caveats. J Clin Neurophysiol 1991;8(4):414–31.

46. Holmes MD, Dodrill CB, Wilensky AJ, et al. Unilateral focal preponderance of interictal epileptiform discharges as a predictor of seizure origin. Arch Neurol 1996;53(3):228–32.

47. Sharbrough FW. Scalp-recorded ictal patterns in focal epilepsy. J Clin Neurophysiol 1993;10(3): 262–7.

Approach to Seizures, Epilepsies, and Epilepsy Syndromes

Martina Vendrame, MD, PhD[a],
Tobias Loddenkemper, MD[b],*

KEYWORDS

• Epilepsy syndromes • Classification • Semiology of seizures

Seizures and epilepsies present with multiple etiologies and multiple clinical features and change across the lifespan. Epilepsy is not a single disease but a diverse group of disorders that have in common an abnormally increased predisposition to epileptic seizures. A systematic approach to epileptic seizures and epilepsies is a first step toward the diagnosis and treatment of these disorders. Determination of clinical seizure type, epilepsy localization, underlying etiology, related medical conditions, and, if possible, epilepsy syndrome follows the general neurologic approach in clinical practice, including description of symptomatic presentation, localization, and etiologic investigation. Description of findings is crucial for selection of the most helpful diagnostic and therapeutic approach, defining relationships to sleep and sleep-related interactions, and comorbidities. For the purposes of this article, the following definitions are used:

Seizure refers to a transient occurrence of signs and/or symptoms due to abnormal excessive or synchronous neuronal activity in the brain.[1] Elements defining an epileptic seizure include mode of onset and termination, clinical manifestations, and abnormal enhanced synchrony.[1]

Epilepsy is a condition characterized by[1] (1) recurrent (2 or more) epileptic seizures, unprovoked by any immediate identified cause; (2) multiple seizures occurring in a 24-hour period that are considered a single event; and (3) an episode of status epilepticus that is considered a single event. Individuals who have had only febrile seizures are excluded from this category.

Epilepsy syndrome refers to a complex of signs and symptoms that define a unique epilepsy condition. This must involve more than just the seizure type; thus, frontal lobe seizures by themselves, for instance, do not constitute a syndrome.[2]

DIAGNOSTIC APPROACH

The diagnostic approach to seizures and epilepsy involves 4 independent steps as follows.[3] These steps have been implemented in the most recent suggestion for a revised epilepsy classification.[4]

1. Clinical presentation (What are the symptoms?)
2. Epilepsy localization (Where is the lesion?)
3. Etiology (What is causing the epilepsy?)
4. Syndrome (other related features that may assist with diagnosis making or fit with known syndromes).

Independent investigational techniques include the collection of a detailed history and clinical course; seizure semiology analysis either by history or video review; physical examination; electrophysiologic studies; structural neuroimaging and

The authors have no conflicts of interest for this article.
^a Division of Clinical Neurophysiology and Sleep, Department of Neurology, Boston University, Neurology C-3, 72 East Concord Street, Boston, MA 02118, USA
^b Division of Epilepsy and Clinical Neurophysiology, Children's Hospital Boston, Harvard Medical School, Fegan 9, 300 Longwood Avenue, Boston, MA 02115, USA
* Corresponding author.
E-mail address: tobias.loddenkemper@childrens.harvard.edu

sleep.theclinics.com

functional and metabolic neuroimaging; and laboratory testing, including genetic and histopathologic studies; these studies aid in answering the questions outlined previously.

Recognizing Nonepileptic Events

When gathering information on events, always consider the option that events may be nonepileptic. In general, when witnesses report the ability to modify or stop a patient's ictal movements during an epileptic seizure, a nonepileptic event should be considered.[5] In **Box 1** some clinical features that may aid the characterization of nonepileptic events, such as psychogenic seizures, parasomnias, and nocturnal panic attacks, are summarized.

The distinction between epileptic and nonepileptic events may represent a significant challenge for clinicians. The most commonly encountered nonepileptic events are the so-called PNES.[6] It is estimated that approximately 70% of PNES cases develop between the second and fourth decades of life, but PNES can also present in children and senior individuals.[6] Patients with PNES may have concurrent epileptic seizures or have had epileptic seizures before presenting with PNES.[6]

Some clinical features can help differentiate PNES from epileptic seizures, but most features are highly nonspecific and no single feature is pathognomonic for PNES.[5,7] When events occur during the night, and out of sleep, this distinction may be even more difficult. Disorders that may present with nocturnal nonepileptic paroxysmal events may include (1) specific sleep-related disorders, such as NREM 3 parasomnias and rapid eye movement (REM) sleep behavior disorder, and (2) psychiatric and behavioral conditions, such as panic attacks[8–10] or PNES, among others. These phenomena usually involve complex motor activity as seen in parasomnias and may have a wide spectrum of alterations of consciousness/awareness, which makes their differentiation from seizures difficult.

An abrupt onset is typically more suggestive of epileptic seizures, although other events, such as cardiac or vasovagal syncope, can also present with rapid onset. Epileptic seizures tend to have a stereotypical pattern, which means that witnesses and patients tend to report events with similar dynamics and features. At times, more than one type of event can be recognized by witnesses/patients and clinician. Ictal activity is also involuntary and uncontrollable, which means that during the seizure the behavior is not goal directed. Some patients during complex partial seizures (especially right temporal in origin) can

---

Box 1
Clinical features that may suggest nonepileptic events

Convulsive Psychogenic Nonepileptic Event

- Less stereotyped
- Does not follow an orderly sequence of a epileptic convulsion
- Long duration (most epileptic convulsions last less than 1–2 minutes; PNES convulsions often last 5–20 minutes or longer)
- Motor movements often are arrhythmic, are asynchronous, and stop then start again
- Eyes closed (eyes usually open with an epileptic convulsion)
- Seems to voluntarily modify or stop movements during the event
- Little or no postictal confusion
- Postictal crying, whispering
- May recall fragments, if gently pressed, with some responsiveness or recall of ictus

NREM Arousal Parasomnias

- 1–2 Episodes per night
- 1–4 Episodes per month
- Episodes occur during NREM 3 sleep
- Episodes occur more likely after 90 minutes of sleep onset
- Episodes can last up to 30 minutes
- Variable movements and actions (less stereotyped)
- Physical and verbal interaction can be seen
- Failure to arouse after the event
- Positive family history is common

Sleep-Related Panic Attacks

- 1–2 Episodes per night
- Episodes lasts 2–8 minutes
- Affective and autonomic features may be predominant
- The patient is aware during the event
- The patient recognizes the event as a panic attack and has a vivid recall
- History of daytime panic attacks is usually present
- Episodes usually occur during transition from NREM 2 to NREM 3

Abbreviations: NREM, non–rapid eye movements of sleep; PNES, psychogenic nonepileptic seizures; SWS, slow wave sleep.

follow commands often then accompanied by automatisms and varying degrees of amnesia. At times, behavior in response to an ictal aura can be seen, which is primarily not ictal in nature but related to the epileptic seizure, such as hand shaking due to a painful aura in the hand. Postictal alterations, including amnesia for the event, lethargy/sleep, and transient neurologic deficits, are also more likely in epileptic seizures and are typically reported with consistency by family members and caretakers.

When typical seizures can be recorded, video-electroencephalogram (EEG) is the gold standard diagnostic tool for nonepileptic events, and a diagnosis of these disorders can be made with high accuracy.[6,11] When video-EEG reveals no ictal epileptic activity before, during, or after the ictus, thorough neurologic, sleep, and psychiatric histories are crucial to confirm the diagnosis of these disorders.

Seizure History and Semiology

Identification and classification of seizures and epilepsies is based on clinical presentation. In epilepsy, semiology refers to the study of the signs and symptoms of seizures. The seizure semiology provides important clues to seizure and epilepsy localization. The collection of information on seizure history and semiology, together with the analysis of seizure semiology with video-EEG data, is essential for understanding the clinical seizure type and provides important information on the type of epilepsy and localization, guiding treatment and addressing prognosis. Furthermore, semiology provides important lateralizing and/or localizing information.[12–14]

The authors find it most useful to analyze the main phases of a seizure along the timeline of occurrence.[15] Simply imagine the timeline of a seizure, and inquire of features in this timeline separately, specifically

1. Seizure setting
2. Seizure onset
3. Seizure presentation and evolution and
4. Postictal symptoms.

Seizure setting

Information on seizure setting requires a reliable witness capable of accurately describing the details of the entire event. If a patient is amnestic for all or part of the seizure, an independent witness is crucial. Circumstances immediately prior to the event should be noted, such as the activity in which the patient was engaged, changes in the environment, changes in the patient's behavior

before seizure onset, and other prodrome (ie, the symptoms reported within minutes, hours, or even days before the seizure onset). The time of day and relationship of the events to sleep may also be elicited. For example, knowing that the events have a specific circadian pattern, arise from a particular sleep/wake state, or occur in the context of sleep deprivation helps distinguish different seizure types and epilepsy syndromes.[16–18] The presence of fever, concomitant illness, occurrence in high-altitude settings, preceding head injury, and perimenstrual timing may be helpful.[19] Information of seizure setting includes also prior medical history, current medical health, cognitive deficits, developmental achievements, and family history.

Seizure onset

Seizure onset in many people with focal epilepsies often is a so-called aura (ie, sensory, gustatory, visual, olfactory, auditory or abdominal, or more complex experiential sensation[s]) experienced by the patient.[20] Auras in some patients occur in combinations. An aura is not necessarily present, however, and other clinical features (described later) may also present as the first seizure symptom depending on the relationship of seizure onset and symptomatogenic cortical areas.

Different clinical phenomena depend on the location and extent of the ictal onset zone and its relationship to symptomatogenic cortical areas (**Fig. 1**).[21] For example, somatosensory auras (such as numbness, tingling, and painful or burning-like sensations) are usually generated from contralateral parietal areas.[22] Visual auras, such as seeing simple and fixed objects, often are related to activation of occipital area (area 17). Complex visual phenomena are more likely to be generated from the right temporo-parieto-occipital junction, and when prominent movement of the visual phenomena is perceived, occipital areas 18 and 19 are frequently involved.[23,24] Auditory auras can arise from the lateral temporal region unilaterally or bilaterally.[25] Olfactory and gustatory auras (ie, smelling of complements that are not present and abnormal tasting) are mostly related to spread into the temporal regions.[26]

The most frequently reported auras are sensations of abdominal discomfort or a rising abdominal sensation located in the epigastric area and are, therefore, named epigastric aura.[27] Some patients report their seizures begin with an unspecific, unexplainable feeling, often localized to the head (cephalic aura).[28] Cephalic auras have been reported when seizure activity spreads into the temporal regions, the parietooccipital areas, and the frontal regions.[29] Autonomic auras that

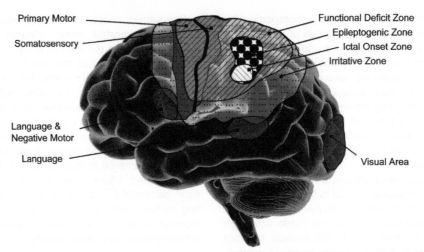

Primary Motor
Somatosensory
Language & Negative Motor
Language

Functional Deficit Zone
Epileptogenic Zone
Ictal Onset Zone
Irritative Zone
Visual Area

Fig. 1. Example of cortical zones in a selected epilepsy patient. The epileptogenic zone is the area of cortex indispensable for the generation of seizures. Within the epileptogenic zone, there is a smaller area, the ictal onset zone, where seizures are generated. The irritative zone is the area producing interictal epileptiform discharges. The symptomatogenic zone is the eloquent region (overlapping with the epileptogenic zone) responsible for the production of the clinical symptoms when activated during a seizure. The functional deficit zone is the area that clinically functions abnormally during periods in between seizures, as illustrated by functional imaging studies. Eloquent cortex is important for generating particular functions, including motor, sensory, language, and memory (ie, motor cortex, somatosensory cortex, visual cortex, and language areas). (*Adapted from* Datta A, Loddenkemper T. The epileptogenic zone. In: Wyllie E, Cascino GD, Gidal BE, et al, editors. Wyllie's treatment of epilepsy. Principles and practice. 5th edition. Philadelphia: Lippincott Williams & Wilkins; 2010; with permission.)

suggest activation of the autonomic system (palpitations, sweating, cold shivers or cold sweats, and piloerection) are most often secondary to symptomatogenic areas in the temporal or insular region.[30] Experiential auras, such as déjà vu (an intense feeling of visual or situational familiarity) or jamais vu (a feeling of visual or situational strangeness), are usually associated with temporal lobe seizures.[21,31,32] Selected auras and their localizing value are listed in **Table 1**.

Seizure presentation and evolution

Seizure presentation and evolution include symptoms and behaviors that a patient displays during the events. For practical purposes of gathering and analyzing reported information, information is presented in the following major categories: (1) motor features, (2) automatisms, (3) language features, (4) autonomic features, and (5) impairment of consciousness.

Symptoms that manifest later in the seizure usually represent spread of the ictal activity to neighboring cortical regions.

Motor features include dystonic posturing; clonic movements; tonic movements; head version; epileptic spasms; eye movements, such as nystagmus or sustained conjugate eye deviation; and other complex motor movements. The types, body site, and lateralization of these motor features can help with localization and lateralization of seizures.[15] For example, unilateral dystonic posturing, unilateral epileptic spasms, unilateral clonic seizures, unilateral tonic seizures, ictal nystagmus, version, or asymmetric tonic posturing (so-called figure 4) are generally indicative of seizure activity from the contralateral side of the brain (compared with the extended arm during the figure 4 prior to secondary generalization).[33–37]

The temporal presentation of the features during a seizure plays a role, however. Late ipsiversion and the last clonic jerk during seizures are frequently related to seizure onset in the ipsilateral brain hemisphere.[36,38] In a patient noted to have right clonic movements followed by right head version, then a generalized tonic clonic seizure, and subsequently several left arm clonic jerks toward the end of a seizure, the seizure may have started in the left hemisphere. Subsequent spread of the seizure into the other hemisphere may explain the late appearance of unilateral motor features ipsilateral to the seizure onset zone.

Automatisms are purposeless movements that may resemble simple repetitive movements or may be a complex sequence of natural-looking movements, such as picking or nestling hand movements or lip smacking, chewing, or tongue-licking movements.[36,39]

Table 1
Common auras and related localization

Aura	Descriptive Seizure Terminology	Brain Localization or Lateralization
Unpleasant or abnormal smell	Olfactory aura	Amygdala in mesial temporal lobe, left or right
Abnormal taste	Gustatory aura	Insula or secondary sensory cortex, left or right
Funny feeling in stomach, which often rises to the chest and neck	Epigastric aura	Insula or superior bank of sylvian fissure, common in mesial temporal lobe epilepsy, left or right
Déjà vu, fear, jamais vu, depersonalization, macropsia, micropsia, autoscopy	Psychic aura	Fear = amygdala Déjà vu or jamais vu = basal temporal lobe Multisensory hallucinations = temporal lobe
Buzzing sound, tone, or other noises	Auditory aura	Primary auditory cortex (Heschl gyrus), left or right
Flashing lights in left visual field	Visual aura	Right primary visual cortex (area 17)
Formed visual hallucinations in left visual field		Right association visual cortex
Left hand pain, tingling, or burning sensation	Somatosensory aura	Right primary somatosensory cortex
Sensation in both shoulders		Supplementary somatosensory cortex, left or right
Sensation in both hands		Superior bank of sylvian fissure of secondary sensory area, left or right

During a seizure, patients may also vocalize (ictal vocalization), verbalize (ictal speech), or have impaired language (ictal aphasia). Ictal speech has been localized to the nondominant temporal region.[40,41] Ictal aphasia usually arises from the dominant lateral temporal but sometimes from dominant frontal areas.[42,43] Ictal vocalization is more often secondary to activity in the dominant hemisphere, involving more frequently the frontal than temporal lobes.[44,45]

Ictal emesis, ictal urinary urge, urge to defecate, and orgasmic auras have been related to seizures in the right/nondominant temporal lobe.[46,47] Ictal sensation of cold has been reported with left temporal (or dominant temporal) lobe symptomatogenic zones. Unilateral piloerection (goose bumps) is generally related to seizures emanating from the ipsilateral hemisphere.[48] Impairment of consciousness can be seen ictally and postictally. Although the exact mechanisms for control of consciousness are not clear, emerging data show that processing of conscious information depends on the involvement of certain cortical and subcortical networks.[49] Recent data have correlated ictal alteration of consciousness with bilateral and/or left temporal lobe seizure activity.[50]

Postictal symptoms

Immediately after the end of a seizure, patients may present with a variety of symptoms that may at times only become obvious during an examination of the patient. These may provide additional important information, because they may indicate the localization of the seizure focus. Todd paresis (or postictal paresis/paralysis) is focal weakness in a part of the body after a seizure.[51] Postictal weakness secondary to a seizure focus is typically contralateral to the localization of the weakness[51] and may affect the arm, leg, and/or face. It usually subsides completely within 24 to 48 hours after the seizure.[51] Similarly, hemianopia (partial vision loss) can also present after a seizure, self-resolves, and is indicative of a contralateral seizure focus.[52] Postictal aphasia and dysphasia are usually suggestive of a seizure arising from the dominant hemisphere.[53] Nose wiping can be observed after a seizure, and it has been seen more frequently ipsilateral to the side of seizure onset.[54,55] Selected questions for history taking in epilepsy patients, including duration and recurrence patterns, are listed in **Box 2**.

Physical Examination

The physical examination provides additional information on the etiology of seizures, type of epilepsy, and epilepsy syndrome. The general physical examination includes the assessment of current health (chronic illnesses, fever, and any change in health conditions), somatic asymmetries, and dysmorphic features. Examination of skin and hair (perhaps with the use of a Wood lamp) and ophthalmologic examination may also provide important details. Neurologic examination can reveal focal abnormalities, such as hemiparesis (details are outlined elsewhere).[56] Under the appropriate supervision and safety measures, selected diagnostic activation procedures (eg, hyperventilation), may be performed.

Investigations: Electrophysiological Studies and Neuroimaging

An EEG is recommended by the American Academy of Neurology in the evaluation of an apparent first unprovoked seizure.[57] It may help in the determination of seizure type and localization, possible identification of an epilepsy syndrome, and estimation of recurrence risk.[58] Activation procedures can be performed with the scope to provoke epileptiform abnormalities and include hyperventilation, photic stimulation, and sleep or sleep deprivation. EEG can be performed in a routine fashion with a minimum of 20 minutes recorded or may be extended to diagnostic ambulatory (home) monitoring and in hospital long-term recordings with the addition of video data in case of frequent events.

Neuroimaging, including MRI, is generally performed and indicated by the American Academy of Neurology (guideline) in the assessment of a patient with new-onset seizures.[57,59] The scope of such imaging is to investigate a possible cause of seizures, such as the identification of a structural abnormality. Abnormalities in such cases are seen in up to one-third of patients, although only in approximately 2% of cases these findings are clinically significant and influence management decisions.[57] In general, as a practical guideline, persistent postictal focal deficits and the lack of return to baseline within a few hours after a seizure should suggest the need of neuroimaging to rule out additional neurologic structural lesions. Further investigations to determine the etiology of seizures, including laboratory blood tests, may also be considered.

Box 2
Selected features of seizure history

Seizure Setting

- Did the seizure occur out wakefulness, sleep, or the transition between wakefulness and sleep?
- Were there other triggers or situational factors (fever, height, menstrual period, light stimulation, sleep deprivation, etc)?

Seizure Onset

- Did the patient have a warning?

Seizure Evolution

- Was consciousness lost or altered? How soon after onset? If consciousness was only altered, were staring and unresponsiveness noted?
- Were motor features or negative motor features seen?
- Were tonic, clonic, myoclonic, dystonic, or other involuntary motor movements observed?
- Was head turning and/or sustained eye deviation noted?
- Did patient have complete loss of muscle tone followed by a fall to ground?
- Were automatisms seen (eg, lip smacking, picking at clothes, or hand wringing)?
- Was there an impairment of language or were there vocalizations?
- Did the patient experience autonomic features, such as increased heart rate or changes in breathing pattern?

Postictal Symptoms

- Did a transient neurologic deficit (eg, aphasia or hemiparesis) or postictal confusion or sleepiness follow after spell ended?
- Did the patient have a tongue bite or urinary/stool incontinence indicating a generalized tonic clonic seizure?

Duration

- How long did each component of episode last?
- How quickly did the patient return to normal after spell ended?

Recurrence

- Has there been more than one spell? If so, what is the frequency and interval between spells?
- Have there been other milder or worse spells?
- Have there been recurrent spells?

The diagnostic approach of seizures rests on basic clinical skills, and it is focused on history taking of seizure type (semiology) and clinical evolution. Approach to investigations should be individualized. EEG provides useful information when incorporated into clinical picture. Careful choice and timing of imaging study are warranted.

CLASSIFICATION APPROACH

To improve communication between providers and to investigate outcome and prognosis, classification of seizures and epilepsies may be helpful. The first classification of seizures and epilepsies released by the International League Against Epilepsy (ILAE) dates back to 1969. Since then, as a consequence of increasing knowledge on seizures and epilepsy and concomitant need of practical clinical applicability of these classifications, multiple revisions have taken place. Revisions of seizure and epilepsy classifications were published, respectively, in 1981[60] and in 1985 and 1989.[60,61] Revised seizure terminology was published in 2001[21] and in 2006[62] and in 2010 additional concepts for seizures and epilepsies were proposed.[4]

In 1969 and 1970, the first ILAE epilepsy classification was suggested by Gastaut.[63,64] Epilepsies were classified as (1) primary or secondary (based on etiology) and (2) partial or generalized (based on seizure localization). The term, *primary epilepsy*, was used to indicate the absence of a known cause for the epilepsy, whereas the term, *secondary epilepsy*, referred to a known cause. *Partial epilepsy* consisted of recurrent seizures which, based on semiological and/or clinical evaluation, were thought to arise from a focal area of the brain. On the contrary, in *generalized epilepsy*, semiology and clinical features were not indicative of a specific brain location.

The 1981 ILAE seizure classification[65] further distinguished seizures into partial or generalized and took into account more 2 types of features for a given partial or generalized seizure. Simply, the classification was as follows:

1. Partial
   a. Simple partial
   b. Complex partial
   c. Secondarily generalized
2. Generalized
   a. Absence
   b. Myoclonic
   c. Atonic
   d. Tonic
   e. Tonic-clonic.

Partial seizures could be simple or complex based on the preservation or loss of consciousness during the events, and secondarily generalized, when a partial seizure spreads and involves the whole brain (and both sides of the body simultaneously with loss of consciousness). Generalized epilepsies were characterized by seizures in the form of absence (ie, staring spells), myoclonic (muscle jerks), loss of tone (atonic), increased tone (tonic), and tonic plus clonic movements.

The ILAE published a revised classification of epilepsies in 1985.[60] Because the term, *secondary generalized epilepsy*, was sometimes confused with the different concept of *secondary* or *secondarily* generalized tonic-clonic seizures, it was abandoned in the subsequent revision. The terms, *primary* and *secondary*, were replaced with *idiopathic* and *symptomatic*, respectively. Both terms were applied to partial and generalized epilepsies. Furthermore, the recognition of *benign rolandic epilepsy* necessitated a category of *primary partial epilepsies*. Furthermore, this publication introduced the new concept of epilepsy syndromes as an "epileptic disorder characterized by a cluster of signs and symptoms customarily occurring together."[60]

The 1989 ILAE epilepsy classification[61] subsequently divided epilepsies in terms of etiology and localization, which is still the current classification system, while all updates since then were proposals. Epilepsies were distinguished as follows[61]:

1. Distinction by etiology
   a. Idiopathic (with age-related onset)
   b. Symptomatic
   c. Cryptogenic (added in order to characterize epilepsy syndromes with a presumed but unknown cause)
2. Distinction by localization
   a. Localization-related (focal, local, partial) epilepsies and syndromes
   b. Generalized epilepsies and syndromes
   c. Epilepsies and syndromes undetermined whether focal or generalized
   d. Special syndromes.

The 1989 ILAE classification of epilepsies by etiology and localization is current and has not yet been replaced, but several revisions have been proposed and entertained. Advantages of the 1989 classification include (1) its simplicity irrespective of exact symptomatology; (2) the categories correlating with seizure types, which are effectively treated with particular types of drugs; (3) separating seizures into *simple partial* and *complex partial*, which distinguishes the putative relationships of these to quality of life; and (4) widely accepted, providing a common language among epileptologists. Disadvantages consist of (1) neglecting conditions on the borderline between generalized and focal epilepsies, (2) the strict one-to-one relationship between clinical seizure type and epilepsy localization, (3) limited description of seizure semiology and evolution, and (4) the inability to accommodate evolving knowledge and working diagnoses.[66]

A seizure classification based only on clinical semiology, so-called semiological seizure classification, was proposed by Lüders and colleagues in the late 1990s.[67–69] According to the semiological seizure classification, seizures are classified as (1) auras, (2) autonomic seizures, (3) dialeptic seizures, (4) motor seizures, or (5) special seizures. Auras are ictal manifestations having sensory, psychosensory, and experiential symptoms. The main ictal manifestation in automotor seizures is automatisms. The main ictal manifestation of a dialeptic seizure is an alteration of consciousness independent of ictal EEG manifestations. The term, dialeptic seizure, has been introduced to distinguish this concept from absence seizures (as dialeptic seizures with a generalized ictal EEG) and complex partial seizures (as dialeptic seizures with a focal ictal EEG).

Motor seizures are subclassified as simple or complex. Simple motor seizures are characterized by simple, unnatural movements that can be triggered by electrical stimulation of the primary and supplementary motor area (such as myoclonic, tonic, clonic and tonic-clonic, and versive seizures). Complex motor seizures are characterized by complex motor movements resembling natural movements but occurring in an inappropriate setting (definition of automatisms). Special seizures include those that are characterized by negative features (so-named atonic, astatic, hypomotor, akinetic, and aphasic seizures). The semiological seizure classification identifies in detail the somatotopic distribution of ictal semiology and seizure evolution.

Many terms from the semiological seizure classification were incorporated in an ILAE glossary of seizure semiology terms in 2001.[21] This glossary delineates descriptive terms that provide additional details on clinical seizure presentation. The glossary contained terms for reference to semiology as well as terms for indicating seizure timing and duration, severity, prodromes, and postictal phenomena. According to this glossary, seizures can be termed, motor, when they involve musculature in any form. The motor event could consist of an increase (positive) or decrease (negative) in muscle contraction to produce a movement.[21]

The semiological seizure classification identifies in detail the somatotopic distribution of ictal semiology and seizure evolution.

The ILAE seizure glossary also contains details on automatisms and associated features of semiology. The term, automatism, is recommended for a more or less coordinated, repetitive motor activity mostly occurring when cognition is impaired. Automatisms often resemble a voluntary movement and may consist of an inappropriate continuation of ongoing preictal motor activity.[21] Lip smacking, lip pursing, chewing, licking, teeth grinding, and swallowing are termed, oroalimentary.[21]

The term, dyscognitive, refers to events in which (1) disturbance of cognition is the predominant feature and (2a) 2 or more of the components of cognition are involved or (2b) involvement of such components is undetermined.[21] Four components of cognition were named and defined as follows[21]: (1) perception—symbolic conception of sensory information; (2) attention—appropriate selection of a principal perception or task; (2) emotion—appropriate affective significance of a perception; (3) memory—ability to store and retrieve percepts or concepts; and (4) executive function—anticipation, selection, monitoring of consequences, and initiation of motor activity, including praxis and/or speech.

In addition to the seizure glossary, the ILAE published a new proposal for classification and terminology of seizures and epilepsies in 2001.[2] The proposal included a classification of seizures by axes. The axes in this proposal were[2]

Axis 1—Ictal seizure semiology
Axis 2—Electroclinical seizure types
Axis 3—Epilepsy syndrome
Axis 4—Etiology of epilepsies
Axis 5—Degree of disability and impairment.

Axis 1 described ictal seizure semiology based on the glossary (described previously). Axis 2 was based on a list of seizure types, which was constructed by the task force. Such seizure types were indicative of specific diagnostic epilepsy entities or etiologies, pathophysiology, or implicated therapy and prognosis. Axis 3 delineated the epilepsy syndromes, which were divided into fully characterized and in development syndromes. Axis 4 referred to pathologic and genetic causes. The 2001 classification also introduced new terminology in reference to epilepsies.[2] The term, symptomatic, was substituted with, known etiology.[2] The term, cryptogenic, was substituted with probably symptomatic, referring to epilepsy of unknown cause.[2] Age-related onset and genetic etiology likely were used to name idiopathic epilepsies.[2]

Due to overlap between axes and limited definitions of categories within axes, a revised 5-D, patient-oriented approach to classifying epilepsies has also been proposed.[3,70] This approach shifts from the syndrome-oriented approach to a neurologic, methodological, patient-oriented approach, using independent criteria for each of the 5 proposed dimensions. The first step in each patient-epileptologist encounter is to take a history of the presenting symptoms and formulate a hypothesis on the localization and etiology of the symptoms. Therefore, the main 5 dimensions of this classification were (1) localization of the epileptogenic zone, (2) clinical seizure presentation, (3) etiology, (4) seizure frequency, and (5) related medical conditions.[3]

Further modifications of seizures and epilepsy classifications were proposed in 2006 in the report of the ILAE classification core group[62] and in the 2010 revised terminology and concepts for organization of seizures and epilepsies.[4] These revisions now also permit further description within each category by other dimensions, including seizure types, localization, cause, or age at onset and other related medical conditions as outlined in the diagnostic approach (discussed previously). Terms, such as complex-partial and simple-partial, were abandoned, and seizures are recognized as "occurring in rapidly engaging bilaterally distributed networks (generalized) and within networks limited to one hemisphere and either discretely localized or more widely distributed (focal)."[4] The terms, focal and generalized, are reused, although it is stressed that generalized seizures may not involve the whole cortex.[4] Epilepsies are distinguished by specificity into 3 major categories: (1) electroclinical syndromes, (2) nonsyndromic epilepsies with structural metabolic causes, and (3) epilepsies of unknown cause.[4] Electroclinical syndromes are again arranged by age at onset or are categorized into epilepsies with structural metabolic and unknown causes and conditions with epileptic seizures traditionally not diagnosed as epilepsy per se.[4]

In the 2010 classification proposal, terminology based on etiology includes genetic, structural-metabolic, and unknown, replacing idiopathic, symptomatic, and cryptogenic.[4] An epilepsy is genetic when "the direct result of a known or presumed genetic defect(s) in which seizures are the core symptom of the disorder."[4] The knowledge regarding the genetic contributions may derive from specific molecular genetic studies that have been well replicated and even become the basis of diagnostic tests (eg,

SCN1A and Dravet syndrome) or the evidence for a central role of a genetic component may come from appropriately designed family studies".[4]

An epilepsy is structural/metabolic when "there is a distinct other structural or metabolic condition or disease that has been demonstrated to be associated with a substantially increased risk of developing epilepsy in appropriately designed studies."[4] Structural lesions include acquired insults, such as stroke, trauma, and sequelae of infection. Structural abnormalities, however, may also be of genetic origin when a separate disorder interposed between the genetic defect and the epilepsy (for example, cases of tuberous sclerosis complex and many malformations of cortical development). Epilepsy has an unknown cause when "the nature of the underlying cause is as yet unknown." In many cases, a genetic basis to their epilepsy is suspected but as-yet unrecognized disorder."[4] Patients are far more able to understand that the cause of their epilepsy is unknown, rather than being told it is idiopathic or cryptogenic, hence the reason that use of these terms are best abandoned.

Selected Epilepsies and Epilepsy Syndromes Presenting in Sleep and on Awakening

The sleep-wake cycle is regulated by different mechanisms that can affect the expression of seizures and epilepsy. During NREM sleep, the thalamus provides bilateral synchronized input to the cortex, potentially leading to the activation of cortical ictal foci and contributing to the generation of seizures in susceptible patients.[71,72] Contrarily, REM sleep is characterized by inhibition of both the thalamocortical synchronization networks and the interhemispheric mechanisms, preventing the spread and generalization of epileptiform activity.[73] It is widely accepted that both interictal epileptiform discharges and ictal epileptiform activity are promoted during NREM sleep.[74] Interictal epileptiform discharges are activated during NREM sleep and seizures are more likely facilitated during NREM 2 sleep.[74,75] Most epileptic seizures and epilepsies (but especially idiopathic/genetic generalized epilepsy syndromes), are suppressed during REM sleep.[75] A certain timing of seizure in relation to sleep-wake cycle and to the night-day circadian rhythms has also been documented.[16] Epilepsy syndromes that are known to be affected by the sleep-wake cycle are listed in Box 3. A few of the sleep-related epilepsies are highlighted.

Box 3
Epilepsies particularly affected by the sleep-wake cycle

- Panayiotopoulos syndrome
- Benign epilepsy with centrotemporal spikes (BECTS)
- Nocturnal frontal lobe epilepsy (NFLE)
- Autosomal-dominant nocturnal frontal lobe epilepsy (ADNFLE)
- Tonic seizures of Lennox-Gastaut syndrome
- Landau-Kleffner syndrome (LKS)
- Encephalopathy of continuous spike-and-wave during sleep (CSWS)

Autosomal-Dominant Nocturnal Frontal Lobe Epilepsy

Frontal lobe seizures are more likely to occur during sleep than seizures from other brain regions. Only 30% of patients with frontal lobe seizures have events during the daytime.[76,77] NFLE is familial and demonstrates an autosomal dominant pattern of inheritance. The mean age of onset of ADNFLE is 14 years.[76] NFLE seizures often occur in clusters, with frequency ranging from 20 per month to 20 events per night.[77] In ADNFLE, seizures have been linked to mutations of the nicotinic acetylcholine receptor.[77] Frontal lobe seizures are characterized by a wide spectrum of manifestations, ranging from brief arousals to complex motor activity and violent outbursts. A choking sensation may also be present. Given these features, frontal lobe seizures may be misdiagnosed with sleep disorders, such as night terrors and REM behavior disorder.[76] Studies have also shown that frontal lobe seizures may often be unrecognized and underreported, because 30% of patients generally have epileptiform abnormalities on routine EEG.[76,77] NFLE is discussed in greater detail elsewhere in this issue in the articles by Provini and colleagues and Derry.

Benign Epilepsy with Centrotemporal Spikes

BECTS, or benign rolandic epilepsy, is the most common focal epilepsy in children. BECTS has a typical onset between age 3 and 13 years with remission during adolescence.[78,79] Seizures occur most often during the night and two-thirds of patients report seizures occur exclusively during sleep.[78] Semiology of seizures in BECTS include "face pulling toward one side" associated with drooling, dysarthria, or subjective paresthesia over the same side, often with preserved consciousness.[79]

BECTS may often be misdiagnosed with other paroxysmal nocturnal events in childhood, including parasomnias. Video-EEG monitoring clearly reveals the diagnosis. BECTS presents with bilateral central and temporal spikes, potentiated during NREM sleep.[78,80] The epileptic discharge rate is higher during drowsiness and light sleep when compared with wakefulness, with no change in spike morphology.[80] Some patients may present with mild neuropsychological deficits.[81] Several studies have shown that despite the increased frequency of seizures and discharges during sleep, there is no disruption of sleep architecture.[78,80] Children typically outgrow BECTS with adolescence, and usually treatment is not needed. Reassurance should be provided to families. BECTS is discussed in greater detail elsewhere in this issue in the article by Bruni and colleagues.

Panayiotopoulos Syndrome

Panayiotopoulos syndrome, or benign epilepsy of childhood with occipital paroxysms (BECOP), presents in children between 2 and 6 years of age.[82] Seizure semiology includes sustained eye deviation and autonomic instability (with dysregulation of temperature, heart rate, respiration, and blood pressure) during sleep, and vomiting at awakening.[83] The semiology of these events in BECOP may resemble nonepileptic paroxysmal attacks, such as panic attacks, sleep terror, and other parasomnias. Routine EEG typically shows discharges in the occipital region may be sufficient for the diagnosis of BECOP.[82,83] BECOP is discussed in greater detail elsewhere in this issue in the article by Bruni and colleagues.

Landau-Kleffner Syndrome and Continuous Spike-and-Wave During Sleep

LKS, also known as epileptic aphasia, is an acquired epilepsy usually presenting at ages 4 to 6 years with language regression (typically a verbal auditory agnosia) and seizures. CSWS is characterized by an electrographic pattern consisting of an almost continuous presence of spike-wave discharges in NREM sleep. Although prognosis in LKS and CSWS for seizure control is positive, cognitive function declines and permanent neuropsychological dysfunction has been seen in several cases.[84] This permanent damage is most evident in those patients who had early-onset EEG abnormality and a prolonged active phase of CSWS.[84] In LKS, the paroxysmal activity permanently affects the posterior temporal area and results in auditory agnosia and language deficits; in CSWS, the frontal lobes are more involved and other cognitive disturbances predominate.[84] Aggressive treatment may include high-dose antiepileptic drugs, corticosteroids, and surgery in specific cases in addition to antiepileptic medications.[85] LKS and CSWS are discussed in greater detail elsewhere in this issue in the articles by Bruni and colleagues and Liukken and colleagues, respectively.

Juvenile Myoclonic Epilepsy

Juvenile myoclonic epilepsy (JME) is an idiopathic generalized epilepsy syndrome, generally presenting during adolescence and early adulthood. Myoclonic seizures, especially after morning awakenings (and breakfast time), are the most common presenting feature.[86] These may be subtle and overlooked for many years as simple clumsiness.[87] Tonic-clonic seizures can occur independently or be associated with myoclonic seizures; they tend to occur in early morning hours or in the early evening. Absence seizures are also present in JME and may look like daytime sleep attacks. Patients with JME are known to be characteristically sensitive to sleep deprivation and excessive alcohol consumption, and they should be educated on avoiding such triggers. There is a strong genetic component to the pathogenesis of JME, and an accurate family history

may particularly help clinicians with the initial diagnosis.[88]

RECONCILING DIAGNOSTIC AND CLASSIFICATION APPROACH

Currently, classifications of seizures and epilepsies are works in progress. The latest 2010 classification proposal permits a diagnostic approach in different dimensions (as outlined previously in this article), with determination of (1) epilepsy localization, (2) clinical seizure presentation, (3) etiology of epilepsy, (4) description of seizure frequency and severity, and (5) inclusion of related medical conditions, paralleling the information acquisition process in clinical practice. It further bridges the gap between a clinically useful classification approach that better adapts to increasing knowledge and a clinical approach. It also provides opportunities to perform research and compare individual patients to similar patient groups in different dimensions.

It not clear whether a single classification may reach a consensus or if multiple classification systems may need to coexist. Different classifications may serve different purposes, at least until there is a better clinical and scientific understanding of certain seizures and epilepsies.[66,89–92]

In practice, clinicians will continue to use these classifications in order to (1) understand the type of seizures and epilepsy affecting a particular

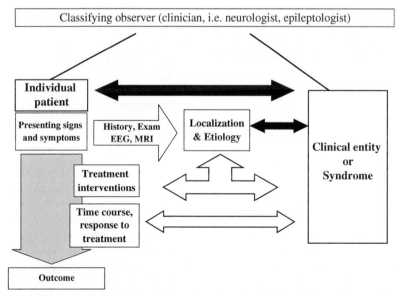

Fig. 2. Approach to seizure and epilepsy diagnosis and management. This diagram shows a general neurologic approach for characterization of seizure etiology and localization as more information becomes available. Information on seizures, other symptoms, and findings from a patient's physical examination are assessed and used to form a localization hypothesis. The validation or rejection of this initial hypothesis evolves over time in light of testing results and patient response to treatment.

patient; (2) identify possible underlying causes and comorbid conditions; (3) better communicate with other clinicians, health care providers, patients, and their families; (4) provide better tailored treatment; and (5) estimate prognosis and outcome. The authors suggest integrating a diagnostic approach with a classification approach.[93] **Fig. 2** presents an overview of the multistep workflow that occurs during this process. Patients present with a specific seizure history and semiology, which is understood by the analysis of the seizure setting, evolution, and postictal signs. The time course and response to treatment, together with the data gathered from investigations (EEG and MRI among other tests), lead to information on localization and etiology, and, in turn, may suggest a specific diagnosis of clinical entity or syndrome. This is used to choose further treatments, medical and surgical, determine further need for testing, and estimate prognosis. Within this evolving diagnostic process, communication between health care providers (ie, pediatricians, neurologists, epileptologists, neuropsychiatrists, and neurosurgeons) is essential.

SUMMARY

Seizures and epilepsies have multiple etiologies, have multiple ways of presentation, and change across lifetime. Future advances in genetics and other diagnostic techniques may make any classification attempt difficult and always limited to its time and current knowledge.[94] Although knowledge of epilepsy increases, clinicians may choose to adapt a basic approach to seizure and epilepsy classifications, in light of their fundamental roles in diagnosis and patient management.

REFERENCES

1. Fisher RS, van Emde Boas W, Blume W, et al. Epileptic seizures and epilepsy: definitions proposed by the International League Against Epilepsy (ILAE) and the International Bureau for Epilepsy (IBE). Epilepsia 2005;46(4):470–2.
2. Engel J Jr. A proposed diagnostic scheme for people with epileptic seizures and with epilepsy: report of the ILAE Task Force on Classification and Terminology. Epilepsia 2001;42(6):796–803.
3. Loddenkemper T, Kellinghaus C, Wyllie E, et al. A proposal for a five-dimensional patient-oriented epilepsy classification. Epileptic Disord 2005;7(4): 308–16.
4. Berg AT, Berkovic SF, Brodie MJ, et al. Revised terminology and concepts for organization of seizures and epilepsies: report of the ILAE Commission on Classification and Terminology, 2005-2009. Epilepsia 2010;51(4):676–85.
5. Syed TU, LaFrance WC Jr, Kahriman ES, et al. Can semiology predict psychogenic nonepileptic seizures? A prospective study. Ann Neurol 2011; 69(6):997–1004.
6. Devinsky O, Gazzola D, LaFrance WC Jr. Differentiating between nonepileptic and epileptic seizures. Nat Rev Neurol 2011;7(4):210–20.
7. An DM, Wu XT, Yan B, et al. Clinical features of psychogenic nonepileptic seizures: a study of 64 cases in southwest China. Epilepsy Behav 2011; 17(3):408–11.
8. Zucconi M, Ferini-Strambi L. NREM parasomnias: arousal disorders and differentiation from nocturnal frontal lobe epilepsy. Clin Neurophysiol 2000; 111(Suppl 2):S129–35.
9. Zucconi M, Manconi M, Bizzozero D, et al. EEG synchronisation during sleep-related epileptic seizures as a new tool to discriminate confusional arousals from paroxysmal arousals: preliminary findings. Neurol Sci 2005;26(Suppl 3):s199–204.
10. Derry CP, Duncan JS, Berkovic SF. Paroxysmal motor disorders of sleep: the clinical spectrum and differentiation from epilepsy. Epilepsia 2006;47(11): 1775–91.
11. Mari F, Di Bonaventura C, Vanacore N, et al. Video-EEG study of psychogenic nonepileptic seizures: differential characteristics in patients with and without epilepsy. Epilepsia 2006;47(Suppl 5):64–7.
12. Datta A, Loddenkemper T. The epileptogenic zone. In: Wyllie E, Cascino GD, Gidal BE, editors. Wyllie's treatment of epilepsy. Principles and practice. 5th edition. Philadelphia: Lippincott Williams & Wilkins; 2010. p. 818–27.
13. Foldvary-Schaefer N, Unnwongse K. Localizing and lateralizing features of auras and seizures. Epilepsy Behav 2010;20(2):160–6.
14. Vendrame M, Zarowski M, Alexopoulos AV, et al. Localization of pediatric seizure semiology. Clin Neurophysiol 2011;122(10):1924–8.
15. Loddenkemper T, Kotagal P. Lateralizing signs during seizures in focal epilepsy. Epilepsy Behav 2005;7(1):1–17.
16. Loddenkemper T, Vendrame M, Zarowski M, et al. Circadian patterns of pediatric seizures. Neurology 2011;76(2):145–53.
17. Kaleyias J, Loddenkemper T, Vendrame M, et al. Sleep-wake patterns of seizures in children with lesional epilepsy. Pediatr Neurol 2011;45(2):109–13.
18. Zarowski M, Loddenkemper T, Vendrame M, et al. Circadian distribution and sleep/wake patterns of generalized seizures in children. Epilepsia 2011; 52(6):1076–83.
19. Jan MM, Girvin JP. Seizure semiology: value in identifying seizure origin. Can J Neurol Sci 2008;35(1): 22–30.

20. Widdess-Walsh P, Kotagal P, Jeha L, et al. Multiple auras: clinical significance and pathophysiology. Neurology 2007;69(8):755–61.

21. Blume WT, Lüders HO, Mizrahi E, et al. Glossary of descriptive terminology for ictal semiology: report of the ILAE task force on classification and terminology. Epilepsia 2001;42(9):1212–8.

22. Mauguiere F, Courjon J. Somatosensory epilepsy. A review of 127 cases. Brain 1978;101(2):307–32.

23. Bien CG, Benninger FO, Urbach H, et al. Localizing value of epileptic visual auras. Brain 2000;123(Pt 2): 244–53.

24. Williamson PD, Thadani VM, Darcey TM, et al. Occipital lobe epilepsy: clinical characteristics, seizure spread patterns, and results of surgery. Ann Neurol 1992;31(1):3–13.

25. Clarke DF, Otsubo H, Weiss SK, et al. The significance of ear plugging in localization-related epilepsy. Epilepsia 2003;44(12):1562–7.

26. Chen C, Shih YH, Yen DJ, et al. Olfactory auras in patients with temporal lobe epilepsy. Epilepsia 2003;44(2):257–60.

27. Henkel A, Noachtar S, Pfander M, et al. The localizing value of the abdominal aura and its evolution: a study in focal epilepsies. Neurology 2002;58(2): 271–6.

28. Palmini A, Gloor P. The localizing value of auras in partial seizures: a prospective and retrospective study. Neurology 1992;42(4):801–8.

29. Canuet L, Ishii R, Iwase M, et al. Cephalic auras of supplementary motor area origin: an ictal MEG and SAM(g2) study. Epilepsy Behav 2008;13(3):570–4.

30. Stefan H, Feichtinger M, Black A. Autonomic phenomena of temperature regulation in temporal lobe epilepsy. Epilepsy Behav 2003;4(1):65–9.

31. Neppe VM. Is deja vu a symptom of temporal lobe epilepsy? S Afr Med J 1981;60(23):907–8.

32. Guedj E, Aubert S, McGonigal A, et al. Deja-vu in temporal lobe epilepsy: metabolic pattern of cortical involvement in patients with normal brain MRI. Neuropsychologia 2010;48(7):2174–81.

33. Wyllie E, Lüders H, Morris HH, et al. The lateralizing significance of versive head and eye movements during epileptic seizures. Neurology 1986;36(5): 606–11.

34. Kernan JC, Devinsky O, Luciano DJ, et al. Lateralizing significance of head and eye deviation in secondary generalized tonic-clonic seizures. Neurology 1993; 43(7):1308–10.

35. Loddenkemper T, Wyllie E, Neme S, et al. Lateralizing signs during seizures in infants. J Neurol 2004; 251(9):1075–9.

36. Bonelli SB, Lurger S, Zimprich F, et al. Clinical seizure lateralization in frontal lobe epilepsy. Epilepsia 2007; 48(3):517–23.

37. Bleasel A, Kotagal P, Kankirawatana P, et al. Lateralizing value and semiology of ictal limb posturing and version in temporal lobe and extratemporal epilepsy. Epilepsia 1997;38(2):168–74.

38. Leutmezer F, Woginger S, Antoni E, et al. Asymmetric ending of secondarily generalized seizures: a lateralizing sign in TLE. Neurology 2002;59(8): 1252–4.

39. Kellinghaus C, Loddenkemper T, Kotagal P. Ictal spitting: clinical and electroencephalographic features. Epilepsia 2003;44(8):1064–9.

40. Yen DJ, Su MS, Yiu CH, et al. Ictal speech manifestations in temporal lobe epilepsy: a video-EEG study. Epilepsia 1996;37(1):45–9.

41. Chee MW, Kotagal P, Van Ness PC, et al. Lateralizing signs in intractable partial epilepsy: blinded multiple-observer analysis. Neurology 1993;43(12): 2519–25.

42. Serafetinides EA, Falconer MA. Speech disturbances in temporal lobe seizures: a study in 100 epileptic patients submitted to anterior temporal lobectomy. Brain 1963;86:333–46.

43. Koerner M, Laxer KD. Ictal speech, postictal language dysfunction, and seizure lateralization. Neurology 1988;38(4):634–6.

44. Penfield W, Rasmussen T. Vocalization and arrest of speech. Arch Neurol Psychiatry 1949;61(1):21–7.

45. Janszky J, Fogarasi A, Jokeit H, et al. Are ictal vocalisations related to the lateralisation of frontal lobe epilepsy? J Neurol Neurosurg Psychiatry 2000; 69(2):244–7.

46. Loddenkemper T, Foldvary N, Raja S, et al. Ictal urinary urge: further evidence for lateralization to the nondominant hemisphere. Epilepsia 2003; 44(1):124–6.

47. Janszky J, Szucs A, Halasz P, et al. Orgasmic aura originates from the right hemisphere. Neurology 2002;58(2):302–4.

48. Loddenkemper T, Kellinghaus C, Gandjour J, et al. Localising and lateralising value of ictal piloerection. J Neurol Neurosurg Psychiatry 2004;75(6):879–83.

49. Yu L, Blumenfeld H. Theories of impaired consciousness in epilepsy. Ann N Y Acad Sci 2009;1157: 48–60.

50. Lux S, Kurthen M, Helmstaedter C, et al. The localizing value of ictal consciousness and its constituent functions: a video-EEG study in patients with focal epilepsy. Brain 2002;125(Pt 12):2691–8.

51. Kellinghaus C, Kotagal P. Lateralizing value of Todd's palsy in patients with epilepsy. Neurology 2004;62(2):289–91.

52. Salmon JH. Transient postictal hemianopsia. Arch Ophthalmol 1968;79(5):523–5.

53. Gabr M, Lüders H, Dinner D, et al. Speech manifestations in lateralization of temporal lobe seizures. Ann Neurol 1989;25(1):82–7.

54. Hirsch LJ, Lain AH, Walczak TS. Postictal nosewiping lateralizes and localizes to the ipsilateral temporal lobe. Epilepsia 1998;39(9):991–7.

55. Leutmezer F, Serles W, Lehrner J, et al. Postictal nose wiping: a lateralizing sign in temporal lobe complex partial seizures. Neurology 1998;51(4): 1175–7.

56. Rowand LP, Pedley TA. Merritt's neurology. 12th edition. Philadelphia: Lippincott Williams & Wilkins; 2009.

57. Krumholz A, Wiebe S, Gronseth G, et al. Practice parameter: evaluating an apparent unprovoked first seizure in adults (an evidence-based review): report of the Quality Standards Subcommittee of the American Academy of Neurology and the American Epilepsy Society. Neurology 2007;69(21):1996–2007.

58. Shinnar S, Kang H, Berg AT, et al. EEG abnormalities in children with a first unprovoked seizure. Epilepsia 1994;35(3):471–6.

59. Gaillard WD, Cross JH, Duncan JS, et al. Epilepsy imaging study guideline criteria: commentary on diagnostic testing study guidelines and practice parameters. Epilepsia 2011;52(9):1750–6.

60. Proposal for classification of epilepsies and epileptic syndromes. Commission on classification and terminology of the international league against epilepsy. Epilepsia 1985;26(3):268–78.

61. Proposal for revised classification of epilepsies and epileptic syndromes. Commission on classification and terminology of the International League Against Epilepsy. Epilepsia 1989;30(4):389–99.

62. Engel J Jr. Report of the ILAE classification core group. Epilepsia 2006;47(9):1558–68.

63. Gastaut H. Classification of the epilepsies. Proposal for an international classification. Epilepsia 1969; 10(Suppl):14–21.

64. Merlis JK. Proposal for an international classification of the epilepsies. Epilepsia 1970;11(1):114–9.

65. Proposal for revised clinical and electroencephalographic classification of epileptic seizures. From the Commission on Classification and Terminology of the International League Against Epilepsy. Epilepsia 1981;22(4):489–501.

66. Loddenkemper T. Classification of the epilepsies. In: Wyllie E, editor. The treatment of epilepsy. Philadelphia: Lippincott Williams and Wilkins; 2010. p. 229–34.

67. Lüders H, Acharya J, Baumgartner C, et al. Semiological seizure classification. Epilepsia 1998;39(9): 1006–13.

68. Lüders H, Acharya J, Baumgartner C, et al. A new epileptic seizure classification based exclusively on ictal semiology. Acta Neurol Scand 1999;99(3): 137–41.

69. Lüders HO, Burgess R, Noachtar S. Expanding the international classification of seizures to provide localization information. Neurology 1993;43(9):1650–5.

70. Kellinghaus C, Loddenkemper T, Najm IM, et al. Specific epileptic syndromes are rare even in tertiary epilepsy centers: a patient-oriented approach to epilepsy classification. Epilepsia 2004;45(3): 268–75.

71. Domich L, Oakson G, Steriade M. Thalamic burst patterns in the naturally sleeping cat: a comparison between cortically projecting and reticularis neurones. J Physiol 1986;379:429–49.

72. Steriade M. Sleep, epilepsy and thalamic reticular inhibitory neurons. Trends Neurosci 2005;28(6): 317–24.

73. Shouse MN, Siegel JM, Wu MF, et al. Mechanisms of seizure suppression during rapid-eye-movement (REM) sleep in cats. Brain Res 1989; 505(2):271–82.

74. Ferrillo F, Beelke M, Nobili L. Sleep EEG synchronization mechanisms and activation of interictal epileptic spikes. Clin Neurophysiol 2000;111(Suppl 2): S65–73.

75. Minecan D, Natarajan A, Marzec M, et al. Relationship of epileptic seizures to sleep stage and sleep depth. Sleep 2002;25(8):899–904.

76. Provini F, Plazzi G, Tinuper P, et al. Nocturnal frontal lobe epilepsy. A clinical and polygraphic overview of 100 consecutive cases. Brain 1999;122(Pt 6): 1017–31.

77. Ryvlin P, Rheims S, Risse G. Nocturnal frontal lobe epilepsy. Epilepsia 2006;47(Suppl 2):83–6.

78. Baglietto MG, Battaglia FM, Nobili L, et al. Neuropsychological disorders related to interictal epileptic discharges during sleep in benign epilepsy of childhood with centrotemporal or Rolandic spikes. Dev Med Child Neurol 2001;43(6):407–12.

79. Wirrell EC. Benign epilepsy of childhood with centrotemporal spikes. Epilepsia 1998;39(Suppl 4): S32–41.

80. Laub MC, Funke R, Kirsch CM, et al. BECT: comparison of cerebral blood flow imaging, neuropsychological testing and long-term EEG findings. Epilepsy Res Suppl 1992;6:95–8.

81. Volkl-Kernstock S, Bauch-Prater S, Ponocny-Seliger E, et al. Speech and school performance in children with benign partial epilepsy with centrotemporal spikes (BCECTS). Seizure 2009;18(5): 320–6.

82. Capovilla G, Striano P, Beccaria F. Changes in Panayiotopoulos syndrome over time. Epilepsia 2009; 50(Suppl 5):45–8.

83. Michael M, Tsatsou K, Ferrie CD. Panayiotopoulos syndrome: an important childhood autonomic epilepsy to be differentiated from occipital epilepsy and acute non-epileptic disorders. Brain Dev 2009; 32(1):4–9.

84. Galanopoulou AS, Bojko A, Lado F, et al. The spectrum of neuropsychiatric abnormalities associated with electrical status epilepticus in sleep. Brain Dev 2000;22(5):279–95.

85. Loddenkemper T, Fernandez IS, Peters JM. Continuous spike and waves during sleep and electrical

status epilepticus in sleep. J Clin Neurophysiol 2011;28(2):154–64.

86. Badawy RA, Macdonell RA, Jackson GD, et al. Why do seizures in generalized epilepsy often occur in the morning? Neurology 2009;73(3): 218–22.

87. Bazil CW. Nocturnal seizures. Semin Neurol 2004; 24(3):293–300.

88. Labate A, Ambrosio R, Gambardella A, et al. Usefulness of a morning routine EEG recording in patients with juvenile myoclonic epilepsy. Epilepsy Res 2007; 77(1):17–21.

89. Wolf P. Of cabbages and kings: some considerations on classifications, diagnostic schemes, semiology, and concepts. Epilepsia 2003;44(1):1–4 [discussion: 4–13].

90. Nicholl JS. Of cabbages and kings: some considerations on classifications, diagnostic schemes, semiology, and concepts. Epilepsia 2003;44(7):988.

91. Avanzini G. A sound conceptual framework for an epilepsy classification is still lacking. Epilepsia 2010;51(4):720–2.

92. Troester M, Rekate HL. Pediatric seizure and epilepsy classification: why is it important or is it important? Semin Pediatr Neurol 2009;16(1):16–22.

93. Loddenkemper T. Criteria for surgery referral. In: Panayiotopoulos T, editor. Atlas of epilepsy. New York: Thieme; 2010. p. 1627–35.

94. Loddenkemper T, Lüders HO. History of seizure and epilepsy classification. In: Lüders HO, editor. Textbook of epilepsy surgery. Abingdon (UK): Taylor & Francis; 2008. p. 160–73.

Primary Sleep Disorders in People with Epilepsy: What We Know, Don't Know, and Need to Know

Madeleine M. Grigg-Damberger, MD[a],*,
Nancy Foldvary-Schaefer, DO, MS[b]

KEYWORDS

- Sleep disorders and epilepsy • Sleep apnea and epilepsy
- Sleepwalking and frontal lobe epilepsy
- Insomnia and epilepsy

Sleep is the golden chain that ties health and our bodies together.

— *Thomas Dekker*

Sleep and epilepsy are common bedfellows. Many sleep disorder symptoms and some primary sleep disorders such as excessive daytime sleepiness (EDS), sleep maintenance insomnia, and obstructive sleep apnea (OSA) are 2 to 3 times more common in people with epilepsy than the general population.[1–14] Adults with epilepsy and sleep complaints have significantly lower quality of life than those without sleep problems.[11–13,15,16] Sleep problems in children with epilepsy are associated with negative effects on daytime behavior and academic performance.[17–19] Recognition of this situation has led to increasing numbers of patients being referred to sleep centers to evaluate whether untreated sleep disorders may be contributing to their seizures. Late-onset or worsening seizure control in older adults may herald OSA.[20,21] Identifying and treating sleep disorders in people with epilepsy improves seizure control and quality of life in some cases. This article reviews the recent evidence for this claim.

QUESTIONNAIRE-BASED STUDIES OF THE PREVALENCE OF PRIMARY SLEEP DISORDERS IN ADULTS WITH EPILEPSY

Sleep disorders are 2 to 3 times more common in adults[11–14] and children[1–10] with epilepsy compared with the general age-matched population, especially when seizures are poorly controlled or complicated by comorbid neurologic conditions.

Most recent studies examining the prevalence of sleep complaints in adults with epilepsy are based on sleep questionnaires, sometimes coupled with structured clinical interviews, neuropsychological testing, or psychiatric evaluation.[11–13,21–24] **Table 1** summarizes these studies. The most common sleep complaints in adults with epilepsy are sleep maintenance insomnia

Financial Disclosure and Conflict of Interest Obligations: We have no conflicts of interest to declare regarding this paper. The use of melatonin to treat insomnia in children with epilepsy is discussed.

[a] Department of Neurology, University of NM School of Medicine, MSC10 5620, One University of NM, Albuquerque, NM 87131-0001, USA

[b] Cleveland Clinic Lerner College of Medicine of Case Western Reserve University, Epilepsy Center, Cleveland Clinic Neurological Institute, 9500 Euclid Avenue, FA 20, Cleveland, OH 44195, USA

* Corresponding author.

E-mail address: mgriggd@salud.unm.edu

Table 1
Questionnaire-based studies evaluating sleep problems in adults with epilepsy

Author, Year	Study Design	Study Population	Findings
Manni et al,[22] 2000	Large case-control	244 focal or generalized epilepsy vs 205 controls	Higher scores on ESS in those with snoring, apneas, or recurrent seizures in past year
Malow et al,[23] 1997	Large case-control	158 with focal or generalized epilepsy vs 68 patients with other neurologic disorders	ESS $\geq$10 in 28% with epilepsy vs 18% controls Symptoms of sleep apnea or RLS independent predictors of ESS >10
Vignatelli et al,[24] 2006	Small case-control	33 with NFLE (36% seizures nightly) vs 27 controls	36% NFLE tired most mornings vs 11% controls; 50% awoke most nights vs 22% controls
De Weerd et al,[11] 2005	Large case-control	492 with epilepsy vs 111controls	39% of people with epilepsy complained of sleep disturbances last 6 months vs 18% controls Quality of life most impaired in epilepsy patients with sleep complaints
Khatami et al,[12] 2006	Prospective large case- control (questionnaire and structured clinical interview)	100 consecutive patients with either generalized or focal epilepsy compared with controls	30% of people with epilepsy had sleep complaints vs 10 controls Loud snoring and restless legs independent predictors of EDS in patients with epilepsy
Xu et al,[15] 2006	Large case series	201 people with refractory partial epilepsy on $\geq$2 AEDS	34% reported sleep disturbances last 6 months 10% prescribed hypnotics Those reporting sleep disturbances more likely to endorse depression or anxiety, have poorer quality of life, and have had a seizure in past week
Piperdou et al,[13] 2008	Large case series	124 consecutive patients with focal or generalized epilepsy: 42% nocturnal seizures	28% had scores suggesting OSA; 25% insomnia and 17% EDS Insomnia independent predictor of reduced quality of life. Insomnia correlated with seizure frequency
Haut et al,[21] 2009	Small case-control retrospective study included extensive neuropsychological testing	31 elders with epilepsy compared with 31 age-matched healthy controls	18% with epilepsy depressed vs 0% controls Poor sleeper associated with more EDS, awakening short of breath, headache

Abbreviations: ESS, Epworth Sleepiness Scale; NFLE, nocturnal frontal lobe epilepsy.

and EDS. A prospective study found 52% of 100 consecutive Greek adults with epilepsy endorsed symptoms of sleep maintenance insomnia versus 38% of 90 age-matched controls,[12] although another study found only 25% of Greek adults with epilepsy reported insomnia.[13] Among 201 adults with medically refractory partial epilepsy, 10% were prescribed hypnotics for complaints of insomnia.[15]

Two questionnaire-based studies have reported that EDS is statistically more common in people with epilepsy versus controls.[13,23] Between 18% and 28% of adults with epilepsy complained of EDS (Epworth Sleepiness Scale [ESS] score >10) compared with 12% to 17% of controls.[13,23] An international cross-sectional survey of 35,327 adults found 24% reported they did not sleep well and 12% complained of severe or dangerous EDS.[25] Although sleepiness in adults with epilepsy is more likely multifactorial, symptoms suggestive of OSA or restless legs syndrome (RLS) were independent predictors of an increased ESS score.[22,23,26]

Several studies find that EDS in people with epilepsy is more likely to be associated with depression or anxiety. Depression and anxiety are more common among adults with epilepsy than healthy controls.[27] Scores on the Beck Depression Inventory suggestive of moderate to severe depression best predicted a complaint of EDS in patients with epilepsy, whereas sleep apnea scores contributed only minor independent effects.[14] Thirty-two percent of 201 patients with refractory partial epilepsy were also taking medications to treat depression, 21% for anxiety; those taking psychotropics were more likely to complain of sleep problems than those not taking them.[15] A retrospective study found 31 mature adults with partial epilepsy endorsed more symptoms of EDS, depression, anxiety, and awakening short of breath or with a headache than age-matched and gender-matched controls.[21] Complaints of EDS reported by 48% of 99 unselected adult patients with epilepsy correlated with anxiety and neck circumference.[28]

Comorbid neurodevelopmental disorders increased the likelihood for sleep complaints in adults with epilepsy. Thirty-one percent of 35 adults with tuberous sclerosis complex (TSC) complained of insomnia, 71% of whom also had a history of epilepsy.[26] Complaints of insomnia were associated with OSA and RLS scores. Daytime sleepiness was associated with depression, antisocial behavior, and psychotropic medications. Patients treated with antiepileptic drugs (AEDs) were more likely to report daytime sleepiness, attention deficits, and anxiety.

Sleep hygiene may contribute to sleep/wake complaints in people with epilepsy. A study examining sleep hygiene in 270 adults with epilepsy compared with controls found that among the individuals with epilepsy: (1) 23% smoked at bedtimes; (2) 29% had irregular sleep/wake schedules or varying degrees of sleep deprivation; and (3) 17% engaged in high-concentration/upsetting activities at bedtime.[22] Controls had many (if not more) poor sleep habits. However, adults with epilepsy were more likely to drink coffee before bedtime (50% of patients with epilepsy vs 30% controls) and nap after dinner (16% epilepsy vs 6% controls). Another study in 108 adults with epilepsy found that many did not practice healthy lifestyle behaviors (including sleep hygiene) even if they were compliant with AED therapy.[29]

Several factors not associated with more sleep complaints in adults with epilepsy have been reported. Most studies did not find gender a risk factor for sleep problems in people with epilepsy,[12,13,22] except one in which women with refractory partial epilepsy reported more severe sleep problems than men.[15] Neither EDS nor insomnia was particularly more common in adults with partial or primary generalized epilepsies.[12,13,22,23] Nocturnal seizures were not more likely to be associated with sleep problems,[15,23] except in people with nocturnal frontal lobe epilepsy (NFLE), who reported only more midsleep awakenings than controls.[24]

IS SLEEP ARCHITECTURE ALTERED IN ADULTS WITH EPILEPSY?

Several older studies reported abnormalities in sleep architecture in adults with epilepsy but few of these controlled either for seizures or medication.[30,31] These studies found: (1) reduced time spent in rapid eye movement (REM) sleep; (2) prolonged REM latency; (3) increased wake after sleep onset (WASO) resulting in reduced total sleep time (TST) and sleep efficiency; and (4) increased number of arousals, awakenings, and stage shifts,[30,31] even in the absence of seizures the night of polysomnography (PSG).[31]

Abnormalities in REM Sleep Often Seen in Adults with Epilepsy

REM sleep may be particularly susceptible to the occurrence of seizures in people with partial epilepsy. One study found that REM sleep time decreased from a mean of 18% to 12% if the patient had a seizure that day and 16% to 7% if the seizure occurred during nighttime sleep.[32] Night seizures (but not day seizures) significantly reduced sleep efficiency, increased REM latency, increased stage 1 sleep, reduced stage 2 and 4 sleep, and increased drowsiness on the Maintenance of Wakefulness test.[32] The reduced sleep efficiency and prolonged REM latency were even greater if the temporal lobe seizure occurred before the first REM period. Both diurnal and nocturnal seizures prolonged REM sleep latency. Nocturnal, but not diurnal, seizures increased stage nonrapid eye movement (NREM) 1 and decreased deeper NREM 3 sleep.

If a motor convulsion occurs during a night of PSG in a person with epilepsy (regardless of whether it is primary generalized or focal in onset), changes in sleep architecture observed may include a prolonged REM latency, decreased TST and REM sleep time and increased WASO, arousals, and NREM 1 and 2 sleep time.[31,33]

Sleep Architecture May Be More Disrupted in People with Temporal Lobe Epilepsy

Some studies suggest that sleep architecture is more disturbed in adults with temporal lobe epilepsy (TLE) compared with those whose seizures emanate from the frontal lobes (frontal lobe epilepsy [FLE]) or who have primary generalized epilepsy (PGE).[31,33,34] In a study involving 15 patients with mesial TLE and 15 with FLE, patients with TLE had reduced sleep efficiency, increased WASO, and more arousals than those with FLE despite their seizures occurring less often in sleep.[34] These differences persisted even after

sleep deprivation or AED withdrawal. **Fig. 1** shows 2 sleep histograms, one from a patient with FLE, the other TLE.

Abnormalities in NREM Sleep Microarchitecture Identified Using Cyclic Alternating Pattern Analysis in People with Epilepsy

For more than 2 decades, sleep researchers have used cyclic alternating pattern (CAP) analysis of NREM sleep microarchitecture to confirm instability of NREM sleep in a variety of sleep disorders, include different epilepsies.[35–45] NREM sleep using CAP analysis can be divided into 2 phases: (A and B. CAPs are periodic cyclic variations in electroencephalographic activity during NREM sleep as the sleeping brain is challenged by the modification of environmental conditions. Close study of several epochs of NREM sleep identified that undisturbed periods of typical NREM sleep (phase B) alternate with phasic events (phase A). The nature of the phasic activity scored as phase A events is further categorized as (1) phase A1: intermittent alpha rhythm in stage NREM; sequences of K-complexes or of delta bursts in NREM 2 or 3; (2) phase A2: periods of desynchronized electroencephalographic activity that follow K-arousals; and (3) phase A3: change in electroencephalogram (EEG) which is scored on arousal following American Academy of Sleep Medicine (AASM) Scoring Manual rules.

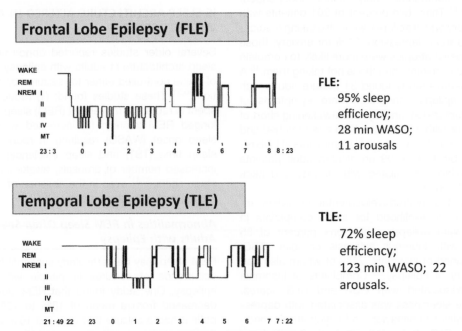

Fig. 1. Two illustrative histograms, one from a patient with FLE, the other with TLE. (*From* Crespel A, Coubes P, Baldy-Moulinier M. Sleep influence on seizures and epilepsy effects on sleep in partial frontal and temporal lobe epilepsies. Clin Neurophysiol 2000;111(Suppl 2):S56–7; with permission.)

In patients with epilepsy, interictal epileptic discharges (IEDs) more often occur in the transition from NREM 1 and 2 to NREM 3, less in NREM 3, and least in REM sleep. Studies evaluating abnormalities in CAP in individuals with different epilepsies compared with controls have shown: (1) most IEDs occur during phase A1 of CAP when NREM sleep was dominated by either K-complexes or delta bursts; (2) studies in primary generalized and frontotemporal partial epilepsies show IEDs are most inhibited during phase B of CAP; (3) nocturnal convulsions or motor seizures most often arise concomitant with phase A of CAP; (4) partial seizures occurring in clusters during sleep more often occurred during CAP; and (5) an increase in CAP rate has been observed during the 30-minute period after a partial seizure in sleep. These findings are nonspecific; similar abnormalities in CAP are seen in patients with OSA, periodic limb movements in sleep (PLMS), RLS, and NREM parasomnias.

SLEEP DISORDERS CONFIRMED BY PSG IN ADULTS WITH EPILEPSY

Sleep studies in adults with epilepsy are most often performed for suspected OSA, occasionally to characterize nocturnal spells, rarely for suspected REM sleep behavior disorder (RBD), or unexplained hypersomnia. Some studies suggest that OSA is found in 10% of unselected adult patients with epilepsy and 30% of patients with medically refractory epilepsy.[19,20,46–48] If an apnea hypopnea index (AHI) of 5 or greater is found in approximately 24% of men and 9% of women in the general adult population (ages 30–60 years),[49,50] then OSA is more prevalent in adults with epilepsy.

OSA in Adults with Epilepsy Often Mild

Using clinical assessment, OSA (AHI $\geq$5) was found in 10% of 283 unselected adults with epilepsy; however, the degree of sleep-disordered breathing (SDB) was mild (AHI 5 to <14) in 67%, moderate (15 to <30) in 22%, and severe ($\geq$30) in only 11%.[46] Using overnight PSG and comparing it with the Sleep Apnea-Sleep Disorders Questionnaire (SA-SDQ), another study found OSA (AHI >5) in 45% of 125 unselected adults with epilepsy.[51] These investigators validated the use of the SA-SDQ: a score of more than 29 on it provided a sensitivity of 75% and a specificity of 65% in men, and 80% and 67%, respectively, in women with epilepsy.

OSA More Likely to be Found in Adults with Medically Refractory, Late-onset, or Worsening Epilepsy

Three recent studies suggest that OSA is more likely to be found in adults with epilepsy who are older, heavier, male, or have late-onset, medically refractory, or worsening epilepsy.[20,46,47] In the first of these groups, OSA was more likely to be found on PSG in adults with epilepsy who were male (15.4% men, 5.4% women), older (46 $\pm$ 15 vs 33 $\pm$ 12 years), sleepier (23% vs 9%), heavier (28.5 $\pm$ 3.6 vs 23.3 $\pm$ 3.7 kg/m^2), and had experienced their first seizure at an older age (32 vs 19 years).[46]

A recent, prospective study compared the prevalence of OSA by PSG in 11 adults with late-onset or worsening seizures with 10 who were seizure free or had improving seizure control at or after the age of 50 years.[20] The group with late-onset or worsening seizures had higher AHI and higher scores on the SA-SDQ and ESS than the group with better-controlled epilepsy. The 2 groups were similar in age, body mass index (BMI, calculated as weight in kilograms divided by the square of height in meters), neck circumference, number of prescribed AEDs, and frequency of nocturnal seizures. The investigators concluded that OSA in older adults is associated with seizure exacerbation in some cases. A retrospective chart review found that the appearance of OSA symptoms in 21 of 29 older adults (median age 56 years, 86% men) coincided with a clear increase in seizure frequency or the first episode of status epilepticus.[47]

OSA (respiratory disturbance index >5) was found in 33% of 39 unselected consecutive adults with medically refractory epilepsy (59% of the men, 19% of the women).[52] Individuals with OSA were more likely to be older, male, have a higher SA-SDQ score, and more likely to have seizures during sleep than those without OSA.[52] A prospective pilot study found OSA (AHI >10) in 46% of 13 adults with refractory epilepsy.[48] Larger prospective studies are needed to confirm these findings.

PLMS and RLS in Adults with Epilepsy

PLMS are common and often nonspecific in adults who do not endorse symptoms of RLS, RBD, narcolepsy with cataplexy, or take psychotropic medications. A few studies have reported PLMS in PSG in adults or children with epilepsy. Sleep studies were most often performed for sleep complaints suggestive of OSA and less often for limb jerking or RLS. In 1 study, complaints of RLS were not more prevalent in adults with epilepsy than healthy controls (18% vs 12%) but RLS was ascertained using a single question.[12]

In a second study involving 158 adults with epilepsy, 35% endorsed symptoms of RLS, but so did 29% of controls with other neurologic disorders.[23] These investigators recorded PSG in 27 of the 42 adults with epilepsy who complained of RLS and found PLMS arousal indexes greater than 10 in only 15%. Another retrospective study by the same group recorded PSG in 63 adults with epilepsy with sleep complaints and found a PLMS index (PLMI) 20 or greater in 17% (45% of whom had PLMI >30).[53] However, most of the PLMS did not cause arousal or need treatment.

RBD Occasionally Found in Older Adults with Epilepsy

Two case series have reported RBD coexisting with epilepsy in older adults. The first described 2 men (ages 60 and 75 years) who developed late-onset sleep-related motor convulsions and who also had symptoms and PSG findings of RBD. RBD preceded the onset of epilepsy by 5 to 10 years.[54] A prospective study found RBD in 10 (12.5%) of 80 older adults (mean age 71 ± 7 years, 47 men) with epilepsy.[55] RBD episodes preceded seizure onset by 4.5 years in 6 individuals and followed it by 9.7 years in 4.

Given the prevalence of OSA in late-onset or worsening epilepsy, RBD needs to be distinguished from pseudo-RBD caused by severe OSA. The term pseudo-RBD was coined by investigators of a study involving 16 adults with severe OSA (mean AHI 68 ± 19) who were believed likely to have RBD because they complained of dream-enacting behaviors and unpleasant dreams.[56] However, skeletal atonia was preserved during REM sleep and continuous positive airway pressure (CPAP) therapy eliminated the abnormal behaviors, unpleasant dreams, daytime sleepiness, and snoring.

QUESTIONNAIRE-BASED STUDIES ON THE PREVALENCE OF SLEEP DISORDERS IN CHILDREN WITH EPILEPSY

Like adults with epilepsy, children with it are more likely to have sleep problems than the general pediatric population.[1–10] Sleep disruption in children with epilepsy is more likely multifactorial, including varying combinations of epilepsy per se, frequent nocturnal seizures disrupting nocturnal sleep organization, effects of AEDs on daytime alertness and nighttime sleep, and treatable primary sleep disorders. Comorbidities such as physical disability,[8] intellectual disability,[2,57,58] neurodevelopmental syndromes,[59,60] autism spectrum disorder,[61] and behavioral disorders[1,7–9,62] may add to the likelihood of sleep disorders in a child with epilepsy.

Sleep complaints in children with epilepsy are rarely reported by patients and caretakers and often misdiagnosed.[63] A case-control parental report study of 43 children with idiopathic benign rolandic epilepsy (ages 6–16 years) found that those with epilepsy had significantly shorter sleep duration and more frequent parasomnias and daytime sleepiness than the controls.[5]

In a prospective study evaluating the prevalence of sleep problems in children with epilepsy, sleep and daytime behavior problems were more common in children with epilepsy than their siblings or healthy age-matched controls.[1] Using post hoc comparisons, 89 children with idiopathic partial or generalized epilepsy had significantly more parasomnias, bedtime difficulties, sleep fragmentation, and daytime drowsiness than their 49 siblings or 321 healthy controls. Using multiple regression analysis, sleep complaints, longer sleep latencies, and shorter sleep times were more likely in children with poor seizure control. Daytime seizures and high nighttime IED discharge rates predicted daytime drowsiness. The presence of behavior problems (inattention, hyperactivity, impulsivity, oppositional defiant disorder) greatly increased the likelihood that sleep problems would be reported in children with epilepsy. Three variables significantly associated with greater sleep problems in these otherwise normal children with epilepsy were length of freedom from seizure, age, and higher rates of IEDs during sleep. The investigators concluded that the presence of epilepsy in a highly selected sample of children (without other comorbidities and whose epilepsy was more often well controlled) was still associated with sleep, behavior, and adjustment problems beyond those seen in their siblings or healthy controls.

A case-control study found that children with epilepsy (n = 79, mean age 10.1 ± 3.1 years) had a mean of 4 ± 3 sleep problems compared with 2 ± 2 in 73 controls matched for age and gender (P<.001).[7] Reports of frequent unsound sleep, snoring, daytime hyperactivity, sudden daytime sleep attacks, limb movements during sleep, and bedtime refusal were more common in children with epilepsy. Mean scores for SDB symptoms were 2 times higher among the children with epilepsy compared with controls (10.5 vs 5.0). Other questionnaire-based studies have found that: (1) symptoms of OSA were 15 times more likely to be reported by the parents of 26 children with epilepsy (mean age 14.6 years) than among an equal number of healthy controls (65% vs 4%)[6]; (2) children with epilepsy compared with control individuals had more daytime sleepiness, less on-task behavior, and less attention[58]; and

(3) children with benign rolandic epilepsy had significantly shorter sleep duration, more frequent parasomnias, and daytime sleepiness than a reference sample of children.[5]

Poor sleep hygiene may also contribute to sleep problems in children with epilepsy. In a prospective study evaluating sleep habits, 121 children with epilepsy were compared with a similar number of healthy Brazilian schoolchildren.[2] Compared with controls, children with epilepsy were more likely to need to be put to bed by their parents, have an afternoon nap, wake during the night, take more than 30 minutes to fall asleep, express fear of the dark, awake with a distressing dream or worry, call out for the parent during the night, or visit the parental bed. Poor seizure control was associated with poorer sleep habits. Compared with the children whose seizures usually occurred when awake, those whose seizures were primarily nocturnal (47%) had significantly more sleep problems. Parental fear and anxiety about seizure recurrence often result in a return to cosleeping in families of children with epilepsy. One study found that 22% of 179 children with epilepsy changed to less independent sleep arrangements after epilepsy onset compared with 8% of 155 children with juvenile diabetes.[10] Cosleeping reduces risk for sudden unexpected death in epilepsy.[64]

IS SLEEP ARCHITECTURE ABNORMAL IN CHILDREN WITH EPILEPSY?

Five case-control studies[35,40,65–67] and 6 case series[62,68–71] have evaluated sleep architecture in children with epilepsy. One case-control study compared 40 children with epilepsy referred for various sleep complaints with 11 children who had moderate OSA (AHI 5–10).[65] These investigators found that the children whose seizures were poorly controlled had significantly lower sleep efficiency, higher arousal indices, and higher REM sleep time compared with children with OSA or those whose epilepsy was controlled. Sleep studies were normal in only 8% of the children with epilepsy and sleep/wake complaints.

A case-control PSG study recording 2 nights of video-PSG with 24-channel EEG in 17 children with partial epilepsy and 11 controls found that children with seizures during PSG had significantly more stage shifts, and less time in bed and sleep time.[66] Other case-control studies report: (1) significantly more NREM 1 and longer REM sleep latency in 11 children with well-controlled PGE than 8 healthy controls[67]; (2) reduced TST, sleep efficiency, and percent REM sleep in 10 children with benign rolandic epilepsy compared with normal controls[35]; (3) reduced sleep efficiency, TST, and

stage 4 sleep in 10 patients with idiopathic generalized epilepsy (most had absence) compared with 10 with idiopathic focal epilepsy and 12 controls[72]; (4) abnormalities in sleep spindles in 15 children with primary generalized epilepsies (9 untreated, 6 treated) and 47 healthy controls.[73] Two other studies[43,74] found no abnormalities in sleep architecture in children with absence seizures.

Abnormal sleep architecture has also been reported in children with epilepsy and other neurodevelopmental disorders. Girls with Rett syndrome (RS) often have epilepsy and severe sleep problems. A study of 202 girls with RS found that more than 80% had sleep problems, and these are more often severe and persistent.[75] Sleep problems in girls with RS include nocturnal laughter (59%), bruxism (55%), long spells of screaming (36%), nocturnal seizures (26%), sleep terrors (18%), and sleep talking (18%). Nocturnal seizures peaked between ages 13 and 17 years, and nocturnal screaming decreased to 30% in those older than 18 years. Frequent nighttime awakenings occurred in 54% up to age 7 years, decreasing to 40% by age 18 years. Compared with age-matched controls, girls with RS did not show the age-related decrease in TST. They also continued to nap during the day: 75% of those 8 years and older took daytime naps and 85% of the over-18-year-olds. Because of their often severe and persistent sleep/wake complaints, girls with RS are often referred to pediatric sleep specialists to determine the cause of abnormal nighttime behaviors. Reduced REM, NREM 2, and NREM 3 sleep time compared with normal controls in 10 children with Lennox-Gastaut syndrome (a medically refractory epilepsy that begins in early childhood with multiple seizure types and intellectual disability).[37]

PREVALENCE OF SLEEP APNEA AND OTHER PRIMARY SLEEP DISORDERS ON SLEEP STUDIES IN CHILDREN WITH EPILEPSY

A retrospective analysis compared PSG findings in 40 children with epilepsy referred for symptoms suggestive of OSA with 11 children with moderate uncomplicated OSA (AHI 5–10).[65] Polysomnographic abnormalities in the children with epilepsy were OSA (AHI >1) in 20%, obstructive hypoventilation in 33%, upper airway resistance syndrome in 8%, primary snoring in 18%, and PLMS in 10%. Children with epilepsy and OSA had significantly higher BMI (29 vs 2), were more often obese (BMI >95th percentile 62% vs 18%), had longer sleep latency (51 vs 16 minutes), higher arousal indices (49 vs 21), and lower nadir SpO_2 (86% vs 90%) despite having a lower mean AHI (3) compared with the nonepilepsy OSA group (7/h). Children with poor seizure control had significantly lower sleep efficiency, higher arousal indices, and a higher percentage of REM sleep compared with children who were seizure free or showed good seizure control. Another study of 30 children with epilepsy recruited for symptoms of OSA found varying degrees of OSA in 80% (AHI $\geq$1.5, mean AHI 8 $\pm$ 9).[62] The mean duration of respiratory events was significantly longer in children with more frequent epileptic seizures.

Several PSG studies have been published screening for OSA and other sleep disorders in children with epilepsy and comorbid neurologic or neurodevelopmental disorders. In a study comparing PSG findings in 11 Italian children with mental retardation and epilepsy (mean age 13 $\pm$ 4 years) and 11 healthy controls without sleep/wake complaints, children with epilepsy had a mean AHI of 5 $\pm$ 3, but only 3 had an AHI greater than 5 (AHI 9–11), and 27% had a PLMI greater than 5.[40] Compared with controls, children with epilepsy had longer sleep latency, higher percentage of WASO and NREM 3 sleep, lower sleep efficiency, more awakenings and stage shifts, higher CAP rate, increased A1 index, and long and less numerous CAP sequences.

In a PSG study involving 10 children (mean age 11 years) with TSC and 10 healthy controls, reduced sleep efficiency (60%–88%) was found in 9 and WASO greater than 10% in 7 TSC children.[76] Frequent nocturnal awakenings occurred in 6 and poorly organized sleep cycles in 3 cases. Compared with controls, the TSC group showed shorter sleep time, lower sleep efficiency, higher number of awakenings and stage shifts, increased NREM 1 and WASO, and decreased REM sleep. Sleep was significantly more disrupted in the 3 children with TSC who had seizures the night of the PSG (sleep efficiency 69%, WASO 24%, mean awakenings 16/h) compared with the TSC children, who did not (sleep efficiency 88%, WASO 5%, and mean awakenings 3/h).

Although girls with RS have peculiar patterns of hyperventilation and apnea awake, they usually do not have OSA. Sleep architecture, sleep efficiency, and breathing were normal in 30 girls with RS (median age 7 years) and age-matched controls.[77] The investigators emphasized that unless there are clinical symptoms suggestive of SDB (such as scoliosis, present in 65% of patients), the diagnostic yield of PSG is low in patients with RS.[77] A particular EEG pattern of rhythmical theta (4–6 Hz) activity over the central regions during NREM sleep often accompanied by central spikes is characteristic of RS.[78] Patients with RS have a higher incidence of sudden unexplained death

(often during sleep) compared with age-matched controls, which may reflect their loss of heart rate variability and impaired cardiac autonomic regulation.[79]

ARE PARASOMNIAS MORE COMMON IN PEOPLE WITH EPILEPSY?

A prospective case-control study found a higher incidence of parasomnias among 89 children with idiopathic epilepsy compared with 49 siblings and 321 healthy control children using parental sleep questionnaires.[1] Parasomnias were not more common in a prospective study of adults with a wide variety of epilepsies and seizure types compared with healthy controls.[12] Sixty percent of adults with epilepsy and 58% of controls complained of at least 1 parasomnia, most often nocturnal leg cramps (25% vs 17%), sleep starts (22% vs 17%), and sleep talking (21% vs 16%). Reports of sleep hallucinations, sleep paralysis, and violent acts during sleep occurred with equal frequency in patients and controls (16%, 4% and 2%, respectively), as were shouting out when sleeping (4% vs 3%). Nightmares and sleep-related bruxism were significantly more common in control individuals (16% vs 6%, and 19% vs 10%, respectively). None of their study individuals reported sleepwalking or bedwetting.

However, NREM arousal disorders (such as sleepwalking, sleep terrors, and confusional arousals) and sleep-related bruxism are significantly more common in patients and their relatives with NFLE.[80] An individual with NFLE has a 6-fold greater lifetime risk for disorders of arousal and 5-fold for sleep-related bruxism compared with controls. The lifetime prevalence of an arousal disorder in relatives of patients with NFLE was 4.7 times greater and nightmares 2.6 times greater compared with relatives of control subjects. As discussed elsewhere in this issue by Guido Rubboli, this situation may be a result of the shared expression of central pattern generators.

DIAGNOSTIC AND TECHNICAL CONSIDERATIONS WHEN PERFORMING SLEEP STUDIES IN PEOPLE WITH EPILEPSY

Comprehensive video-PSG is most often performed in people with epilepsy for suspected OSA or to identify primary sleep disorders contributing to complaints of EDS. Sometimes, sleep clinicians are asked to determine the etiology of paroxysmal nocturnal events (PNEs). The AASM clinical practice parameters recommend in-laboratory video-PSG in the evaluation of parasomnias that are unusual or atypical because of the patient's age at onset; the time, duration, or frequency of occurrence of the behavior; or the specifics of the particular motor patterns in question (eg, stereotypical, repetitive, or focal).[81]

PSG is not needed if the nocturnal behavior events are typical, noninjurious, infrequent, and not disruptive to the child or family.[81] However, in children with sleep terrors or sleepwalking events occurring more than 2 to 3 times per week (and symptoms suggestive of OSA or PLMS), PSG should be considered. Obstructive SDB was found in 58% of 84 children with frequent arousal parasomnias[82]; tonsillectomy eliminated OSA and arousals. A detailed discussion of the differentiation of seizures and other types of PNEs can be found elsewhere.

If sleep-related epilepsy is suspected in patients with PNEs and no known diagnosis of epilepsy, EEG with sleep is recommended. If nocturnal events occur only at night and are frequent, video-PSG with expanded EEG before prolonged inpatient video-EEG monitoring may be appropriate, especially if concomitant OSA or RBD is suspected. If the first (or second with 24 hours of sleep deprivation) routine EEG with sleep is normal and the clinical suspicion for a sleep-related epilepsy remains, long-term video-EEG monitoring is recommended. **Table 2** summarizes studies evaluating the diagnostic yield of IEDs with clinical neurophysiology tests in children with sleep-related seizures.

Is One Night of PSG Sufficient to Confirm or Exclude OSA in People with Epilepsy?

Usually 1 night of PSG is sufficient to confirm OSA in people with epilepsy. Two studies have evaluated first-night effects, recording 2 consecutive nights of comprehensive in-laboratory PSG in adults with epilepsy. One study found the only significant difference in sleep architecture was increased NREM 3 time and percent on the second night in 53 adults with medically refractory epilepsies.[92] Another study compared median AHI recording on 2 consecutive nights of PSG in 29 adults with epilepsy and OSA (AHI >5).[93] These investigators found that (1) time spent in REM and NREM 3, and the percent time in REM sleep was greater on night 2; (2) median difference in AHI between nights 1 and 2 was 3.25; and (3) the first PSG confirmed (or excluded) OSA (AHI $\geq$5) in all but 1 patient.

Table 2
Likelihood of detecting interictal epileptiform discharges on a clinical neurophysiology test in children

Clinical Test	Diagnostic Yield
Routine EEG recording 20–30 min	IEDs found on initial EEG in 37% of children with definite epilepsy, and 13% suspected epilepsy (n = 534)[83]; Initial EEG normal in 50% of children with clinically diagnosed epilepsy[84,85]
Routine EEG with video recording 25–30 min	Diagnosis determined in 45% referred for frequent paroxysmal events; 55% in the developmentally challenged[86] Confirmed staring spells, tics, stereotypias, tremor, paroxysmal eye movements, breath holding, or cyanotic spells[86]
Sleep-deprived EEG	Sleep deprivation increased likelihood NREM sleep observed NREM sleep observed in 57% of sleep-deprived, 44% partially sleep-deprived, and 21% nonsleep-deprived (n = 820 pediatric EEGs)[87] No increase in odds ratio of finding IEDs whether sleep occurred, partial or total sleep deprivation[87] Need to test 11 children with sleep-deprived EEG to identify 1 additional child with IEDs[87]
Overnight diagnostic video-PSG	35% have event recorded during 1 night of PSG, often need 2 nights to confirm diagnosis 41% of patients referred for minor events, 78% of 36 patients with known epilepsy
Daytime video-EEG recording for 4–8 h	80% diagnostic yield if spells occur daily (n = 230)[88] Best reserved for children whose events occur daily[88,89]
Long-term video-EEG monitoring for 2–5 d	45%–80% of patients who have $\geq$1 event per wk[88,90,91] Diagnostic in 53%, confirming epilepsy in 34%; nonepileptic behaviors in 96%[91] Likelihood of capturing an event was greater if a patient had an event frequency of at least 1 per wk

Recognizing the Effects of Vagal Nerve Stimulation on Respiration During Sleep

Vagal nerve stimulation (VNS, a treatment of medically refractory epilepsy) often alters the rate and amplitude of breathing when it activates during sleep. Numerous small case series describe this effect. Decreases in airflow and respiratory effort (and rarely frank obstructive events) are observed during the period of stimulation. These findings have been observed in adults[94–96] and children.[68,70,97–101] Most often, the respiratory change is an increase in the respiratory rate and decrease in respiratory amplitude when the device fires, which usually does not cause an arousal or desaturation.

Studies of the effects of VNS in children with epilepsy[97,98,100,101] describe: (1) the respiratory effort and tidal volume decrease when the VNS activates, which usually causes an increase in the respiratory rate, rarely a decrease, but no arousal or desaturation[97]; (2) the reductions in the amplitude of the respiratory effort were most pronounced in the first 15 seconds (maximal decrease 47% ± 17%) although it persisted throughout in a few[100]; (3) a rebound increase in respiratory amplitude is sometimes seen after the activation[100]; (4) the effects are often more pronounced during NREM sleep compared with REM sleep[100]; and (6) greater than 1% decreases in arterial oxygen saturation have been observed in a few children beginning 10 seconds after it fires, resolving quickly. Frank obstructive events with significant desaturation are uncommon. When this situations is observed, consider reducing the VNS signal frequency, which may lessen the effect. This strategy often suppresses the effect of VNS on respiration. The effects of VNS on breathing in sleep do not usually warrant its removal.

CLINICAL IMPACT OF TREATING SLEEP DISORDERS IN PEOPLE WITH EPILEPSY

A paucity of studies have examined the effects of treating primary sleep disorders on seizure control in people with epilepsy. Large prospective trials of the impact of treating primary sleep disorders in people with epilepsy are needed.

Treating OSA in People with Epilepsy

One prospective study examined the effects of treating OSA with CPAP in adults with medically refractory epilepsy.[102] Investigators found seizures were reduced 50% or more compared with their baseline in 28% of patients treated with CPAP versus 15% treated with sham CPAP, although the study was not powered to detect significant differences between groups.[102] Seven other small retrospective case series reported that CPAP improved epilepsy control in some (but not all) cases.[20,47,103–107]

In 1 study,[47] CPAP in 12 adults with epilepsy led to a significant reduction in EDS and seizure frequency in 4. In another study,[104] 3 of 10 adults with epilepsy became seizure free after their OSA was treated; 1 had a greater than 95% reduction in seizure frequency and 3 others greater than 50% (2 with positional therapy to avoid sleep supine and 8 with CPAP). In a third study,[103] 4 patients with medically refractory epilepsy had a greater than 50% reduction in their seizure frequency after CPAP use for 6 to 24 months, and AEDs were discontinued in 2 cases. In a study investigating the impact of OSA therapy on spike rate in 6 patients with epilepsy with OSA treated with CPAP, and 2 treated with supplemental oxygen for snoring and chronic obstructive pulmonary disease, reduced interictal spiking during sleep was observed, especially those who had high spike rates before treatment.[106] Another study[48] found a 45% or greater reduction in seizure frequency in 3 of 6 adults with epilepsy who used CPAP, and 60% or greater in 1 of 3 children who tolerated it. Compliant use of CPAP for 6 months or longer reduced seizure frequency by more than 150% in a retrospective study of 41 adults with OSA and epilepsy who had no change in their AEDs.[107] Seizure frequency decreased from 1.8 to 1 per month in the CPAP adherent group, whereas seizure frequency was 2.1 per month at baseline and 1.8 per month at follow-up in the group who were not adherent.

Melatonin to Treat Sleep Disorders in Children with Epilepsy

Alterations in the circadian secretion of melatonin and lower nocturnal melatonin levels have been reported in children with epilepsy, especially those with medically resistant seizures.[108,109] Melatonin may have anticonvulsant effects, shown in several animal models of epilepsy.[4,89,110–120] Mechanisms by which melatonin may improve seizure control include its ability to reduce the electrical activity of neurons secreting glutamate (the primary central nervous system [CNS] excitatory neurotransmitter) while enhancing neuronal release of neurons that secrete γ-aminobutyric acid (the primary CNS inhibitory neurotransmitter). Moreover, melatonin is metabolized to kynurenic acid (an endogenous anticonvulsant). Melatonin and its metabolites may have neuroprotective effects in that they can act as a free radical scavenger and antioxidant. However, relatively high doses of melatonin are needed to inhibit experimental seizures, and such doses are more likely to produce undesirable adverse effects of decreased body temperature, and even cognitive and motor impairment.

Four randomized double-blind, placebo-controlled studies of bedtime oral melatonin in children with epilepsy have shown positive effects on sleep.[4,112,121,122] These studies found that: (1) oral melatonin improved sleep latency and quality and reduced parasomnias by a mean of 60% in 31 children with epilepsy (ages 3–12 years)[121]; (2) nightly oral melatonin in 23 children with medically refractory epilepsy resulted in significant improvements in bedtime resistance, sleep duration, sleep latency, nocturnal arousals, sleepwalking, nocturnal enuresis, daytime sleepiness, and even seizure frequency[4]; (3) nightly use of oral melatonin (3 mg increased weekly to 9 mg as needed) in 25 children with epilepsy, mental retardation, and sleep/wake disorders (mean age 10.5 years) resulted in significant subjective improvements in sleep[122]; and (4) there were significantly fewer nocturnal awakenings and better control of convulsions in 10 children with severe medically intractable epilepsy given 3 mg of oral melatonin before bed nightly for 3 months followed by placebo for 3 months.[112] In humans, melatonin has relatively low toxicity, rare reports of nightmares, hypotension, and daytime sleepiness.

SUMMARY

The relationship between sleep and epilepsy is a fruitful and rewarding area for research. More research and knowledge are needed to better understand: (1) why is sleep macroarchitecture and microarchitecture altered in patients with epilepsy; (2) whether treating primary sleep disorders in patients with epilepsy improves seizure control; (3) the influence of circadian rhythms and chronotypes on different epilepsy syndromes; and (4) whether frequent IEDs during sleep with few or no seizures should be treated. A better understanding of the link between particular epilepsies, nonepileptic parasomnias, sleep fragmentation, and arousals is needed to optimize quality of life in patients with epilepsy.

REFERENCES

1. Cortesi F, Giannotti F, Ottaviano S. Sleep problems and daytime behavior in childhood idiopathic epilepsy. Epilepsia 1999;40(11):1557–65.

2. Batista BH, Nunes ML. Evaluation of sleep habits in children with epilepsy. Epilepsy Behav 2007;11(1): 60–4.

3. Ong LC, Yang WW, Wong SW, et al. Sleep habits and disturbances in Malaysian children with epilepsy. J Paediatr Child Health 2010;46(3): 80–4.

4. Elkhayat HA, Hassanein SM, Tomoum HY, et al. Melatonin and sleep-related problems in children with intractable epilepsy. Pediatr Neurol 2010; 42(4):249–54.

5. Tang SS, Clarke T, Owens J, et al. Sleep behavior disturbances in rolandic epilepsy. J Child Neurol 2011;26(2):239–43.

6. Maganti R, Hausman N, Koehn M, et al. Excessive daytime sleepiness and sleep complaints among children with epilepsy. Epilepsy Behav 2006;8(1): 272–7.

7. Stores G, Wiggs L, Campling G. Sleep disorders and their relationship to psychological disturbance in children with epilepsy. Child Care Health Dev 1998;24(1):5–19.

8. Wirrell E, Blackman M, Barlow K, et al. Sleep disturbances in children with epilepsy compared with their nearest-aged siblings. Dev Med Child Neurol 2005;47(11):754–9.

9. Byars AW, Byars KC, Johnson CS, et al. The relationship between sleep problems and neuropsychological functioning in children with first recognized seizures. Epilepsy Behav 2008;13(4):607–13.

10. Williams J, Lange B, Sharp G, et al. Altered sleeping arrangements in pediatric patients with epilepsy. Clin Pediatr (Phila) 2000;39(11):635–42.

11. de Weerd A, de Haas S, Otte A, et al. Subjective sleep disturbance in patients with partial epilepsy: a questionnaire-based study on prevalence and impact on quality of life. Epilepsia 2004;45(11): 1397–404.

12. Khatami R, Zutter D, Siegel A, et al. Sleep-wake habits and disorders in a series of 100 adult epilepsy patients–a prospective study. Seizure 2006;15(5): 299–306.

13. Piperidou C, Karlovasitou A, Triantafyllou N, et al. Influence of sleep disturbance on quality of life of patients with epilepsy. Seizure 2008;17(7): 588–94.

14. Jenssen S, Gracely E, Mahmood T, et al. Subjective somnolence relates mainly to depression among patients in a tertiary care epilepsy center. Epilepsy Behav 2006;9(4):632–5.

15. Xu X, Brandenburg NA, McDermott AM, et al. Sleep disturbances reported by refractory partial-onset epilepsy patients receiving polytherapy. Epilepsia 2006;47(7):1176–83.

16. Manni R, Tartara A. Evaluation of sleepiness in epilepsy. Clin Neurophysiol 2000;111(Suppl 2): S111–4.

17. Chan S, Baldeweg T, Cross JH. A role for sleep disruption in cognitive impairment in children with epilepsy. Epilepsy Behav 2011;20(3): 435–40.

18. Parisi P, Bruni O, Pia Villa M, et al. The relationship between sleep and epilepsy: the effect on cognitive functioning in children. Dev Med Child Neurol 2010; 52(9):805–10.

19. Manni R, Terzaghi M. Comorbidity between epilepsy and sleep disorders. Epilepsy Res 2010; 90(3):171–7.

20. Chihorek AM, Abou-Khalil B, Malow BA. Obstructive sleep apnea is associated with seizure occurrence in older adults with epilepsy. Neurology 2007;69(19):1823–7.

21. Haut SR, Katz M, Masur J, et al. Seizures in the elderly: impact on mental status, mood, and sleep. Epilepsy Behav 2009;14(3):540–4.

22. Manni R, Politini L, Sartori I, et al. Daytime sleepiness in epilepsy patients: evaluation by means of the Epworth sleepiness scale. J Neurol 2000; 247(9):716–7.

23. Malow BA, Bowes RJ, Lin X. Predictors of sleepiness in epilepsy patients. Sleep 1997;20(12): 1105–10.

24. Vignatelli L, Bisulli F, Naldi I, et al. Excessive daytime sleepiness and subjective sleep quality in patients with nocturnal frontal lobe epilepsy: a case-control study. Epilepsia 2006;47(Suppl 5):73–7.

25. Soldatos CR, Allaert FA, Ohta T, et al. How do individuals sleep around the world? Results from a single-day survey in ten countries. Sleep Med 2005;6(1):5–13.

26. van Eeghen AM, Numis AI, Staley BA, et al. Characterizing sleep disorders of adults with tuberous sclerosis complex: a questionnaire-based study and review. Epilepsy Behav 2011;20(1):68–74.

27. Stefanello S, Marin-Leon L, Fernandes PT, et al. Depression and anxiety in a community sample with epilepsy in Brazil. Arq Neuropsiquiatr 2011; 69(2B):342–8.

28. Giorelli AS, Neves GS, Venturi M, et al. Excessive daytime sleepiness in patients with epilepsy: a subjective evaluation. Epilepsy Behav 2011; 21(4):449–52.

29. Kobau R, DiIorio C. Epilepsy self-management: a comparison of self-efficacy and outcome expectancy for medication adherence and lifestyle behaviors among people with epilepsy. Epilepsy Behav 2003;4(3):217–25.

30. Manni R, Galimberti CA, Zucca C, et al. Sleep patterns in patients with late onset partial epilepsy receiving chronic carbamazepine (CBZ) therapy. Epilepsy Res 1990;7(1):72–6.

31. Touchon J, Baldy-Moulinier M, Billiard M, et al. Sleep organization and epilepsy. Epilepsy Res Suppl 1991;2:73–81.

32. Bazil CW, Castro LH, Walczak TS. Reduction of rapid eye movement sleep by diurnal and nocturnal seizures in temporal lobe epilepsy. Arch Neurol 2000;57(3):363–8.

33. Montplaisir J, Laverdiere M, Saint-Hilaire JM, et al. Nocturnal sleep recording in partial epilepsy: a study with depth electrodes. J Clin Neurophysiol 1987;4(4):383–8.

34. Crespel A, Baldy-Moulinier M, Coubes P. The relationship between sleep and epilepsy in frontal and temporal lobe epilepsies: practical and physiopathologic considerations. Epilepsia 1998;39(2): 150–7.

35. Bruni O, Novelli L, Luchetti A, et al. Reduced NREM sleep instability in benign childhood epilepsy with centro-temporal spikes. Clin Neurophysiol 2010; 121(5):665–71.

36. De Gennaro L, Ferrara M, Spadini V, et al. The cyclic alternating pattern decreases as a consequence of total sleep deprivation and correlates with EEG arousals. Neuropsychobiology 2002; 45(2):95–8.

37. Eisensehr I, Parrino L, Noachtar S, et al. Sleep in Lennox-Gastaut syndrome: the role of the cyclic alternating pattern (CAP) in the gate control of clinical seizures and generalized polyspikes. Epilepsy Res 2001;46(3):241–50.

38. Gigli GL, Calia E, Marciani MG, et al. Sleep microstructure and EEG epileptiform activity in patients with juvenile myoclonic epilepsy. Epilepsia 1992; 33(5):799–804.

39. Manni R, Zambrelli E, Bellazzi R, et al. The relationship between focal seizures and sleep: an analysis of the cyclic alternating pattern. Epilepsy Res 2005;67(1–2):73–80.

40. Miano S, Bruni O, Arico D, et al. Polysomnographic assessment of sleep disturbances in children with developmental disabilities and seizures. Neurol Sci 2010;31(5):575–83.

41. Parrino L, Halasz P, Tassinari CA, et al. CAP, epilepsy and motor events during sleep: the unifying role of arousal. Sleep Med Rev 2006; 10(4):267–85.

42. Parrino L, Smerieri A, Spaggiari MC, et al. Cyclic alternating pattern (CAP) and epilepsy during sleep: how a physiological rhythm modulates a pathological event. Clin Neurophysiol 2000;111(Suppl 2):S39–46.

43. Terzano MG, Parrino L, Anelli S, et al. Effects of generalized interictal EEG discharges on sleep stability: assessment by means of cyclic alternating pattern. Epilepsia 1992;33(2):317–26.

44. Terzano MG, Parrino L, Garofalo PG, et al. Activation of partial seizures with motor signs during cyclic alternating pattern in human sleep. Epilepsy Res 1991;10(2–3):166–73.

45. Zucconi M, Oldani A, Smirne S, et al. The macrostructure and microstructure of sleep in patients

with autosomal dominant nocturnal frontal lobe epilepsy. J Clin Neurophysiol 2000;17(1):77–86.

46. Manni R, Terzaghi M, Arbasino C, et al. Obstructive sleep apnea in a clinical series of adult epilepsy patients: frequency and features of the comorbidity. Epilepsia 2003;44(6):836–40.

47. Hollinger P, Khatami R, Gugger M, et al. Epilepsy and obstructive sleep apnea. Eur Neurol 2006; 55(2):74–9.

48. Malow BA, Weatherwax KJ, Chervin RD, et al. Identification and treatment of obstructive sleep apnea in adults and children with epilepsy: a prospective pilot study. Sleep Med 2003;4(6): 509–15.

49. Young T, Palta M, Dempsey J, et al. The occurrence of sleep-disordered breathing among middle-aged adults. N Engl J Med 1993;328(17):1230–5.

50. Young T, Peppard P, Palta M, et al. Population-based study of sleep-disordered breathing as a risk factor for hypertension. Arch Intern Med 1997;157(15):1746–52.

51. Weatherwax KJ, Lin X, Marzec ML, et al. Obstructive sleep apnea in epilepsy patients: the Sleep Apnea scale of the Sleep Disorders Questionnaire (SA-SDQ) is a useful screening instrument for obstructive sleep apnea in a disease-specific population. Sleep Med 2003;4(6):517–21.

52. Malow BA, Levy K, Maturen K, et al. Obstructive sleep apnea is common in medically refractory epilepsy patients. Neurology 2000;55(7):1002–7.

53. Malow BA, Fromes GA, Aldrich MS. Usefulness of polysomnography in epilepsy patients. Neurology 1997;48(5):1389–94.

54. Manni R, Terzaghi M. REM behavior disorder associated with epileptic seizures. Neurology 2005; 64(5):883–4.

55. Manni R, Terzaghi M, Zambrelli E. REM sleep behaviour disorder in elderly subjects with epilepsy: frequency and clinical aspects of the comorbidity. Epilepsy Res 2007;77(2–3):128–33.

56. Iranzo A, Santamaria J. Severe obstructive sleep apnea/hypopnea mimicking REM sleep behavior disorder. Sleep 2005;28(2):203–6.

57. Didden R, Korzilius H, van Aperlo B, et al. Sleep problems and daytime problem behaviours in children with intellectual disability. J Intellect Disabil Res 2002;46(Pt 7):537–47.

58. Didden R, de Moor JM, Korzilius H. Sleepiness, on-task behavior and attention in children with epilepsy who visited a school for special education: a comparative study. Res Dev Disabil 2009; 30(6):1428–34.

59. Conant KD, Thibert RL, Thiele EA. Epilepsy and the sleep-wake patterns found in Angelman syndrome. Epilepsia 2009;50(11):2497–500.

60. Segawa M, Nomura Y. Polysomnography in the Rett syndrome. Brain Dev 1992;14(Suppl):S46–54.

61. Liu X, Hubbard JA, Fabes RA, et al. Sleep disturbances and correlates of children with autism spectrum disorders. Child Psychiatry Hum Dev 2006;37(2):179–91.

62. Becker DA, Fennell EB, Carney PR. Daytime behavior and sleep disturbance in childhood epilepsy. Epilepsy Behav 2004;5(5):708–15.

63. Nunes ML. Sleep disorders. J Pediatr (Rio J) 2002; 78(Suppl 1):S63–72 [in Portuguese].

64. Nobili L, Proserpio P, Rubboli G, et al. Sudden unexpected death in epilepsy (SUDEP) and sleep. Sleep Med Rev 2011;15(4):237–46.

65. Kaleyias J, Cruz M, Goraya JS, et al. Spectrum of polysomnographic abnormalities in children with epilepsy. Pediatr Neurol 2008;39(3):170–6.

66. Nunes ML, Ferri R, Arzimanoglou A, et al. Sleep organization in children with partial refractory epilepsy. J Child Neurol 2003;18(11):763–6.

67. Maganti R, Sheth RD, Hermann BP, et al. Sleep architecture in children with idiopathic generalized epilepsy. Epilepsia 2005;46(1):104–9.

68. Zaaimi B, Grebe R, Berquin P, et al. Vagus nerve stimulation induces changes in respiratory sinus arrhythmia of epileptic children during sleep. Epilepsia 2009;50(11):2473–80.

69. Hallbook T, Lundgren J, Rosen I. Ketogenic diet improves sleep quality in children with therapy-resistant epilepsy. Epilepsia 2007;48(1):59–65.

70. Pruvost M, Zaaimi B, Grebe R, et al. Cardiorespiratory effects induced by vagus nerve stimulation in epileptic children. Med Biol Eng Comput 2006; 44(4):338–47.

71. Koh S, Ward SL, Lin M, et al. Sleep apnea treatment improves seizure control in children with neurodevelopmental disorders. Pediatr Neurol 2000; 22(1):36–9.

72. Barreto JR, Fernandes RM, Sakamoto AC. Correlation of sleep macrostructure parameters and idiopathic epilepsies. Arq Neuropsiquiatr 2002; 60(2-B):353–7.

73. Myatchin I, Lagae L. Sleep spindle abnormalities in children with generalized spike-wave discharges. Pediatr Neurol 2007;36(2):106–11.

74. Sato S, Dreifuss FE, Penry JK. The effect of sleep on spike-wave discharges in absence seizures. Neurology 1973;23(12):1335–45.

75. Young D, Nagarajan L, de Klerk N, et al. Sleep problems in Rett syndrome. Brain Dev 2007; 29(10):609–16.

76. Bruni O, Cortesi F, Giannotti F, et al. Sleep disorders in tuberous sclerosis: a polysomnographic study. Brain Dev 1995;17(1):52–6.

77. Marcus CL, Carroll JL, McColley SA, et al. Polysomnographic characteristics of patients with Rett syndrome. J Pediatr 1994;125(2):218–24.

78. Niedermeyer E, Naidu SB, Plate C. Unusual EEG theta rhythms over central region in Rett

syndrome: considerations of the underlying dysfunction. Clin Electroencephalogr 1997;28(1): 36–43.

79. Sekul EA, Moak JP, Schultz RJ, et al. Electrocardiographic findings in Rett syndrome: an explanation for sudden death? J Pediatr 1994;125(1):80–2.

80. Bisulli F, Vignatelli L, Naldi I, et al. Increased frequency of arousal parasomnias in families with nocturnal frontal lobe epilepsy: a common mechanism? Epilepsia 2010;51(9):1852–60.

81. Kushida CA, Littner MR, Morgenthaler T, et al. Practice parameters for the indications for polysomnography and related procedures: an update for 2005. Sleep 2005;28(4):499–521.

82. Guilleminault C, Palombini L, Pelayo R, et al. Sleepwalking and sleep terrors in prepubertal children: what triggers them? Pediatrics 2003;111(1):e17–25.

83. Aydin K, Okuyaz C, Serdaroglu A, et al. Utility of electroencephalography in the evaluation of common neurologic conditions in children. J Child Neurol 2003;18(6):394–6.

84. Camfield P, Gordon K, Camfield C, et al. EEG results are rarely the same if repeated within six months in childhood epilepsy. Can J Neurol Sci 1995;22(4):297–300.

85. Gilbert DL, Gartside PS. Factors affecting the yield of pediatric EEGs in clinical practice. Clin Pediatr (Phila) 2002;41(1):25–32.

86. Watemberg N, Tziperman B, Dabby R, et al. Adding video recording increases the diagnostic yield of routine electroencephalograms in children with frequent paroxysmal events. Epilepsia 2005;46(5): 716–9.

87. Gilbert DL. Interobserver reliability of visual interpretation of electroencephalograms in children with newly diagnosed seizures. Dev Med Child Neurol 2006;48(12):1009–10 [author reply: 1010–1].

88. Chen LS, Mitchell WG, Horton EJ, et al. Clinical utility of video-EEG monitoring. Pediatr Neurol 1995;12(3):220–4.

89. Valente KD, Freitas A, Fiore LA, et al. The diagnostic role of short duration outpatient V-EEG monitoring in children. Pediatr Neurol 2003;28(4):285–91.

90. Bye AM, Kok DJ, Ferenschild FT, et al. Paroxysmal non-epileptic events in children: a retrospective study over a period of 10 years. J Paediatr Child Health 2000;36(3):244–8.

91. Mohan KK, Markand ON, Salanova V. Diagnostic utility of video EEG monitoring in paroxysmal events. Acta Neurol Scand 1996;94(5):320–5.

92. Marzec ML, Selwa LM, Malow BA. Analysis of the first night effect and sleep parameters in medically refractory epilepsy patients. Sleep Med 2005;6(3): 277–80.

93. Selwa LM, Marzec ML, Chervin RD, et al. Sleep staging and respiratory events in refractory epilepsy patients: is there a first night effect? Epilepsia 2008; 49(12):2063–8.

94. Malow BA, Edwards J, Marzec M, et al. Effects of vagus nerve stimulation on respiration during sleep: a pilot study. Neurology 2000;55(10):1450–4.

95. Marzec M, Edwards J, Sagher O, et al. Effects of vagus nerve stimulation on sleep-related breathing in epilepsy patients. Epilepsia 2003;44(7):930–5.

96. Holmes MD, Miller JW, Voipio J, et al. Vagal nerve stimulation induces intermittent hypocapnia. Epilepsia 2003;44(12):1588–91.

97. Nagarajan L, Walsh P, Gregory P, et al. Respiratory pattern changes in sleep in children on vagal nerve stimulation for refractory epilepsy. Can J Neurol Sci 2003;30(3):224–7.

98. Hsieh T, Chen M, McAfee A, et al. Sleep-related breathing disorder in children with vagal nerve stimulators. Pediatr Neurol 2008;38(2):99–103.

99. Zaaimi B, Grebe R, Berquin P, et al. Vagus nerve stimulation therapy induces changes in heart rate of children during sleep. Epilepsia 2007;48(5): 923–30.

100. Zaaimi B, Heberle C, Berquin P, et al. Vagus nerve stimulation induces concomitant respiratory alterations and a decrease in SaO2 in children. Epilepsia 2005;46(11):1802–9.

101. Khurana DS, Reumann M, Hobdell EF, et al. Vagus nerve stimulation in children with refractory epilepsy: unusual complications and relationship to sleep-disordered breathing. Childs Nerv Syst 2007;23(11):1309–12.

102. Malow BA, Foldvary-Schaefer N, Vaughn BV, et al. Treating obstructive sleep apnea in adults with epilepsy: a randomized pilot trial. Neurology 2008;71(8):572–7.

103. Beran RG, Holland GJ, Yan KY. The use of CPAP in patients with refractory epilepsy. Seizure 1997;6(4): 323–5.

104. Vaughn BV, D'Cruz OF, Beach R, et al. Improvement of epileptic seizure control with treatment of obstructive sleep apnoea. Seizure 1996;5(1):73–8.

105. Devinsky O, Ehrenberg B, Barthlen GM, et al. Epilepsy and sleep apnea syndrome. Neurology 1994;44(11):2060–4.

106. Oliveira AJ, Zamagni M, Dolso P, et al. Respiratory disorders during sleep in patients with epilepsy: effect of ventilatory therapy on EEG interictal epileptiform discharges. Clin Neurophysiol 2000; 111(Suppl 2):S141–5.

107. Vendrame M, Auerbach S, Loddenkemper T, et al. Effect of continuous positive airway pressure treatment on seizure control in patients with obstructive sleep apnea and epilepsy. Epilepsia 2011;52(11): e168–71.

108. Paprocka J, Dec R, Jamroz E, et al. Melatonin and childhood refractory epilepsy–a pilot study. Med Sci Monit 2010;16(9):CR389–96.

109. Ardura J, Andres J, Garmendia JR, et al. Melatonin in epilepsy and febrile seizures. J Child Neurol 2010;25(7):888–91.

110. Scorza FA, Colugnati DB, Arida RM, et al. Cardiovascular protective effect of melatonin in sudden unexpected death in epilepsy: a hypothesis. Med Hypotheses 2008;70(3):605–9.

111. Sanchez-Forte M, Moreno-Madrid F, Munoz-Hoyos A, et al. The effect of melatonin as anticonvulsant and neuron protector. Rev Neurol 1997;25(144):1229–34 [in Spanish].

112. Uberos J, Augustin-Morales MC, Molina Carballo A, et al. Normalization of the sleep-wake pattern and melatonin and 6-sulphatoxy-melatonin levels after a therapeutic trial with melatonin in children with severe epilepsy. J Pineal Res 2011;50(2):192–6.

113. Fenoglio-Simeone K, Mazarati A, Sefidvash-Hockley S, et al. Anticonvulsant effects of the selective melatonin receptor agonist ramelteon. Epilepsy Behav 2009;16(1):52–7.

114. Molina-Carballo A, Munoz-Hoyos A, Sanchez-Forte M, et al. Melatonin increases following convulsive seizures may be related to its anticonvulsant properties at physiological concentrations. Neuropediatrics 2007;38(3):122–5.

115. Yahyavi-Firouz-Abadi N, Tahsili-Fahadan P, Riazi K, et al. Melatonin enhances the anticonvulsant and proconvulsant effects of morphine in mice: role for nitric oxide signaling pathway. Epilepsy Res 2007;75(2–3):138–44.

116. Yildirim M, Marangoz C. Anticonvulsant effects of melatonin on penicillin-induced epileptiform activity in rats. Brain Res 2006;1099(1):183–8.

117. Yahyavi-Firouz-Abadi N, Tahsili-Fahadan P, Riazi K, et al. Involvement of nitric oxide pathway in the acute anticonvulsant effect of melatonin in mice. Epilepsy Res 2006;68(2):103–13.

118. Ray M, Mediratta PK, Reeta K, et al. Receptor mechanisms involved in the anticonvulsant effect of melatonin in maximal electroshock seizures. Methods Find Exp Clin Pharmacol 2004;26(3):177–81.

119. Mevissen M, Ebert U. Anticonvulsant effects of melatonin in amygdala-kindled rats. Neurosci Lett 1998;257(1):13–6.

120. Lapin IP, Mirzaev SM, Ryzov IV, et al. Anticonvulsant activity of melatonin against seizures induced by quinolinate, kainate, glutamate, NMDA, and pentylenetetrazole in mice. J Pineal Res 1998;24(4):215–8.

121. Gupta M, Aneja S, Kohli K. Add-on melatonin improves sleep behavior in children with epilepsy: randomized, double-blind, placebo-controlled trial. J Child Neurol 2005;20(2):112–5.

122. Coppola G, Iervolino G, Mastrosimone M, et al. Melatonin in wake-sleep disorders in children, adolescents and young adults with mental retardation with or without epilepsy: a double-blind, cross-over, placebo-controlled trial. Brain Dev 2004;26(6):373–6.

Diagnostic Yield of Sleep and Sleep Deprivation on the EEG in Epilepsy

Madeleine M. Grigg-Damberger, MD[a],*,
Nancy Foldvary-Schaefer, DO, MS[b]

KEYWORDS

- Sleep and epilepsy • Sleep deprivation
- Electroencephalogram • Polysomnogram • Lunar cycle

Sleep is the interest we have to pay on the capital which is called in at death; and the higher the rate of interest and the more regularly it is paid, the further the date of redemption is postponed.

—Arthur Schopenhauer

Sufficient sleep is highly important for optimal cognitive performance and learning.[1] Sleep deprivation is associated with impairments in sustained attention,[2] executive function,[3] learning,[4] memory,[1] glucose metabolism,[5] and appetite regulation.[6] Effects of sleep deprivation are summarized in **Box 1**. Definitions of sleep deprivation and short or insufficient sleep vary greatly.[7] In this review, total sleep deprivation (TSD) is defined as no sleep for 24 hours or more and partial sleep deprivation as up to 5 hours of sleep time within a 24-hour period. Insufficient sleep is a reduction in sleep time of a magnitude to be associated with negative outcomes.[8]

Observational and epidemiologic studies report that optimal sleep duration of 7 to 8 hours is associated with maintenance of good health.[9] The risk of death is increased by more than 15% in those who report sleeping more than 8.5 hours or less than 3.5 to 4.5 hours per night.[10] The United States has become a nation at war with sleep. Chronic sleep loss and sleep disorders are estimated to affect 70 million Americans.[11] Sleep duration of adults and adolescents in the United States has declined by 1.5 to 2 hours over the last half century.[12] From 2004 to 2006, 63% of adults in the United States usually slept 7 to 8 hours during a 24-hour period, 21% slept 6 hours, 8% less than 6 hours, and 9% 9 or more hours.[13] More than a third of adolescents averaged only 6.5 to 7 hours of sleep on school nights; their chronic sleep debt (and needs) is confirmed by sleeping 8 to 8.5 hours when allowed. Chronic short sleep (variably defined as <6 or <7 hours of sleep per 24 hours) is associated with a higher relative risk of all-cause mortality,[14] obesity,[15,16] increased risk for hypertension,[17,18] eating more fat,[19] and lower self-reported overall health[20] in young and middle-aged adults.

Certain types of seizures and epilepsy syndromes are likely to occur primarily during sleep and are particularly vulnerable to the effects of sleep deprivation. Many people with epilepsy have insufficient sleep, which can contribute to the severity of their epilepsy. Sleep deprivation can activate seizures in people with epilepsy and in a few without it. Interictal epileptiform

The authors have no conflicts of interest to declare regarding this article.
[a] Department of Neurology, University of New Mexico School of Medicine, MSC10 5620, One University of NM, Albuquerque, NM 87131-0001, USA
[b] Cleveland Clinic Lerner College of Medicine of Case Western Reserve University, Epilepsy Center, Cleveland Clinic Neurological Institute, 9500 Euclid Avenue, FA 20, Cleveland, OH 44195, USA
* Corresponding author.
E-mail address: mgriggd@salud.unm.edu

Box 1
Effects of sleep deprivation

- Impairs creative thinking and verbal fluency
- Slowed reaction times and reasoning
- More mistakes and omissions
- Difficulty memorizing new information and working memory
- Slows computational problem-solving speed
- Decreased ability to estimate performance
- Microsleeps cause lapses in attention
- Reduced ability to appreciate a complex situation while avoiding distraction
- More difficulty controlling mood and avoiding inappropriate behavior

discharges (IEDs) are also activated by sleep. Electroencephalograms (EEGs) are most often ordered to evaluate, diagnose, and manage epileptic seizures and epilepsy. The presence, type, and location of IEDs on an EEG can help characterize the type of epilepsy and location of the epileptic focus, as well as predict whether seizures are likely to recur. Sleep, particularly non–rapid eye movement (NREM) sleep, activates IEDs. In many patients with epilepsy, IEDs are often seen only during sleep. Recording sleep on an EEG (with or without sleep deprivation or sedation) can increase the likelihood that IEDs will be found. This review provides a summary of research related to these issues.

EARLY BELIEFS AND RESEARCH ON SLEEP, SLEEP DEPRIVATION, SEIZURES, EPILEPSY, AND THE MOON

Since antiquity, physicians have cautioned their patients with epilepsy to avoid sleep deprivation.[21] Hippocrates (fifth century BC) emphasized that a patient prone to epileptic seizures should "spend the day awake and the night asleep. If this habit be disturbed, it is not so good…worst of all when one sleeps neither night nor day."[22] To avoid recurrence of seizures, Soranus (second century) cautioned his patients "sleep must be undisturbed" because "on slight impulse the body repeats what it just seems to have abandoned."[23]

By late antiquity and the early Middle Ages, little distinction was made between epilepsy, sleepwalking, madness, and demonic possession. Those with such symptoms were lunatics, suffering from "diseases of the moon," and prone to attacks recurring at periodic intervals, particularly at night (descriptively called *mondsüchtig* in

German).[24] The waxing moon heated the atmosphere, melted the brain, and provoked these attacks.[24]

Physicians of the nineteenth century continued to debate the susceptibility of epileptics to the moon and its cycles. The German physician Romberg[25] (1853) argued for the planetary influence of the moon (especially the new and full phases) on epilepsy. Lunar cycles of the moon as the cause for epileptic seizures was largely laid to rest in 1854 after Moreau showed that daily seizure frequencies for more than 5 years among institutionalized epileptic patients were unrelated. However, research and speculation on the full moon as a causative factor for epileptic seizures has waxed again. Recent studies ponder whether the brightness of a full moon disturbs nighttime sleep, shortening sleep duration and quality, thus provoking seizures. Roosli and colleagues[26] (2006) found average nocturnal sleep duration was 19 minutes less and subjects felt more tired when the moon was full compared with the new moon in 31 healthy Swiss adult volunteers who kept sleep diaries for 6 weeks. Baxendale and Fisher[27] (2008) found a significant correlation between the mean number of seizures and the fullness of the moon in 1571 seizures recorded in a dedicated epilepsy inpatient unit over 341 days. However, the correlation disappeared when they controlled for the local clarity of the night sky, prompting the investigators to suggest that the brightness of the sky rather than the fullness of the moon is the pathologic factor.

Artificial nighttime light pollution and stellar visibility may lessen nocturnal sleep duration and quality.[28] Sixty percent of the world population now sleep under light-polluted skies (>90% in the United States and Europe).[28] The nighttime sky on a moonless night far from the city lights has an illuminance ranging from 1 to 5×10^{-4} lux, in contrast to 0.1 to 0.3 lux when the moon is full. Artificial lighting of the infrastructures we build lights our nighttime skies far more than a full moon. Artificial lighting of shopping centers is often 10 to 20 lux (200 times brighter than natural night illuminance). Research has shown as little as 1.5 lux can affect circadian rhythms. Even a bedroom nightlight, particularly of blue light at a wavelength of 460 nm, has been shown to reduce and delay nocturnal pineal melatonin production.

On the subject of environmental stimuli that reduce nocturnal sleep quality and duration, noise exposure should be considered.[29] Studies have shown that sleeping in a very noisy environment can lead to increases in time in bed awake, the number of awakenings, sleep stage shifts, and

NREM 1 and 2 (at the expense of NREM 3 and rapid eye movement).[29,30] Noise exposure during sleep may increase heart rate, blood pressure, and body movements.[30] The World Health Organization guidelines recommend a maximum sound level of 30 dB for continuous background noise, and 45 dB for individual noise events, to promote good sleep. Reducing nighttime noise to 35 to 45 dB (from 60 to 80 dB) and sound masking in intensive care units have been shown to lead to better outcomes and shorter hospital stays.[31]

PATIENTS WITH EPILEPSY OFTEN COMPLAIN OF INSUFFICIENT OR POOR-QUALITY NOCTURNAL SLEEP

Patients with epilepsy are much more likely to complain of insufficient or poor-quality nocturnal sleep than sex-matched and gender-matched healthy controls.[32–42] Inadequate sleep may lead patients with epilepsy to a state of chronic partial sleep deprivation. Many, but not all, studies report that sleep maintenance insomnia and excessive daytime sleepiness (EDS) occur more frequently in adults with epilepsy than in the general population.[36–40] A prospective study using a clinical interview and a standardized sleep questionnaire found 30% of 100 adults with epilepsy to report sleep complaints compared with 10% of 90 controls.[38] The adults with epilepsy were more likely to report symptoms suggestive of sleep maintenance insomnia (52% vs 38%), sleep-onset insomnia (34% vs 28%), EDS (19% vs 14%), restless legs (18% vs 12%), and sleep apnea (9% vs 3%) than were controls.[38] Similarly, sleep complaints were 2-fold higher (39% vs 18%, $P<.0001$) among 486 adults with partial (localization-related, focal) epilepsy who responded to a mailed questionnaire in comparison with controls.[36] Another prospective case series found that 25% of 124 consecutive adults with epilepsy who visited an outpatient epilepsy clinic over a 10-month period complained of insomnia and 17% complained of EDS.[39]

DIAGNOSTIC YIELD OF SLEEP DEPRIVATION AS AN ACTIVATION MANEUVER ON EEG

Whether the IED activation produced by TSD is due to sleep itself (greater amounts of sleep recorded, sampling effects) or because TSD exerts an independent activating effect has been intensely debated for more than half a century. Some have argued that TSD does not offer greater activation than sleep alone, whereas others think TSD activates IEDs independent of sleep induction.

Mattson and colleagues[43] (1965) were the first to systematically study this process. After 26 to 28 hours of wakefulness, IEDs were seen in 34% of 89 subjects who had at least 1 seizure and a normal routine EEG, 56% of 34 patients with convulsive epilepsy and IEDs on routine EEGs, and 0% of 20 patients with neurologic disorders other than epilepsy.[43] Rowan and colleagues[44] (1982) found a significantly greater IED yield after TSD compared with routine wake and drug-induced sleep EEGs; IEDs were recorded in 28% of their subjects only after TSD and activated a new epileptic focus in 7%. Degen and Degen,[45] who spent years studying the effects of sleep deprivation on IEDs, found that (1) for most seizure types, spontaneous sleep and sleep-deprived recordings produced similar activation rates; and (2) seizures were more likely to be activated by sleep or sleep deprivation in patients who had idiopathic primary generalized epilepsy rather than partial focal (localization-related) epilepsy. A prospective study of 721 subjects who had a second EEG after the first was inconclusive found a significantly greater percentage containing IEDs after TSD as compared with a second routine record (23% vs 10%).[46]

Studies in adults suggest that sleep deprivation remains an easy and cost-effective strategy to increase the likelihood of recording IEDs. Leach and colleagues[47] (2006) systematically evaluated the diagnostic yield of sleep deprivation in 85 patients. Generalized spike-wave discharges were seen in 36 patients (43%) on at least 1 EEG, and focal discharges in 15 (18%) patients. The sensitivity of sleep deprivation was 92%, 58% for drug-induced EEG and 44% for routine EEG. Among the 15 patients showing focal discharges, sleep-deprived EEG provoked abnormalities in 11 (73%) patients. Routine and drug-induced EEG produced abnormalities in 40% and 27%, respectively. Seven (47%) patients had changes seen only after sleep deprivation. Only 2 (13%) patients had IEDs only on the routine EEG, and 1 patient had IEDs only on the drug-induced sleep recording. The authors argued that sleep deprivation was an easy and inexpensive way of increasing the yield of IEDs in young patients presenting with epilepsy.

Gandelman-Marton and Theitler[48] (2011) found that IEDs were recorded far more often if a sleep-deprived EEG was done within 3 days after a first seizure in 78 adults whose first routine EEG showed no IEDs. Oldani and colleagues[49] (1998) evaluated the reliability of routine EEG, daytime EEG after sleep deprivation, and nocturnal video-polysomnography (PSG), to diagnose nocturnal frontal lobe epilepsy in 23 patients. All patients had normal video-EEG when awake. Nocturnal video-PSG confirmed the diagnosis in 87% of patients and daytime video-EEG, with sleep deprivation in 52%. Labate and colleagues[50] (2007) found that generalized IEDs were much more likely to occur on the routine non–sleep-deprived EEG if the study was recorded at 9 AM rather than 3 PM in 29 patients with juvenile myoclonic epilepsy (JME).

YIELD OF SLEEP DEPRIVATION ON THE EEG IN CHILDREN DIFFERS FROM THAT IN ADULTS

Age of the patient (child or adult) may significantly affect the diagnostic yield of sleep and/or sleep deprivation for activating IEDs in EEG. The initial routine EEG will be normal in approximately one-half of children with clinically diagnosed epilepsy.[51,52] A prospective study by Aydin and colleagues[53] (2003) on 534 children referred for EEG for possible epilepsy found IEDs in 37% of the children with definite epilepsy, and in 13% of clinically suspected cases. Depriving a child of sleep for an EEG can challenge the child and his or her parents, and may not be needed.[54]

A prospective study by Gilbert[55] (2006) evaluated the diagnostic utility of sleep or varying degrees of sleep deprivation for activation of IEDs in 820 pediatric EEGs. NREM 2 sleep was observed in 57% of sleep-deprived, 44% of partially sleep-deprived, and 21% of non–sleep-deprived pediatric EEGs. Partial sleep deprivation was defined as 5 hours of sleep the night before for children aged 11 to 15 years and 7 hours for children aged 3 to 10 years. Sleep deprivation increased the likelihood that NREM 2 sleep would be recorded by 6-fold, and partial sleep deprivation by nearly 3-fold. However, the odds ratio that IEDs would be found was not increased by the presence of sleep, TSD, or partial sleep deprivation. The investigators concluded that the only significant effect of sleep deprivation was to increase the odds of sleep occurring.

CONSIDER ORAL MELATONIN TO INDUCE SLEEP IN CHILDREN DURING EEG

Given the likelihood IEDs are found in a routine EEG in a child even awake and the challenges of depriving young patients of sleep, alternative strategies for activating the EEG should be considered. Oral melatonin has been used to induce sleep in this population. Eisermann and colleagues[56] (2010) reported their experience using melatonin while recording a sleep EEG in 70 children. Sleep was obtained in 56 (80%) children, with a mean (standard deviation) sleep latency of 25 (8) minutes (range 15–45 minutes)

after melatonin administration and mean duration of 17 (9) minutes (5–55 minutes). Half of the children woke up spontaneously after 13 (8) minutes (5–40 minutes). Among 18 children with severe behavior problems that made interpretable EEG recording in the awake state impossible, sleep was obtained in 13 (72%) children. The rare symptoms reported (4%) after melatonin use were not reliably related to the drug.

Ashrafi and colleagues[57] (2010) compared melatonin with chloral hydrate for recording sleep on EEG in 348 children aged 1 month to 6 years. The investigators partially deprived the children of sleep the night before, and randomly administered chloral hydrate and melatonin on an alternative-day basis. The investigators found: (1) sleep-onset latency in the chloral hydrate and melatonin groups to be similar, but sleep duration and drowsiness time to be significantly shorter when melatonin was used; (2) more children in the melatonin group required a second dose of sedative to induce sleep compared with those in the chloral hydrate group (11% vs 3%); and (3) IEDs were significantly more likely to be observed in children sedated with melatonin (53% vs 46%).

ISOLATED CONVULSIONS FOLLOWING SLEEP DEPRIVATION

How often does prolonged TSD trigger a convulsion in people *without* epilepsy? Most of these reports and research come from sleep-deprived military personnel. Bennett[58] (1963) described 3 Air Force pilots who had a single generalized convulsive motor seizure following prolonged TSD, which prompted them to record EEGs 24 hours apart before and after 24 to 36 hours of TSD in 129 healthy aviators and 29 controls, and found that none had activation of epileptiform activity on the EEG when deprived of sleep.[59]

Gunderson and colleagues[60] (1973) reported that 38 soldiers had a single witnessed generalized convulsion while returning or en route to Vietnam. The investigators found that a majority of soldiers before they left had "a large amount of alcohol but little or no sleep," and estimated that the risk of a sleep-deprived seizure was 1 in 10,000 after 24 to 36 hours of TSD and 1 in 2500 after 2 or more days of sleep loss.

Friis and Lund[61] (1974) reported that 37 (2.9%) of 1250 patients seen over a 13-year period had isolated convulsions most often triggered by lack of sleep, and less often by somatic overexertion or emotional strain. Most were men, aged 20 to 50 years. Twenty-nine percent had recurrent stress convulsions triggered by the same factors when followed over 5 to 12 years. IEDs were seen in the initial EEGs of 10 patients (generalized 7, focal 3), but EEG abnormalities tended to disappear with time. Febrile convulsions were common in the offspring of patients with stress convulsions (6 times greater than expected). The authors estimated that the prevalence of isolated stress convulsions in the general adult population was 1 per 100,000.

More recently, sleep deprivation was identified as a risk factor for seizures of poorly slept Japanese tourists who arrived in Hawaii in the evening.[62] A large case-control study by Leone and colleagues[63] (2002) found that sleep deprivation increased the risk for a first generalized tonic-clonic (GTC) seizure by 2.4 times. Seventy-seven percent of 44 patients with a first-ever seizure within 24 hours of illicit use of amphetamine or relative analogues reported concomitant sleep deprivation.[64]

SLEEP DEPRIVATION AS A TRIGGER FOR SEIZURES IN PEOPLE WITH EPILEPSY

Many patients with partial seizures report partial sleep deprivation (sleeping less than their habitual sleep time) as a major seizure trigger.[65–69] A study evaluated the effects of sleeping 1.5 hours less than usual (partial sleep deprivation) or 1.5 hours longer than usual (oversleeping) on the probability a seizure would occur in 14 subjects with temporal lobe epilepsy.[68] Patients kept seizure and sleep diaries for 2 years, logging 682 seizures. The probability a seizure would occur was significantly greater for partial sleep deprivation (0.58) than normal sleep (0.09) and oversleeping (0.28). Eight (57%) subjects were particularly vulnerable to partial sleep deprivation as a seizure trigger, and 3 others to oversleeping.

The 3 most frequently cited seizure triggers in 223 adults with partial epilepsy were worry and stress (31%), sleep deprivation (27%), and missed medication (25%).[65] Another study found the most common seizure triggers reported by 400 adults with epilepsy were stress (30%), sleep deprivation (18%), sleep (14%), and fatigue (13%).[70] Stress, fatigue, and sleep deprivation correlated positively, whereas sleep more often correlated negatively with the occurrence of seizures.

Haut and colleagues[66] (2007) found that the relative odds a partial seizure would occur the next day decreased by 0.91 for each increased hour of sleep the preceding night in 71 patients with partial epilepsy who kept seizure/sleep diaries for 12 months. Pratt and colleagues[69] (1968) found 37% of patients with epilepsy to report that 2 hours of sleep loss or more activated or at least contributed to seizures. Fang and colleagues[71]

(2008) found that sleep deprivation was cited as a seizure trigger in 13% of 120 children with medically intractable epilepsy. Some studies doubt sleep deprivation to be the main trigger of seizures, especially in patients with partial seizures. Instead, stress (often leading to sleep deprivation) is proposed to be the more likely trigger.[70]

JME is characterized by myoclonic jerks and GTC seizures on awakening, especially in sleep-deprived individuals. One-third of patients with JME also have absence seizures. Patients with JME are unlikely to outgrow their need for antiepileptic medication.[72] Sleep deprivation was the most common trigger for generalized motor convulsions in 15 patients with JME.[73] Sleep deprivation, often coupled with acute drug withdrawal and/or alcohol use, was often the cause of recurrence of seizures after a long period of remission in 105 patients with JME.[74] Another study found that 77% of 75 patients with JME reported that sleep deprivation triggered their seizures.[75] Given this, lifestyle advice emphasizing the importance of sufficient sleep is crucial in maintaining seizure freedom in patients with JME and in many patients with other epilepsies.[72]

SLEEP DEPRIVATION ENHANCES CORTICAL EXCITABILITY, MORE SO IN PEOPLE WITH EPILEPSY

Experimental studies in humans have used transcranial magnetic stimulation (TMS) to assess excitability of the cerebral motor cortex and responsiveness of corticospinal pathways during sleep. Single or paired-pulse TMS paradigms have been used to test reactivity and excitability of the parts of the cerebral cortex during different sleep states and wakefulness. Several studies using TMS during sleep in normal young adult volunteers suggest that corticospinal excitability is reduced during sleep in comparison with wakefulness.[76,77] Sleep deprivation in normal young adult subjects is associated with enhanced cortical excitation by reduction of intracortical inhibition.[78,79]

Several studies have been done using TMS in people with epilepsy to evaluate whether they have increased cortical excitability during sleep as compared with normal controls, and whether sleep deprivation enhances this. Salih and colleagues[80] (2006) used paired-pulse TMS to test intracortical inhibition and facilitation in the hemisphere of the epileptic focus in 3 patients with untreated nonlesional, nongenetic frontal lobe epilepsy. All 3 patients showed a major decrease of intracortical inhibition in NREM sleep. The investigators hypothesized that decreased intra-cortical inhibition during NREM sleep might explain how NREM sleep could promote seizures. Badawy and colleagues[81] (2006) found that 30 patients with idiopathic generalized or focal epilepsies had a significant increase in cortical excitability when deprived of sleep, compared with normal controls. Increased cortical excitability in the patients with generalized epilepsies was bilateral, lateralized to the hemisphere containing the epileptic focus in the patients with focal epilepsies. Manganotti and colleagues[82] (2006) found higher levels of cortical excitability in 10 patients with JME when deprived of sleep, significantly greater than a similar number of healthy controls. Del Felice and colleagues[83] (2011) found higher cortical excitability, which localized to the frontal and prefrontal regions in 12 patients with JME when deprived of sleep or during rebound sleep. Sleep deprivation reduces cortical responsiveness to incoming stimuli and is associated with increased levels of adenosine.[3]

SUMMARY

Clinicians should question patients with epilepsy regarding the impact of varying degrees of sleep deprivation on their seizures. If sleep deprivation triggers seizures in a particular patient, he or she should be counseled on avoiding it and on preemptive treatment.

REFERENCES

1. Chee MW, Chuah LY. Functional neuroimaging insights into how sleep and sleep deprivation affect memory and cognition. Curr Opin Neurol 2008; 21(4):417–23.
2. Lim J, Dinges DF. Sleep deprivation and vigilant attention. Ann N Y Acad Sci 2008;1129:305–22.
3. Boonstra TW, Stins JF, Daffertshofer A, et al. Effects of sleep deprivation on neural functioning: an integrative review. Cell Mol Life Sci 2007;64(7–8):934–46.
4. Curcio G, Ferrara M, De Gennaro L. Sleep loss, learning capacity and academic performance. Sleep Med Rev 2006;10(5):323–37.
5. Spiegel K, Tasali E, Leproult R, et al. Effects of poor and short sleep on glucose metabolism and obesity risk. Nat Rev Endocrinol 2009;5(5):253–61.
6. Morselli L, Leproult R, Balbo M, et al. Role of sleep duration in the regulation of glucose metabolism and appetite. Best Pract Res Clin Endocrinol Metab 2010;24(5):687–702.
7. Grandner MA, Patel NP, Gehrman PR, et al. Problems associated with short sleep: bridging the gap between laboratory and epidemiological studies. Sleep Med Rev 2010;14(4):239–47.

8. Strine TW, Chapman DP. Associations of frequent sleep insufficiency with health-related quality of life and health behaviors. Sleep Med 2005;6(1):23–7.
9. Bixler E. Sleep and society: an epidemiological perspective. Sleep Med 2009;10(Suppl 1):S3–6.
10. Kripke DF, Garfinkel L, Wingard DL, et al. Mortality associated with sleep duration and insomnia. Arch Gen Psychiatry 2002;59(2):131–6.
11. National Heart, Lung and Blood Institute, US Department of Health and Human Services. Your guide to healthy sleep. Bethesda (MD): National Institutes of Health; 2005.
12. Van Cauter E, Spiegel K, Tasali E, et al. Metabolic consequences of sleep and sleep loss. Sleep Med 2008;9(Suppl 1):S23–8.
13. Schoenborn CA, Adams PF. Sleep duration as a correlate of smoking, alcohol use, leisure-time physical inactivity, and obesity among adults: United States, 2004-2006, 2008. NCHS Health and Stats: Health E-Stat; May 2008. 2011 (September 1, 2011).
14. Gallicchio L, Kalesan B. Sleep duration and mortality: a systematic review and meta-analysis. J Sleep Res 2009;18(2):148–58.
15. Buxton OM, Marcelli E. Short and long sleep are positively associated with obesity, diabetes, hypertension, and cardiovascular disease among adults in the United States. Soc Sci Med 2010;71(5): 1027–36.
16. Nielsen LS, Danielsen KV, Sorensen TI. Short sleep duration as a possible cause of obesity: critical analysis of the epidemiological evidence. Obes Rev 2011;12(2):78–92.
17. Cappuccio FP, Stranges S, Kandala NB, et al. Gender-specific associations of short sleep duration with prevalent and incident hypertension: the Whitehall II Study. Hypertension 2007;50(4): 693–700.
18. Gottlieb DJ, Redline S, Nieto FJ, et al. Association of usual sleep duration with hypertension: the Sleep Heart Health Study. Sleep 2006;29(8):1009–14.
19. Grandner MA, Kripke DF, Naidoo N, et al. Relationships among dietary nutrients and subjective sleep, objective sleep, and napping in women. Sleep Med 2010;11(2):180–4.
20. Steptoe A, Peacey V, Wardle J. Sleep duration and health in young adults. Arch Intern Med 2006; 166(16):1689–92.
21. Grigg-Damberger MM, Damberger SJ. Historical aspects of sleep and epilepsy. In: Bazil CW, Malow BA, Sammaritano MR, editors. Sleep and epilepsy: the clinical spectrum. New York: Elsevier; 2002. p. 3–16.
22. Hippocrates. 'The sacred disease', 'Aphorisms' and 'Prognosis'. In: Lloyd GE, editor. Hippocratic writings. Boston: Penguin; 1983. p. 170–85, 206–51.
23. Temkin O. The falling sickness: a history of epilepsy from the Greeks to the beginnings of modern

neurology. Revised 2nd edition. Baltimore (MD): Johns Hopkins Press; 1994.

24. Stahl WH. Moon madness. Ann Med Hist New Ser 1937;9:248–63.

25. Romberg MH. A manual of the nervous diseases of man, vol. 2. 1853.

26. Roosli M, Juni P, Braun-Fahrlander C, et al. Sleep-less night, the moon is bright: longitudinal study of lunar phase and sleep. J Sleep Res 2006;15(2): 149–53.

27. Baxendale S, Fisher J. Moonstruck? The effect of the lunar cycle on seizures. Epilepsy Behav 2008;13(3): 549–50.

28. Falchi F, Cinzano P, Elvidge CD, et al. Limiting the impact of light pollution on human health, environment and stellar visibility. J Environ Manage 2011; 92(10):2714–22.

29. Zaharna M, Guilleminault C. Sleep, noise and health: review. Noise Health 2010;12(47):64–9.

30. Stansfeld SA, Matheson MP. Noise pollution: non-auditory effects on health. Br Med Bull 2003;68: 243–57.

31. Xie H, Kang J, Mills GH. Clinical review: the impact of noise on patients' sleep and the effectiveness of noise reduction strategies in intensive care units. Crit Care 2009;13(2):208.

32. Chan B, Cheong EY, Ng SF, et al. Evaluation of sleep disturbances in children with epilepsy: a question-naire-based case-control study. Epilepsy Behav 2011;21(4):437–40.

33. van Golde EG, Gutter T, de Weerd AW. Sleep disturbances in people with epilepsy; prevalence, impact and treatment. Sleep Med Rev 2011;15(6):357–68.

34. Ong LC, Yang WW, Wong SW, et al. Sleep habits and disturbances in Malaysian children with epilepsy. J Paediatr Child Health 2010;46(3):80–4.

35. Batista BH, Nunes ML. Evaluation of sleep habits in children with epilepsy. Epilepsy Behav 2007;11(1): 60–4.

36. de Weerd A, de Haas S, Otte A, et al. Subjective sleep disturbance in patients with partial epilepsy: a questionnaire-based study on prevalence and impact on quality of life. Epilepsia 2004;45(11): 1397–404.

37. Soldatos CR, Allaert FA, Ohta T, et al. How do individuals sleep around the world? Results from a single-day survey in ten countries. Sleep Med 2005;6(1):5–13.

38. Khatami R, Zutter D, Siegel A, et al. Sleep-wake habits and disorders in a series of 100 adult epilepsy patients—a prospective study. Seizure 2006;15(5):299–306.

39. Piperidou C, Karlovasitou A, Triantafyllou N, et al. Influence of sleep disturbance on quality of life of patients with epilepsy. Seizure 2008;17(7):588–94.

40. Jenssen S, Gracely E, Mahmood T, et al. Subjective somnolence relates mainly to depression among

patients in a tertiary care epilepsy center. Epilepsy Behav 2006;9(4):632–5.

41. Xu X, Brandenburg NA, McDermott AM, et al. Sleep disturbances reported by refractory partial-onset epilepsy patients receiving polytherapy. Epilepsia 2006;47(7):1176–83.

42. Wirrell E, Blackman M, Barlow K, et al. Sleep disturbances in children with epilepsy compared with their nearest-aged siblings. Dev Med Child Neurol 2005; 47(11):754–9.

43. Mattson RH, Pratt KL, Calverley JR. Electroencephalograms of epileptics following sleep deprivation. Arch Neurol 1965;13(3):310–5.

44. Rowan AJ, Veldhuisen RJ, Nagelkerke NJ. Comparative evaluation of sleep deprivation and sedated sleep EEGs as diagnostic aids in epilepsy. Electroencephalogr Clin Neurophysiol 1982;54(4):357–64.

45. Degen R, Degen HE. Sleep and sleep deprivation in epileptology. Epilepsy Res Suppl 1991;2:235–60.

46. Roupakiotis SC, Gatzonis SD, Triantafyllou N, et al. The usefulness of sleep and sleep deprivation as activating methods in electroencephalographic recording: contribution to a long-standing discussion. Seizure 2000;9(8):580–4.

47. Leach JP, Stephen LJ, Salveta C, et al. Which electroencephalography (EEG) for epilepsy? The relative usefulness of different EEG protocols in patients with possible epilepsy. J Neurol Neurosurg Psychiatry 2006;77(9):1040–2.

48. Gandelman-Marton R, Theitler J. When should a sleep-deprived EEG be performed following a presumed first seizure in adults? Acta Neurol Scand 2011;124(3):202–5.

49. Oldani A, Zucconi M, Smirne S, et al. The neurophysiological evaluation of nocturnal frontal lobe epilepsy. Seizure 1998;7(4):317–20.

50. Labate A, Ambrosio R, Gambardella A, et al. Usefulness of a morning routine EEG recording in patients with juvenile myoclonic epilepsy. Epilepsy Res 2007; 77(1):17–21.

51. Camfield P, Gordon K, Camfield C, et al. EEG results are rarely the same if repeated within six months in childhood epilepsy. Can J Neurol Sci 1995;22(4):297–300.

52. Gilbert DL, Gartside PS. Factors affecting the yield of pediatric EEGs in clinical practice. Clin Pediatr (Phila) 2002;41(1):25–32.

53. Aydin K, Okuyaz C, Serdaroglu A, et al. Utility of electroencephalography in the evaluation of common neurologic conditions in children. J Child Neurol 2003;18(6):394–6.

54. Nijhof SL, Bakker AL, Van Nieuwenhuizen O, et al. Is the sleep-deprivation EEG a burden for both child and parent? Epilepsia 2005;46(8):1328–9.

55. Gilbert DL. Interobserver reliability of visual interpretation of electroencephalograms in children with newly diagnosed seizures. Dev Med Child Neurol 2006;48(12):1009–10 [author reply: 1010–1].

56. Eisermann M, Kaminska A, Berdougo B, et al. Melatonin: experience in its use for recording sleep EEG in children and review of the literature. Neuropediatrics 2010;41(4):163–6.

57. Ashrafi MR, Mohammadi M, Tafarroji J, et al. Melatonin versus chloral hydrate for recording sleep EEG. Eur J Paediatr Neurol 2010;14(3):235–8.

58. Bennett DR. Sleep deprivation and major motor convulsions. Neurology 1963;13:953–8.

59. Bennett DR, Mattson RH, Ziter FA, et al. Sleep deprivation: neurological and electroencephalographic effects. Aerosp Med 1964;35:888–90.

60. Gunderson CH, Dunne PB, Feyer TL. Sleep deprivation seizures. Neurology 1973;23(7):678–86.

61. Friis ML, Lund M. Stress convulsions. Arch Neurol 1974;31(3):155–9.

62. Mullins ME, Elias MF. Seizures in east-bound visitors to Hawaii. Hawaii Med J 1998;57(2):408–11.

63. Leone M, Bottacchi E, Beghi E, et al. Risk factors for a first generalized tonic-clonic seizure in adult life. Neurol Sci 2002;23(3):99–106.

64. Brown JW, Dunne JW, Fatovic DM, et al. Amphetamine-associated seizures: clinical features and prognosis. Epilepsia 2011;52(2):401–4.

65. Dionisio J, Tatum WO. Triggers and techniques in termination of partial seizures. Epilepsy Behav 2010;17(2):210–4.

66. Haut SR, Hall CB, Masur J, et al. Seizure occurrence: precipitants and prediction. Neurology 2007;69(20):1905–10.

67. Pinikahana J, Dono J. The lived experience of initial symptoms of and factors triggering epileptic seizures. Epilepsy Behav 2009;15(4):513–20.

68. Rajna P, Veres J. Correlations between night sleep duration and seizure frequency in temporal lobe epilepsy. Epilepsia 1993;34(3):574–9.

69. Pratt KL, Mattson RH, Weikers NJ, et al. EEG activation of epileptics following sleep deprivation: a prospective study of 114 cases. Electroencephalogr Clin Neurophysiol 1968;24(1):11–5.

70. Frucht MM, Quigg M, Schwaner C, et al. Distribution of seizure precipitants among epilepsy syndromes. Epilepsia 2000;41(12):1534–9.

71. Fang PC, Chen YJ, Lee IC. Seizure precipitants in children with intractable epilepsy. Brain Dev 2008; 30(8):527–32.

72. Mantoan L, Walker M. Treatment options in juvenile myoclonic epilepsy. Curr Treat Options Neurol 2011;13(4):355–70.

73. Dhanuka AK, Jain BK, Daljit S, et al. Juvenile myoclonic epilepsy: a clinical and sleep EEG study. Seizure 2001;10(5):374–8.

74. Sokic D, Ristic AJ, Vojvodic N, et al. Frequency, causes and phenomenology of late seizure recurrence in patients with juvenile myoclonic epilepsy after a long period of remission. Seizure 2007; 16(6):533–7.

75. da Silva Sousa P, Lin K, Garzon E, et al. Self-perception of factors that precipitate or inhibit seizures in juvenile myoclonic epilepsy. Seizure 2005; 14(5):340–6.

76. Manganotti P, Fuggetta G, Fiaschi A. Changes of motor cortical excitability in human subjects from wakefulness to early stages of sleep: a combined transcranial magnetic stimulation and electroencephalographic study. Neurosci Lett 2004;362(1): 31–4.

77. Grosse P, Khatami R, Salih F, et al. Corticospinal excitability in human sleep as assessed by transcranial magnetic stimulation. Neurology 2002;59(12): 1988–91.

78. Scalise A, Desiato MT, Gigli GL, et al. Increasing cortical excitability: a possible explanation for the proconvulsant role of sleep deprivation. Sleep 2006;29(12):1595–8.

79. Kreuzer P, Langguth B, Popp R, et al. Reduced intracortical inhibition after sleep deprivation: a transcranial magnetic stimulation study. Neurosci Lett 2011; 493(3):63–6.

80. Salih F, Khatami R, Steinheimer S, et al. A hypothesis for how non-REM sleep might promote seizures in partial epilepsies: a transcranial magnetic stimulation study. Epilepsia 2007;48(8):1538–42.

81. Badawy RA, Curatolo JM, Newton M, et al. Sleep deprivation increases cortical excitability in epilepsy: syndrome-specific effects. Neurology 2006;67(6): 1018–22.

82. Manganotti P, Bongiovanni LG, Fuggetta G, et al. Effects of sleep deprivation on cortical excitability in patients affected by juvenile myoclonic epilepsy: a combined transcranial magnetic stimulation and EEG study. J Neurol Neurosurg Psychiatry 2006; 77(1):56–60.

83. Del Felice A, Fiaschi A, Bongiovanni GL, et al. The sleep-deprived brain in normals and patients with juvenile myoclonic epilepsy: a perturbational approach to measuring cortical reactivity. Epilepsy Res 2011;96(1–2):123–31.

Seizures, Epilepsy, and Circadian Rhythms

Wytske A. Hofstra-van Oostveen, MD, PhD[a,b,*],
Al W. de Weerd, MD, PhD[b]

KEYWORDS

- Circadian rhythmicity • Seizures • Epilepsy • Melatonin

Several studies have shown that sleep and sleep restriction can influence epilepsy and trigger epileptic seizures. Circadian rhythmicity plays an important role in sleep physiology. Knowledge of the influence of circadian rhythmicity on epilepsy and seizures, and vice versa, is scarce. Greater knowledge of the interactions between circadian rhythm and epilepsy may be of value for understanding the pathophysiology of epilepsy, especially for the timing of diagnostic procedures and therapy to improve seizure control.

CIRCADIAN RHYTHMS IN EPILEPSY
Twenty-Four Hour Rhythmicity in (Human) Seizure Occurrence

In animal studies, clear diurnal (ie, 24-hour) seizure patterns in various epilepsy models have been observed. For example, studies in rodents with limbic epilepsy have shown that more spontaneous seizures occurred and seizure latency was shorter under light than during darkness. Quigg and colleagues[1] used continuous electroencephalogram (EEG) recordings to confirm the clock timing of seizures in epileptic rats. The animals were first entrained to a 12-hour/12-hour light-dark cycle then exposed to constant darkness to unmask their free-running circadian rhythmicity. During light-dark exposure, spontaneous limbic seizures occurred nearly twice as often during the light period. Seizures continued to occur in the same pattern during constant darkness after correcting for the core body temperature (CBT) rhythm. These findings show that spontaneous limbic seizures in rats occur in a true endogenously mediated circadian pattern.[1]

More than a century ago, Gowers[2] classified human seizure occurrence into 3 categories: diurnal, nocturnal, and diffuse. Later studies have confirmed and extended his findings. Examples of such are the hypermotor seizures of some frontal lobe epilepsies that occur preferentially during sleep (nocturnal frontal lobe epilepsy), and the myoclonic seizures in juvenile myoclonic epilepsy (JME) that occur most often shortly after awakening in the morning.[3,4]

Only a few studies provide detailed information about temporal distribution (clock timing) of seizures over the 24-hour day. One case report based on a seizure diary maintained for 5 years by a subject with 2 epileptic foci showed that temporal and parietal seizures occurred independently from each other in nonrandom daily patterns.[5] For temporal seizures, a peak incidence was found at 1210 hours, and for parietal seizures the peak was at 0250 hours.

Three retrospective studies used continuous EEG monitoring to confirm the clock timing of seizures.[6–8] Quigg and colleagues[8] studied the clock timing of seizures in 64 patients with mesial

Financial disclosure and conflict of interest statement: None of the authors has any conflict of interest to disclose.

[a] Department of Neurology, Medisch Spectrum Twente Hospital, Postbus 50 000, 7500 KA Enschede, The Netherlands

[b] Department of Clinical Neurophysiology and Sleep Centre SEIN, Dokter Denekampweg 20, 8025 BV, Zwolle, The Netherlands

* Corresponding author. Department of Neurology, Medisch Spectrum Twente Hospital, Postbus 50 000, 7500 KA Enschede, The Netherlands.

E-mail address: w.hofstra@mst.nl

Sleep Med Clin 7 (2012) 99–104
doi:10.1016/j.jsmc.2011.12.005

temporal lobe epilepsy (MTLE), 26 with extra–temporal lobe epilepsy (XTLE), and 8 with lesional temporal lobe epilepsy (LTLE). The investigators found that seizures in LTLE and XTLE occur randomly, but seizures in the patients with MTLE had a distinct nonrandom pattern with a peak incidence at approximately 1500 hours. Quigg and colleagues further found that patients with MTLE had a similar circadian cycle of seizures to that observed in a rat model of limbic epilepsy. Pavlova and colleagues[7] found that nonrandom timing to seizures varied in the patients with TLE and XTLE in 26 patients with epilepsy. The peak incidence was between 1500 and 1900 hours in the patients with TLE, and between 1900 and 2300 hours in those with XTLE.

Hofstra and colleagues[6] recently evaluated the temporal distribution of 808 clinical seizures in 100 adults and 76 children with partial epilepsies seen in the authors' tertiary epilepsy center. This study found nonrandom daytime peaks in all types of seizures, with significantly more seizures than expected occurring from 1100 to 1700 hours and fewer seizures from 2300 to 0500 hours. The investigators found clear daytime peak incidences in seizures, especially for extratemporal seizures in children and temporal lobe seizures in adults. Lowest incidences and numbers of seizures, especially complex partial seizures, were seen in the adults between 2300 and 0500 hours, and the children with either tonic, TLE, or XTLE seizures also had significantly fewer seizures in this time period.

Karafin and colleagues[9] analyzed the circadian timing of seizures in 60 patients with MTLE for 2 to 16 days who had a mean of 11 seizures per patient. Patients showed a bimodal pattern of seizure occurrence, with peak seizure frequencies occurring between 0600 and 0800 hours and between 1500 and 1700 hours. Loddenkemper and colleagues[10] evaluated the diurnal incidence of seizures in 332 consecutive children with lesional focal epilepsy who had inpatient video-EEG monitoring at their institution over a 3-year period. Data were analyzed in relation to clock time, wakefulness/sleep, and seizure localization. Seizures in patients with frontal lesions occurred mostly during sleep (72%). Seizures in mesial temporal (64%), neocortical temporal (71%), and occipital (66%) lesional epilepsy occurred mostly during wakefulness. Temporal lobe seizures occurred more frequently during wakefulness (66%) compared with extratemporal seizures (32%) (odds ratio, 2.7). Temporal lobe seizures peaked between 0900 and 1200 hours as well as from 1500 to 1800 hours, whereas extratemporal seizures peaked between 0600 and 0900 hours. Sleep, not clock time, provides a more robust

stimulus for seizure onset, especially for frontal lobe seizures. Temporal lobe seizures are more frequent during wakefulness than are extratemporal seizures.

Two published studies have evaluated the timing of seizures in patients undergoing intracranial EEG monitoring (a gold standard for confirming the location of seizures). Daruzzo and colleagues[11] found that seizures from the parietal, occipital, mesial temporal, and neocortical temporal lobes were non-uniformly distributed when they analyzed the timing of 669 seizures of 131 adult patients with different focal epilepsies. Occipital seizures were seen most frequently between 1600 and 1900 hours, whereas parietal and frontal lobe seizures peaked between 0400 and 0700 hours. Two peaks were found in the occurrence of seizures from the mesial temporal lobe (1600–1900 hours and 0700–1000 hours). Seizures from the neocortical temporal lobe also had a peak incidence between 1600 and 1900 hours. Hofstra and colleagues[12] analyzed the temporal distribution of 450 spontaneous seizures in 33 patients with epilepsy who underwent long-term intracranial EEG and video monitoring. The investigators found that seizures showed an uneven distribution over the day, depending on lobe of origin: temporal lobe seizures occurred preferentially between the hours of 1100 and 1700 hours, frontal seizures between 2300 and 0500 hours, and parietal seizures between 1700 and 2300 hours.[12]

A significant limitation of all the aforementioned studies is that they analyzed the time of day, not circadian rhythmicity. To further study the interaction between circadian rhythmicity and seizure occurrence, Hofstra and colleagues[13] performed a prospective pilot study in the authors' tertiary epilepsy center, analyzing 124 seizures of 21 patients admitted for long-term video-EEG monitoring. The investigators found that temporal lobe seizures occurred most often between 1100 and 1700 hours and frontal seizures primarily between 2300 and 0500 hours. The investigators also measured dim light melatonin onset (DLMO) in each patient and correlated it with the clock timing of their seizures, and found that temporal seizures occurred most frequently in the 6 hours before DLMO and frontal seizures in the 6 to 12 hours after the DLMO. These results suggest that temporal and frontal seizures not only occur in diurnal patterns, but also are truly time-locked to the circadian phase. More research with larger sample sizes is needed to confirm these results.

Twenty-Four Hour Rhythmicity in the Occurrence of Interictal EEG Activity

The preferential timing of interictal epileptic discharges (IEDs) during seizure-free periods has been studied extensively in humans. In several studies, it has been found that the number of IEDs increases significantly during sleep, in parallel with ultradian 100-minute cycles of rapid eye movement (REM)/non–rapid eye movement (NREM).[14] During NREM sleep (especially NREM 1 and 2), focal and generalized IEDs are common. Although attenuated, focal IEDs persist in REM sleep, but generalized IEDs are rare in REM sleep. However, none of the aforementioned studies evaluated the pure influence of circadian rhythmicity, and their results may be masked by the sleep-wake cycle. These studies give an insight into the influence of sleep on IEDs, but not the contribution of the endogenous 24-hour circadian rhythm.

To date, only one study has focused on circadian rhythmicity in IEDs using a forced desynchrony protocol. Pavlova and colleagues[15] measured hourly plasma melatonin levels in 5 patients with generalized epilepsy undergoing continuous video-EEG monitoring according to a protocol whereby their sleep/wake schedule was evenly distributed across the circadian cycle. Patients were studied in dim light (<8 lux) to prevent circadian entrainment. The investigators found that all 5 subjects had normal circadian rhythmicity of plasma melatonin relative to their habitual sleep times. In the 3 patients with sufficient IEDs to assess circadian variability, IEDs most often occurred during NREM sleep (NREM/wake ratio = 14:1). Two patients had NREM sleep in all circadian phases and apparent circadian variation in IEDs, but with different phases relative to peak melatonin.

Clock Genes

Several groups have studied the genetics of circadian rhythmicity, and have found various genes that are at least partly responsible for the characteristic activity of the individual suprachiasmatic nucleus and the interindividual differences. The activity depends on the expression of the so-called autoregulatory translation-transcription feedback loops of genes including the Period genes (Per1, Per2, Per3), the Clock gene, and the 2 Cryptochrome genes (Cry 1, Cry2). Several animal studies have demonstrated that deletion or mutation of these clock genes can lead to rhythms with abnormal periods or even arrhythmic phenotypes. It would be interesting to study clock genes in relation to epilepsy and seizures.

The loss of circadian PAR bZIP transcription factors in mice may cause severe epilepsy.[16] These factors are transcriptionally controlled by the circadian molecular oscillator and are thought to be influenced by the circadian clock. Although this is a very interesting finding for insight into the interaction between the circadian rhythm and epilepsy, the precise relevance of this study for human epilepsies remains to be elucidated. No studies have yet been published regarding clock genes in epilepsy patients.

THE INFLUENCE OF EPILEPSY AND SEIZURES ON CIRCADIAN RHYTHMICITY

There are few data on the circadian rhythm in human epilepsy. Far more is known on the influence of epilepsy and seizures on several body functions mediated by the circadian rhythm.

Sleep and Sleep-Wake Cycle

The interaction of sleep and epilepsy has been studied extensively. Several studies have observed that the occurrence of seizures differs in different sleep stages: NREM (especially NREM 2) facilitates partial seizures, whereas seizures are typically inhibited during REM sleep. Furthermore, partial seizures tend to generalize more often during sleep than when a patient is awake.[17] Epilepsy and seizures are also known to have considerable influence on sleep and sleep quality. The effects of recent seizures, antiepileptic drugs, and severity of the epilepsy syndrome may result in disorganized sleep in epileptic patients. The various epilepsy syndromes and types of seizures can influence sleep to a different extent.[18] This aspect is discussed in greater detail elsewhere in this issue.

Chronotypes

The term chronotype refers to the preferred phase of an individual for timing his or her daily activities, sleep, and wakefulness. Distribution of chronotypes is based on the interindividual variation in the endogenous phase of the circadian clock under entrained conditions (ie, when circadian rhythmicity is synchronized to the 24-hour day). Morning types tend to adopt an earlier sleep schedule than do evening types, and peaks in performance and alertness are seen earlier in the day in morning types than in evening types.[19–21]

Very little is known about the distribution of chronotypes in epilepsy. In 2 studies of rodent epilepsy models, patterns of daily activity were studied. One study showed marked changes in the patterns of daily activity and motor hyperactivity in rats after pilocarpine-induced status epilepticus. The acrophase (rhythm peak) was delayed for more than 4 hours for up to 12 weeks in the rats after a single episode of status epilepticus.[22] In another study by the same investigators, behavioral rhythms of a rodent model of chronic atypical absence seizures found that the mice had increased motor hyperactivity but no phase shift.[23]

Pung and Schmitz[24] compared chronotypes of 20 patients with JME with those of 20 patients with TLE using standardized chronotype questionnaires. The patients with JME tended to have a characteristic circadian rhythm comparable with an extreme eveningness type (going to bed later at night, getting up later in the morning, and feeling fit at a later time during the day) in comparison with the patients with TLE.

Hofstra and colleagues[25] recently performed a large study evaluating whether patients with different types of epilepsy could be distinguished from the general population by their chronotypes and subjective sleep parameters. The investigators compared the distribution of chronotypes and subjective sleep parameters (sleep duration and time of midsleep on free days) in 200 patients with epilepsy with those in the general population (N = 4012).[25] Patients with epilepsy were evaluated using the morningness-eveningness and the Munich Chronotype questionnaires. Significant differences were found in morningness-eveningness distribution, timing of midsleep (corrected for sleep duration), and total sleep time on free days between the patients with epilepsy and the healthy controls. The patients with epilepsy were more often morning-oriented, had earlier midsleep, and had longer sleep duration on free days. However, no differences were observed in the distribution of chronotypes or subjective sleep parameters between the groups of patients with specific epilepsy syndromes (TLE, frontal lobe epilepsy, JME). These results suggest that epilepsy itself (rather than seizure timing) has a significant influence on chronotype behavior and subjective sleep parameters in individuals with epilepsy. However, further studies are needed to determine whether certain chronotypes influence epilepsy and timing of seizures (ie, the other way around).

Melatonin

Melatonin is an intensively studied hormone as regards epilepsy and epileptic seizures. Its precise value is still disputed because results are very inconsistent. Some investigators have described low melatonin levels in patients with epilepsy, whereas others have observed normal or even elevated levels.[26–29] Some studies describe elevated levels following complex partial seizures, whereas others report no changes in melatonin levels after complex partial or generalized tonic-clonic seizures.[26,28]

The effects of melatonin on seizure frequency have also been studied. In studies using several different animal models, melatonin has been shown to have a depressive effect on brain excitability and to prevent seizures.[30–32] Furthermore, removal of the pineal gland leads to seizure activity, which can be counteracted by administration of exogenous melatonin.[33] Results in humans are again conflicting. Some studies report reduced seizure frequency in patients with epilepsy when given melatonin,[34–36] and seizure rates increasing to pretreatment levels after stopping melatonin.[35] However, other studies have found no clear group effect of melatonin on seizure frequency or even have observed increased seizure activity.[37,38] With all these conflicting results, further research is necessary to define the precise effects on epileptic seizures of melatonin as well as its role in seizure prevention and epilepsy.

Core Body Temperature

The effects of epilepsy and seizures on CBT rhythmicity have rarely been studied in either animal models or people with epilepsy. Quigg and colleagues[39] studied whether CBT was altered in an electrically induced limbic status epilepticus model of MTLE by measuring CBT in the animals during light-entrained and free-running constant dark conditions. The investigators found that the circadian component of CBT was preserved in all animals; however, in the free-running condition, the CBT of the epileptic animals was more complex and even polyrhythmic compared with the normal animals. Furthermore, neuronal density was decreased in regions of the anterior and posterior hypothalamus but not in the suprachiasmatic nuclei of the epileptic rats. The investigators concluded that the alterations in CBT are due to the epileptic state and are independent of isolated seizures, arguing that the altered circadian thermoregulation in epileptic rats might be related to seizure-induced regional hypothalamic neuronal loss. Whether this relationship exists in humans with MTLE needs to be studied. Another study by the same investigators found that changes are observed in CBT after seizures in experimental rat models, including postictal phase shifts and more complex CBT rhythms.[40]

Body temperature can also affect seizures. For instance, fever can act as a trigger to induce seizures. Data from an epileptic rat model show that body temperature recorded in 10-minute epochs during which seizures occurred was slightly lower than in seizure-free epochs.[1] These data support the hypothesis that physiologic elevations in CBT are not associated with (more frequent) seizure occurrence.

SUMMARY AND DISCUSSION

It can be concluded that various studies have focused on the interaction between circadian rhythmicity and (human) epilepsy. From studies in humans as well as animals we now understand that seizure occurrence seems to have 24-hour rhythmicity, depending on the type of seizure and lobe of origin. A pilot study in humans suggested that temporal and frontal seizures not only occur in diurnal patterns but also are time-locked to the circadian phase. A study in rats showed a true endogenous-mediated circadian rhythm in seizure occurrence in a rodent model of limbic epilepsy. Only one study has been published on circadian rhythmicity in interictal discharges, which provided evidence for such a rhythm in IEDs in a small number of patients with generalized epilepsy.

More is known on the influence of epilepsy and seizures on circadian rhythms. Numerous studies have focused on sleep in epilepsy, and describe significant influences of epilepsy and seizures on sleep. Only 2 studies have focused on chronotypes, 1 of which found significant differences in chronotypes between patients with TLE and JME. The other study found no differences between patients with different epilepsy syndromes, but did observe significant differences in morningness/eveningness distribution, timing of midsleep, and sleep duration on free days between epilepsy patients and healthy controls. Even less is known about CBT in people with epilepsy. Several hormones falling under the influence of the circadian clock have also been studied. Results on the interaction of melatonin (the most intensively studied hormone) and seizures are far from conclusive, as differences in baseline levels and postictal levels have been found.

Although there are still many questions to be answered, it can be concluded from the studies described herein that there is proof that circadian rhythm and epilepsy at least interact. There are considerable gaps in the knowledge of this interaction, especially in humans. Thus far, all but one of the studies in humans have been performed in daily life, meaning that subjects are entrained by zeitgeber and that true endogenous circadian patterns cannot be observed. To explore endogenous rhythmicity, constant routines and trials are needed in studies. Such trials have often been performed in healthy subjects, but it can be ethically challenging to perform such trials in epilepsy patients, as sleep deprivation enhances seizures.

It is easier to explore true circadian rhythmicity in animals. More elaborate trials with animal epilepsy models could be performed, including for instance phase shifting of the circadian rhythm, to study the effects on seizure frequency and temporal distribution of seizures. In humans, it would be interesting to study the correlation between seizure occurrence and individual circadian rhythmicity. Furthermore, more extensive studies on the distribution of chronotypes in various epilepsy syndromes would be informative. Adjustment of antiepileptic treatment to the individual's circadian rhythmicity may improve seizure control, and deserves to be studied. As mentioned, this may be of great value for better timing of diagnostic procedures and therapeutic options in epilepsy.

REFERENCES

1. Quigg M, Clayburn H, Straume M, et al. Effects of circadian regulation and rest-activity state on spontaneous seizures in a rat model of limbic epilepsy. Epilepsia 2000;41(5):502–9.
2. Gowers W. Course of epilepsy. Epilepsy and other chronic convulsive diseases: their causes, symptoms and treatment. New York: William Wood; 1885. p. 157–64.
3. Panayiotopoulos CP, Obeid T, Tahan AR. Juvenile myoclonic epilepsy: a 5-year prospective study. Epilepsia 1994;35(2):285–96.
4. Scheffer IE, Bhatia KP, Lopes-Cendes I, et al. Autosomal dominant nocturnal frontal lobe epilepsy. A distinctive clinical disorder. Brain 1995;118(Pt 1): 61–73.
5. Quigg M, Straume M. Dual epileptic foci in a single patient express distinct temporal patterns dependent on limbic versus nonlimbic brain location. Ann Neurol 2000;48(1):117–20.
6. Hofstra WA, Grootemarsink BE, Dieker R, et al. Temporal distribution of clinical seizures over the 24 hour day: a retrospective observational study in a tertiary epilepsy clinic. Epilepsia 2009;50(9): 2019–26.
7. Pavlova MK, Shea SA, Bromfield EB. Day/night patterns of focal seizures. Epilepsy Behav 2004; 5(1):44–9.
8. Quigg M, Straume M, Menaker M, et al. Temporal distribution of partial seizures: comparison of an animal model with human partial epilepsy. Ann Neurol 1998;43(6):748–55.
9. Karafin M, St Louis EK, Zimmerman MB, et al. Bimodal ultradian seizure periodicity in human mesial temporal lobe epilepsy. Seizure 2010;19(6): 347–51.
10. Loddenkemper T, Vendrame M, Zarowski M, et al. Circadian patterns of pediatric seizures. Neurology 2011;76(2):145–53.

11. Durazzo TS, Spencer SS, Duckrow RB, et al. Temporal distributions of seizure occurrence from various epileptogenic regions. Neurology 2008; 70(15):1265–71.

12. Hofstra WA, Spetgens WP, Leijten FS, et al. Diurnal rhythms in seizures detected by intracranial ECoG-monitoring: an observational study. Epilepsy Behav 2009;14(4):617–21.

13. Hofstra WA, Gordijn MC, Van der Palen J, et al. Timing of temporal and frontal seizures in relation to the circadian phase: a prospective pilot study. Epilepsy Res 2011;94(3):158–62.

14. Shouse MN, da Silva AM, Sammaritano M. Circadian rhythm, sleep, and epilepsy. J Clin Neurophysiol 1996;13(1):32–50.

15. Pavlova MK, Shea SA, Scheer FA, et al. Is there a circadian variation of epileptiform abnormalities in idiopathic generalized epilepsy? Epilepsy Behav 2009;16(3):461–7.

16. Gachon F, Fonjallaz P, Damiola F, et al. The loss of circadian PAR bZip transcription factors results in epilepsy. Genes Dev 2004;18(12):1397–412.

17. Bazil CW, Walczak TS. Effects of sleep and sleep stage on epileptic and nonepileptic seizures. Epilepsia 1997;38(1):56–62.

18. Sammaritano MR, Therrien M. Epilepsy and the "sleep-wake cycle". In: Bazil CW, Malow BA, Sammaritano MR, editors. Sleep and epilepsy: the clinical spectrum. 2nd edition. Amsterdam: Elsevier Science; 2002. p. 145–56.

19. Kerkhof GA, Van Dongen HP. Morning-type and evening-type individuals differ in the phase position of their endogenous circadian oscillator. Neurosci Lett 1996;218(3):153–6.

20. Roenneberg T, Kuehnle T, Pramstaller PP, et al. A marker for the end of adolescence. Curr Biol 2004;14(24):R1038–9.

21. Roenneberg T, Merrow M. Entrainment of the human circadian clock. Cold Spring Harb Symp Quant Biol 2007;72:293–9.

22. Stewart LS, Leung LS. Temporal lobe seizures alter the amplitude and timing of rat behavioral rhythms. Epilepsy Behav 2003;4(2):153–60.

23. Stewart LS, Bercovici E, Shukla R, et al. Daily rhythms of seizure activity and behavior in a model of atypical absence epilepsy. Epilepsy Behav 2006;9(4):564–72.

24. Pung T, Schmitz B. Circadian rhythm and personality profile in juvenile myoclonic epilepsy. Epilepsia 2006;47(Suppl 2):111–4.

25. Hofstra WA, Gordijn MC, van Hemert-van der Poel JC, et al. Chronotypes and subjective sleep parameters in epilepsy patients: a large question-naire study. Chronobiol Int 2010;27(6):1271–86.

26. Bazil CW, Short D, Crispin D, et al. Patients with intractable epilepsy have low melatonin, which increases following seizures. Neurology 2000; 55(11):1746–8.

27. Laakso ML, Leinonen L, Hatonen T, et al. Melatonin, cortisol and body temperature rhythms in Lennox-Gastaut patients with or without circadian rhythm sleep disorders. J Neurol 1993;240(7):410–6.

28. Rao ML, Stefan H, Bauer J. Epileptic but not psychogenic seizures are accompanied by simultaneous elevation of serum pituitary hormones and cortisol levels. Neuroendocrinology 1989;49(1):33–9.

29. Schapel GJ, Beran RG, Kennaway DL, et al. Melatonin response in active epilepsy. Epilepsia 1995; 36(1):75–8.

30. Champney TH, Hanneman WH, Legare ME, et al. Acute and chronic effects of melatonin as an anticonvulsant in male gerbils. J Pineal Res 1996; 20(2):79–83.

31. Lapin IP, Mirzaev SM, Ryzov IV, et al. Anticonvulsant activity of melatonin against seizures induced by quinolinate, kainate, glutamate, NMDA, and pentylenetetrazole in mice. J Pineal Res 1998;24(4):215–8.

32. Mevissen M, Ebert U. Anticonvulsant effects of melatonin in amygdala-kindled rats. Neurosci Lett 1998;257(1):13–6.

33. Rudeen PK, Philo RC, Symmes SK. Antiepileptic effects of melatonin in the pinealectomized Mongolian gerbil. Epilepsia 1980;21(2):149–54.

34. Fauteck J, Schmidt H, Lerchl A, et al. Melatonin in epilepsy: first results of replacement therapy and first clinical results. Biol Signals Recept 1999; 8(1–2):105–10.

35. Molina-Carballo A, Munoz-Hoyos A, Reiter RJ, et al. Utility of high doses of melatonin as adjunctive anticonvulsant therapy in a child with severe myoclonic epilepsy: two years' experience. J Pineal Res 1997; 23(2):97–105.

36. Peled N, Shorer Z, Peled E, et al. Melatonin effect on seizures in children with severe neurologic deficit disorders. Epilepsia 2001;42(9):1208–10.

37. Coppola G, Iervolino G, Mastrosimone M, et al. Melatonin in wake-sleep disorders in children, adolescents and young adults with mental retardation with or without epilepsy: a double-blind, crossover, placebo-controlled trial. Brain Dev 2004; 26(6):373–6.

38. Sheldon SH. Pro-convulsant effects of oral melatonin in neurologically disabled children. Lancet 1998; 351(9111):1254.

39. Quigg M, Clayburn H, Straume M, et al. Hypothalamic neuronal loss and altered circadian rhythm of temperature in a rat model of mesial temporal lobe epilepsy. Epilepsia 1999;40(12):1688–96.

40. Quigg M, Straume M, Smith T, et al. Seizures induce phase shifts of rat circadian rhythms. Brain Res 2001;913(2):165–9.

Nocturnal Frontal Epilepsies: Diagnostic and Therapeutic Challenges for Sleep Specialists

Federica Provini, MD*, Francesca Bisulli, MD,
Paolo Tinuper, MD

KEYWORDS

- Nocturnal frontal lobe seizures • Paroxysmal arousal
- Nocturnal paroxysmal dystonia
- Epileptic nocturnal wandering • Limbic system
- Video-polysomnography

Nocturnal frontal lobe epilepsy (NFLE) is a particular form of partial epilepsy in which seizures appear almost exclusively during sleep and are characterized by complex and bizarre motor behaviors. NFLE was originally described by Lugaresi and Cirignotta in 1981.[1] The investigators coined the term nocturnal paroxysmal dystonia (NPD), underlying the peculiar motor pattern of these paroxysmal nocturnal events characterized by ballistic movements, bimanual-bipedal activity, rocking axial and pelvic torsion, and/or sustained dystonic posturing or tremor of the limbs.[1,2] The clinical and polysomnographic (PSG) features (stereotypic motor pattern of the episodes, their short duration and good response to low doses of carbamazepine) suggested an epileptic origin of the events. However, in the absence of concomitant electroencephalographic (EEG) epileptic discharges, the investigators posed the question whether these episodes constituted hitherto unrecognized epileptic seizures or a new kind of movement sleep disorder. Subsequently, Tinuper and colleagues,[3] reported two of three patients with NPD whose typical short-lasting NPD progressed to a convulsion. Subdural electrodes confirmed these were associated with ictal epileptic discharges arising from the frontal lobes. In all three patients, attacks occurred repeatedly with different intensity, representing "fragments" of the same seizure. They concluded that short-lasting attacks of NPD truly represent sleep-related frontal lobe seizures.

In subsequent years, all-night PSG recordings performed under audiovisual control documented that NFLE seizures form a wide spectrum of motor manifestations varying in complexity and duration.[4–9]

NFLE is currently considered a syndrome characterized by 3 main types of seizures: paroxysmal arousals (PAs, the simplest kind of seizure), NPD, and epileptic nocturnal wandering (ENW, the most complex type of seizure).

PAs are brief simple motor phenomena, similar to an apparent sudden awakening. During a PA, the patient displays stereotyped movements such as suddenly sitting up on the bed and raising head and trunk bringing the arms forward, with

Disclosure: Dr Provini has consulted for Sanofi-Aventis. Prof Tinuper has consulted for Cyberonics, Eisai, GSK, Janssen-Cilag, Novartis, Sanofi-Aventis, and UCB.
Financial disclosure: This study is supported by University of Bologna RFO 2010 grant.
Department of Neurological Sciences, IRCCS Istituto delle Scienze Neurologiche, University of Bologna, Via Ugo Foscolo 7, 40123 Bologna, Italy
* Corresponding author.
E-mail address: federica.provini@unibo.it

Sleep Med Clin 7 (2012) 105–112
doi:10.1016/j.jsmc.2011.12.007

a frightened expression (**Fig. 1**). In other cases, the patient can present dystonic postures and/or dyskinetic movements (choreoathetosic or ballistic) of a limb, typically the arm, or rhythmic movements of the pelvis and/or limbs, sometimes with vocalization. PA lasts for less than 20 seconds, is highly stereotyped and very frequent, and occurs repetitively (up to hundreds of times) throughout the night (see **Fig. 1**).

Patients are usually unaware of their behaviors during the night, but if PAs are very frequent, patients may feel exhausted on awakening in the morning and could present excessive daytime sleepiness.[6,10,11]

Major attacks, NPD, begin like PA, with a sudden arousal associated with complex, stereotyped, often violent motor behavior, with repetitive or rhythmic trunk and limb movements, rocking (coital-like) movements of the pelvis, vocalization, and screaming. In addition, patients may emit guttural sounds, curse, or swear, or they may even whistle or spit. In other episodes, a dystonic-dyskinetic component prevails and seizures may be characterized by asymmetric bilateral tonic postures with head deviation to one side, extension of the ipsilateral limbs, and flexion of the contralateral limbs (**Fig. 2**). In these cases, attacks resemble supplementary motor area seizures. NPD lasts longer (30–50 seconds) than PA.

ENW is the most complex and longest NFLE seizure type, lasting up to several minutes.[12,13] At the onset of the episodes, patients suddenly present dystonic posturing and dyskinetic movements. Then, they get out of bed and wander around, often maintaining dystonic postures, repeatedly jumping around and changing direction in a sort of grotesque dance.[13] They can vocalize unintelligibly and scream with a terrified expression. ENW can mimic sleepwalking, the well-known arousal parasomnia, but the agitated and violent motor behavior of ENW is quite different from the calmer physiologic motor pattern in sleepwalking patients.[13] ENW in patients examined by us was associated with more frequent PA and with NPD, the PA representing the initial features of the more complex long-lasting episodes. This association and the orderly complexity of the attacks suggested a progressive spread of the ictal discharge to involve wider brain

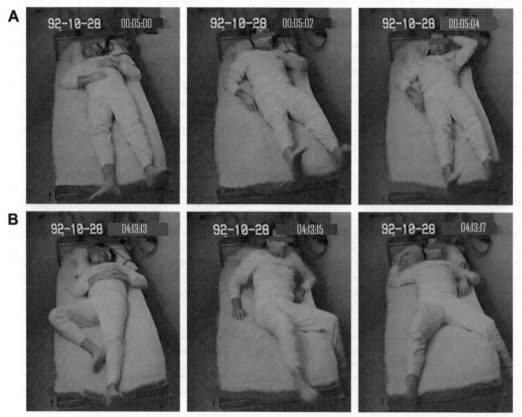

Fig. 1. Two PAs recorded in the same patient during the same night. The 2 photographic sequences (*A, B*) show the characteristic recurrent stereotyped semiology of PA. The patient abruptly sits up in bed, raising head and trunk, bringing the arms forward, with eyes open and a frightened expression.

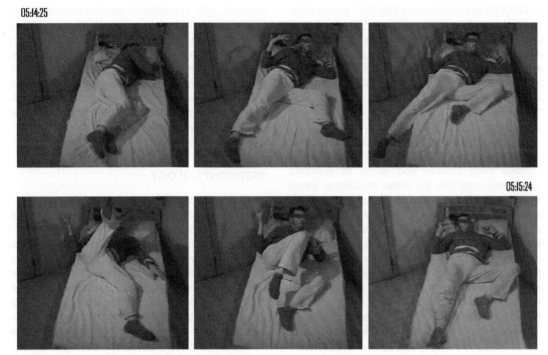

05:14:25

05:15:24

Fig. 2. Patient with NFLE displaying an NPD attack. Photographic sequences (excerpts taken at regular intervals) show the semiology of the episode characterized by violent movements of the trunk and limbs, in particular the legs, and dystonic asymmetric posturing.

regions in a graded manner.[5,14] Less than 10% of patients have only PA seizures; most have different types of seizures which tend to overlap in the same patient, the briefest episodes form the initial fragment of more prolonged attacks.[5,6]

CLINICAL FEATURES

NFLE affects both sexes, with a higher prevalence in men (women:men ratio is 3:7). Seizures appear more frequently during adolescence (mean age at onset, 14 ± 10 years) but can affect any age (until 64 years) and tend to increase in frequency during life.[6]

Neurologic examination is normal in most cases. Causative factors (such as birth anoxia, febrile convulsions, head injury) are present in only 10% of cases. Brain computed tomography/magnetic resonance imaging shows negative results in about 90% of cases.

Seizures are frequent, occurring every night or almost every night, usually many times per night (mean 3 ± 3 attacks nightly in our population), increasing in frequency over the years, without a spontaneous improvement.[6] Secondarily generalized seizures and/or seizures during wakefulness are rare, often appearing for limited periods.

A quarter of our patients had a positive family history for epilepsy, but the same seizure type,

consistent with a possible autosomal dominant pattern, was established in only a few cases. Nearly half of our patients had a positive family history for 1 or more parasomnias, and a third of our patients presented in their personal history taking, mostly in infancy, sleep disorders resembling parasomnias. This frequency is much higher than that reported for large control populations. This is not a mere coincidence because the data were confirmed in our recent prospective familial aggregation study in which statistical analysis showed that probands with NFLE had a higher lifetime prevalence of some parasomnias, namely, the arousal parasomnias and bruxism, than controls.[15] The higher frequency of arousal disorders in families with NFLE suggests an intrinsic link between parasomnias and NFLE. Several, not mutually exclusive, explanations for this link are possible, and, probably, an abnormal cholinergic system and related pathways could represent a model unifying the pathogenesis of NFLE and parasomnias.[16]

AUTOSOMAL DOMINANT NFLE

In 1994, Scheffer and colleagues[17,18] demonstrated that NFLE can be inherited as an autosomal dominant disorder, naming the condition autosomal dominant NFLE (ADNFLE). In 1995, Phillips and colleagues[19] mapped the locus responsible for ADNFLE to chromosome 20q13.2, and, subsequently, mutations in the gene encoding for the α4 subunit of the Ach neuronal receptor (CHRNA4) were demonstrated.[20] Further linkage sites were later described at chromosomes 15q24,[21] 3p22-24, and 8q11.2-q21.1,[22] and other mutations were reported in genes encoding for the α2 and β2 subunits of the Ach receptor (CHRNA2 and CHRNB2).[23–25]

Even though mutations in Ach nicotinic neuronal receptors remain a rare cause of ADNFLE, because most families and nearly all sporadic cases were negative for these mutations, these receptors do seem to be responsible for ADNFLE. In vitro analyses of the functional properties of nAChR disclosed a gain of function of these mutant receptors associated with ADNFLE[26] that may underlie the neuronal dysfunction responsible for the epileptic seizures. In addition, a recent positron emission tomography study comparing 8 nonsmoking patients with ADNFLE with 7 controls demonstrated a regional nAChR density decrease in the prefrontal cortex, despite the known distribution of these receptors throughout the cerebral cortex.[27]

EEG AND PSG FINDINGS

NFLE seizures appear almost exclusively during sleep, especially during non–rapid eye movement (NREM) sleep, in 60% of the cases during stage 2.[6]

Interictal wake and sleep EEG are often normal. Ictal EEG can be normal even during the episodes in almost half the cases. In some patients, special electrodes are needed to detect EEG epileptic abnormalities. In nearly all patients, seizure onset is characterized by autonomic manifestations involving heart rate, breathing, vasomotor tone, and sympathetic skin response.

By evaluating the autonomic response using a time-variant spectral analysis technique in 45 seizures in 10 patients with NFLE, we recently demonstrated a significant shift in autonomic cardiac control toward a sympathetic predominance in the 10 seconds preceding motor manifestation of seizures, with a further increase after seizure onset.[28] This autonomic activation resembles that observed before physiologic arousal from sleep and could therefore represent the autonomic expression of arousal, which in turn may facilitate seizure occurrence. Other neurophysiologic data support the involvement of an abnormal activation of the arousal system in the pathophysiology of NFLE and may trigger the onset of the epileptic discharge by modulating cortical excitability.[16]

A remarkable periodicity of the nocturnal attacks, in particular PA, could be detected in some patients, with stereotyped attacks occurring with a characteristic interval of 20 to 40 seconds for long stretches during NREM sleep, reflecting the pulsatility of arousal mechanisms.[29,30] A K complex often coincides or immediately precedes seizure onset, suggesting K complexes may provoke a cortical arousal mainly in the frontal cortex, facilitating a paroxysmal discharge in a predisposed subject, giving rise to repetitive seizures.[31]

PATHOPHYSIOLOGY

EEG and neuroradiologic and neurosurgical observations suggest that NFLE originates from foci in the mesio-orbital surface of the frontal lobe.[5,6] More recent neurosurgical studies in selected (pharmacoresistant) cases found that the epileptogenic focus was often located in extrafrontal areas, but even in these patients the ictal discharge seems to arise from the prefrontal allocortex.[32,33] According to Devinsky and colleagues,[34] the prefrontal allocortical regions, anterior cingulate gyrus, anterior insula, and orbitofrontal cortex belong to the so-called rostral limbic system.[34] Unlike the caudal limbic system (hippocampus, parahippocampal gyrus, and posterior cingulate gyrus), its rostral counterpart has mainly executive (motor) functions.[34] This view supports the finding that NFLE seizures originating from the prefrontal regions are mainly characterized by motor (somatomotor and visceromotor) manifestations. The ictal discharge arising in the frontal limbic cortex (mesio-orbital cortex) spreads to the adjacent areas of the frontal lobe (premotor and supplementary motor area), basal ganglia, basal forebrain, hypothalamus, and midbrain and, through a subset of parallel pathways, to the hindbrain and spinal cord. The limbic system makes use of this pathway known as the "emotional motor system" to modulate the somatomotor and visceromotor responses integrating instinctive behavior (**Fig. 3**).[35]

These multiple bonds linking the rostral limbic system to the prefrontal cortex, basal nuclei, hindbrain, and spinal cord would explain why a sudden arousal during a seizure lasting less than 2 minutes is accompanied by major autonomic manifestations, dystonic posturing, choreoathetosic and rhythmic dyskinetic movements, and, in many cases, abnormal emotional disorders such as shouting, swearing, whistling, spitting, and uttering obscenities.

Acknowledging that the limbic system comprises 2 anatomofunctionally different parts, it should be emphasized that the anterior region, the rostral limbic system, is involved in the physiopathology of NFLE seizures.

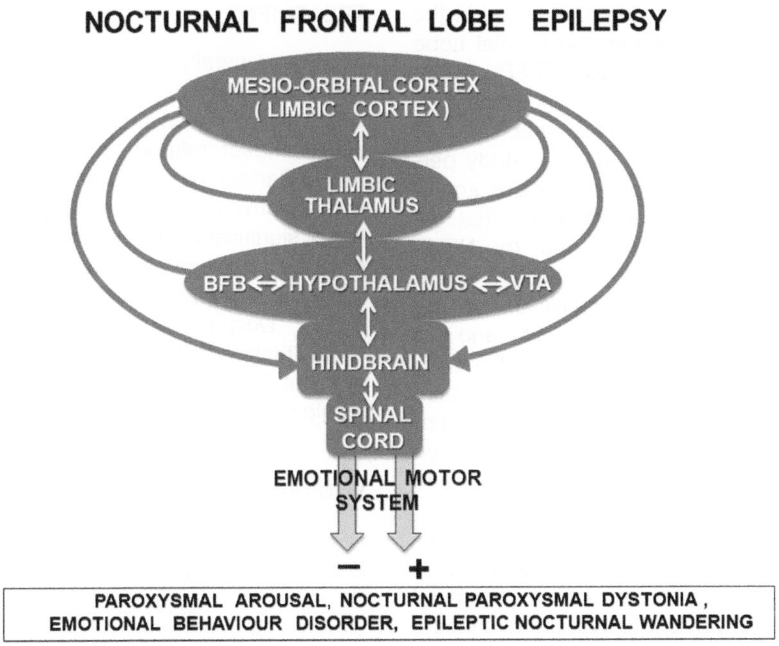

NOCTURNAL FRONTAL LOBE EPILEPSY

Fig. 3. Main anatomic structures involved in the manifestation of NFLE.

DIAGNOSIS PROCEDURES

Evaluation of NFLE seizures begins with an in-depth clinical interview with the patient but, most importantly, with family members, especially if they sleep in the same bed or room.[36,37] Detailed history taking elucidates the motor characteristics, frequency, duration, and timing of episodes. Prompting the patient to make audio-video recordings at home may often add details that are missed in verbal descriptions given by relatives. NFLE is much more likely than sleep arousal disorder if attacks arise or persist into childhood recurring several times during the same night. Moreover, NFLE seizures occur in a stereotyped manner, and tremor, dystonia, ballism, or abnormal movements are present during the attack.

Video-PSG (VPSG) monitoring for the diagnosis of NFLE remains necessary in complex cases or in cases in which there is doubt. In these patients, VPSG should include standard bipolar EEG (according to the International 10–20 System), electro-oculogram, electrocardiography, chin and limb electromyography (ie, of the right and left deltoid and tibialis anterior muscles), chest and abdominal respirogram. VPSG documents the abnormal motor aspect of the seizures with dystonic-dyskinetic postures or ballic components, the semiological features specific for NFLE. If doubts remain, it is useful to repeat the VPSG to demonstrate the stereotypy of the attacks.[38] Clearly, the more

frequent the events, the more likely VPSG will be of value.[37] In distinguishing NFLE from non-epileptic events, it is important to remember that the absence of scalp-recorded ictal EEG activity in no way rules out that the events are epileptic in nature since many NFLE seizures have no scalp-recorded ictal EEG activity or even postictal slowing.[6]

DIFFERENTIAL DIAGNOSIS

Distinguishing NFLE seizures from nonepileptic sleep-related events, in particular arousal disorders, is often difficult and sometimes impossible by history taking alone.[36,37] For this reason, before the advent of the audiovisual recordings, NFLE could be confused with arousal disorders.

Because of the nocturnal occurrence of NFLE, it is difficult to collect a reliable semiological description of the seizures from the bed partner, and crucial diagnostic features (dystonic posturing, hypermotor movements) are missed. In addition to clinical difficulties, ictal and interictal EEG discharges often fail to disclose epileptiform abnormalities in a substantial percentage of patients with NFLE so that diagnosis cannot be based on EEG findings. Sleep VPSG is the gold standard diagnostic test, but it is expensive and does not always capture the event in a single-night recording.

Alternative tools for establishing the diagnosis of NFLE, and distinguishing these seizures from NREM arousal disorders or REM sleep behaviour disorder (RBD) are still lacking. Discussed in the article elsewhere in this issue, the Frontal Lobe Epilepsy and Parasomnia scale (FLEP) developed by Derry and colleagues[39] is limited by contradictory diagnostic accuracy data.[40]

Recently a case-control diagnostic study performed by our group disclosed 2 major anamnestic patterns and 4 minor features that we called SINFLE (structured interview for NFLE) with unsatisfactory sensitivity but high specificity.[41] A positive history of dystonic or hyperkinetic pattern had a specificity of 91.5%, and this percentage improved if at least 1 of the following 4 minor anamnestic features was added: duration of the episode for less than 2 minutes, unstructured vocalization during the episode, experience of an aura preceding the motor attack, and a history of tonic-clonic seizures during sleep.[41]

In addition, episodes of sleep terror and sleepwalking are isolated and rare (1 episode every 1–4 months), without any stereotypic extrapyramidal patterns (dystonic posturing, ballic movements, tremor, choreoathetosis), and tend to disappear with time.

RBD can usually be differentiated from NFLE; RBD primarily affects elder males and episodes prevail in the second half of the night, unlike arousal disorders and ENW. Patients exhibit dream enactment and the PSG during these shows REM sleep without atonia. Nocturnal panic attacks are also characterized by a sudden awakening from sleep with dramatic autonomic activation and a sensation of imminent death but these episodes often recur only once per night and are prolonged (many minutes).[42]

Differential diagnosis of NFLE must include attacks described under the terms of NPD of intermediate and long duration.[5,43] NPD of intermediate duration (3–5 minutes) triggered by arousal during sleep and by protracted exercise during wakefulness differs from NFLE in duration because of the triggering effect of exercise and, above all, the peculiar motor pattern, characterized by asynchronous jerks of the head, trunk, and limbs, making the patient look like a puppet on strings. NPD with long-lasting (2–50 minutes) dystonic-dyskinetic attacks, arising from light sleep, recurring several times per night and resistant to antiepileptic drugs was observed in 2 patients. One of them developed Huntington disease 20 years after onset of the nocturnal attacks. The long duration of the attacks, the inefficacy of anticonvulsants, and the link with Huntington disease in 1 patient suggest a basal ganglia involvement. Long- and intermediate-duration dystonic-dyskinetic attacks are, however, extremely rare.

TREATMENT

NFLE is generally considered a benign disorder. Some patients decline therapy because their seizures are not disturbing and have a limited social impact related to their nocturnal occurrence. Carbamazepine, often at very low dosages, was effective in most patients with NFLE, controlling or significantly reducing seizures in about 70% of cases.[6] The same efficacy was reported for oxcarbazepine, especially in children,[44] and topiramate.[45] Despite the generally benign nature of NFLE, therapy failed to modify seizure frequency in about 30% of patients. In some of these cases, surgical treatment can provide excellent results.[32]

SUMMARY

NFLE is a more common epileptic syndrome than is currently believed, and its apparent rarity may be because diagnosis is seldom made without audiovisual recording. NFLE should always be suspected when paroxysmal nocturnal motor events arise or persist into adulthood and recur several times during the same night. To date, an international consensus on valid and reliable diagnostic procedures for NFLE is lacking. Future efforts must focus on developing a reliable algorithm to aid physicians in the differential diagnosis of paroxysmal motor sleep disorders.

ACKNOWLEDGMENTS

We thank Elena Zoni for photographic assistance and Anne Collins for assistance in preparing the manuscript.

REFERENCES

1. Lugaresi E, Cirignotta F. Hypnogenic paroxysmal dystonia: epileptic seizures or a new syndrome? Sleep 1981;4:129–38.
2. Lugaresi E, Cirignotta F, Montagna P. Nocturnal paroxysmal dystonia. J Neurol Neurosurg Psychiatry 1986;49:375–80.
3. Tinuper P, Cerullo A, Cirignotta F, et al. Nocturnal paroxysmal dystonia with short-lasting attacks: three cases with evidence for an epileptic frontal lobe origin of seizures. Epilepsia 1990;31:549–56.
4. Montagna P, Sforza E, Tinuper P, et al. Paroxysmal arousals during sleep. Neurology 1990;40:1063–6.
5. Montagna P. Nocturnal paroxysmal dystonia and nocturnal wandering. Neurology 1992;42:61–7.
6. Provini F, Plazzi G, Tinuper P, et al. Nocturnal frontal lobe epilepsy. A clinical and polygraphic overview of 100 consecutive cases. Brain 1999;122:1017–31.

7. Provini F, Montagna P, Plazzi G, et al. Nocturnal frontal lobe epilepsy: a wide spectrum of seizures. Mov Disord 2000;15:1264.

8. Provini F, Plazzi G, Lugaresi E. From nocturnal paroxysmal dystonia to nocturnal frontal lobe epilepsy. Clin Neurophysiol 2000;111(Suppl 2):S2–8.

9. Provini F, Plazzi G, Montagna P, et al. The wide clinical spectrum of nocturnal frontal lobe epilepsy. Sleep Med Rev 2000;4:375–86.

10. Peled R, Lavie P. Paroxysmal awakenings from sleep associated with excessive daytime somnolence: a form of nocturnal epilepsy. Neurology 1986;36:95–8.

11. Vignatelli L, Bisulli F, Naldi I, et al. Excessive daytime sleepiness and subjective sleep quality in patients with nocturnal frontal lobe epilepsy: a case-control study. Epilepsia 2006;47:73–7.

12. Pedley TA, Guilleminault C. Episodic nocturnal wanderings responsive to anticonvulsant drug therapy. Ann Neurol 1977;2:30–5.

13. Plazzi G, Tinuper P, Montagna P, et al. Epileptic nocturnal wanderings. Sleep 1995;18:749–56.

14. Nobili L, Francione S, Mai R, et al. Nocturnal frontal lobe epilepsy: intracerebral recordings of paroxysmal motor attacks with increasing complexity. Sleep 2003;26:883–6.

15. Bisulli F, Vignatelli L, Naldi I, et al. Increased frequency of arousal parasomnias in families with nocturnal frontal lobe epilepsy: a common mechanism? Epilepsia 2010;51:1852–60.

16. Montagna P, Provini F, Bisulli F, et al. Nocturnal epileptic seizures versus the arousal parasomnias. Somnologie 2008;12:25–37.

17. Scheffer IE, Bhatia KP, Lopes-Cendes I, et al. Autosomal dominant frontal epilepsy misdiagnosed as sleep disorder. Lancet 1994;343:515–7.

18. Scheffer IE, Bhatia KP, Lopes-Cendes I, et al. Autosomal dominant frontal epilepsy. A distinctive clinical disorder. Brain 1995;118:61–3.

19. Phillips HA, Scheffer IE, Berkovic SF, et al. Localization of a gene for autosomal dominant nocturnal frontal lobe epilepsy to chromosome 20q 13.2. Nat Genet 1995;10:117–8.

20. Steinlein OK, Mulley JC, Propping P, et al. A missense mutation in the neuronal nicotinic acetylcholine receptor alpha 4 subunit is associated with autosomal dominant nocturnal frontal lobe epilepsy. Nat Genet 1995;11:201–3.

21. Phillips HA, Scheffer IE, Crossland KM, et al. Autosomal dominant nocturnal frontal-lobe epilepsy: genetic heterogeneity and evidence for a second locus at 15q24. Am J Hum Genet 1998;63:1108–16.

22. Combi R, Ferini-Strambi L, Montruccoli A, et al. Two new putative susceptibility loci for ADNFLE. Brain Res Bull 2005;67:257–63.

23. De Fusco M, Becchetti A, Patrignani A, et al. The nicotinic receptor beta 2 subunit is mutant in nocturnal frontal lobe epilepsy. Nat Genet 2000;26:275–6.

24. Phillips HA, Favre I, Kirkpatrick M, et al. CHRNB2 is the second acetylcholine receptor subunit associated with autosomal dominant nocturnal frontal lobe epilepsy. Am J Hum Genet 2011;68:225–31.

25. Aridon P, Marini C, Di Resta C, et al. Increased sensitivity of the neuronal nicotinic receptor alpha 2 subunit causes familial epilepsy with nocturnal wandering and ictal fear. Am J Hum Genet 2006; 79:342–50.

26. Marini C, Guerrini R. The role of the nicotinic acetylcholine receptors in sleep-related epilepsy. Biochem Pharmacol 2007;74:1308–14.

27. Picard F, Bruel D, Servent D, et al. Alteration of the in vivo nicotinic receptor density in ADNFLE patients: a PET study. Brain 2006;129:2047–60.

28. Calandra-Buonaura G, Toschi N, Provini F, et al. Physiologic autonomic arousal heralds motor manifestations of seizures in nocturnal frontal lobe epilepsy: implications for pathophysiology. Sleep Med 2012, in press.

29. Lugaresi E, Coccagna G, Mantovani M, et al. Some periodic phenomena arising during drowsiness and sleep in man. Electroencephalogr Clin Neurophysiol 1972;32:701–5.

30. Sforza E, Montagna P, Rinaldi R, et al. Paroxysmal periodic motor attacks during sleep: clinical and polygraphic features. Electroencephalogr Clin Neurophysiol 1993;86:161–6.

31. Tinuper P, Bisulli F, Provini F, et al. Nocturnal frontal lobe epilepsy: new pathophysiological interpretations. Sleep Med 2011;12(Suppl 2):S39–42.

32. Nobili L, Francione S, Mai R, et al. Surgical treatment of drug-resistant nocturnal frontal lobe epilepsy. Brain 2007;139:561–73.

33. Proserpio P, Cossu M, Francione S, et al. Epileptic motor behaviors during sleep: anatomo-electroclinical features. Sleep Med 2011;12(Suppl 2):S33–8.

34. Devinsky O, Morrell MJ, Vogt BA. Contributions of anterior cingulate cortex to behaviour. Brain 1995; 118:279–306.

35. Holstege G, Bandler R, Saper CB. The emotional motor system. Prog Brain Res 1996;107:3–6.

36. Tinuper P, Provini F, Bisulli F, et al. Movement disorders in sleep: guidelines for differentiating epileptic from non-epileptic motor phenomena arising from sleep. Sleep Med Rev 2007;11:255–67.

37. Bisulli F, Vignatelli L, Provini F, et al. Parasomnias and nocturnal frontal lobe epilepsy (NFLE): lights and shadows—controversial points in the differential diagnosis. Sleep Med 2011;12(Suppl 2):S27–32.

38. Tinuper P, Grassi C, Bisulli F, et al. Split-screen synchronized display. A useful video-EEG technique for studying paroxysmal phenomena. Epileptic Disord 2004;6:27–30.

39. Derry CP, Davey M, Johns M, et al. Distinguishing sleep disorders from seizures: diagnosing bumps in the night. Arch Neurol 2006;63:705–9.

40. Manni R, Terzaghi M, Repetto A. The FLEP scale in diagnosing nocturnal frontal lobe epilepsy, NREM and REM parasomnias: data from a tertiary sleep and epilepsy unit. Epilepsia 2008;49:1581–5.

41. Bisulli F, Vignatelli L, Naldi I, et al. Diagnostic accuracy of a structured interview for nocturnal frontal lobe epilepsy (SINFLE): a proposal for developing diagnostic criteria. Sleep Med 2012;13:81–7.

42. Plazzi G, Montagna P, Provini F, et al. Sudden arousals from slow-wave sleep and panic disorder. Sleep 1998;21:548–51.

43. Lugaresi E, Cirignotta F. Two variants of nocturnal paroxysmal dystonia with attacks of short and long duration. In: Degen R, Niedermeyer E, editors. Epilepsy, sleep and sleep deprivation. Amsterdam: Elsevier; 1984. p. 169–73.

44. Raju GP, Sarco DP, Poduri A, et al. Oxcarbazepine in children with nocturnal frontal-lobe epilepsy. Pediatr Neurol 2007;37:345–9.

45. Oldani A, Manconi M, Zucconi M, et al. Topiramate treatment for nocturnal frontal lobe epilepsy. Seizure 2006;15:649–52.

Differentiating Seizures from Other Paroxysmal Nocturnal Events in Young and Older Adults

Christopher P. Derry, MB BS, MRCP, PhD

KEYWORDS

- Parasomnia • Nocturnal frontal lobe epilepsy • Sleep
- Epilepsy • EEG • Video

One of the important questions sleep clinicians and technologists ask when observing paroxysmal motor events during a polysomnogram (PSG) is whether this could be an epileptic seizure. Answering this question is often not straightforward. Clear descriptions of events are often lacking, because witness accounts are often absent or incomplete. Although nocturnal tonic-clonic seizures have characteristic features and are usually not difficult to diagnose (particularly if witnessed), partial seizures may cause more problems. Frontal lobe partial seizures during sleep are most likely to cause diagnostic confusion, especially when these occur predominantly or exclusively from sleep (so-called nocturnal frontal lobe epilepsy [NFLE]). Distinguishing them from nonepileptic parasomnias can be challenging.

An appreciation of the range of epileptic and nonepileptic sleep disorders, their clinical characteristics, and the use and limitations of investigations in this setting assists the clinician in reaching the correct diagnosis; these are reviewed in this article.

PAROXYSMAL NOCTURNAL EVENTS: THE DIFFERENTIAL DIAGNOSIS

There are several epileptic and nonepileptic conditions that should be considered in the patient with paroxysmal events in sleep.

Sleep-Related Seizures

Four main seizure types may occur predominantly or exclusively from sleep: generalized tonic-clonic, complex partial seizures of frontal lobe onset, complex partial seizures of temporal lobe onset, and tonic seizures. The characteristic features of these are discussed later.

Tonic-clonic seizures

Tonic-clonic seizures from sleep are usually easily diagnosed if collateral history is available from a bed partner or another witness. The characteristic progression of a tonic-clonic seizure is well described.[1] There may be an initial cry, followed by jaw clenching and cessation of respiration associated with tonic limb extension in which the limbs are usually extended. This tonic phase is followed by clonic jerking of the limbs, usually symmetric in nature, ending with a deep inspiration and subsequent stertorous breathing. A tonic-clonic seizure usually lasts 1.5 to 2.5 minutes. After the seizure, there is initially stupor, followed by confusion lasting minutes. Often this is followed by a return to sleep.

Even if no witness account is available, tonic-clonic seizures may be associated with tongue biting (usually on the lateral aspect) and urinary incontinence; evidence of such features on waking should raise the suspicion that a tonic-clonic

Conflicts of interest: The author has none to disclose.
Financial disclosures: The author has none to disclose.
Department of Clinical Neurosciences, Western General Hospital, Crewe Road, Edinburgh, EH4 2XU, UK
E-mail address: cderry@nhs.net

Sleep Med Clin 7 (2012) 113–123
doi:10.1016/j.jsmc.2011.12.006
1556-407X/12/$ – see front matter © 2012 Elsevier Inc. All rights reserved.

seizure occurred, particularly if associated with generalized myalgias and unusual fatigue, headache, amnesia, or malaise.

Frontal lobe seizures

Complex partial seizures arising from the frontal lobes can cause diagnostic confusion, because the features range from subtle to dramatic or bizarre.[2] Most individuals with frontal lobe epilepsy (FLE) have a significant proportion or all of their events during sleep. NFLE is the diagnosis if 90% or more of the seizures arise from sleep. Frontal lobe complex partial seizures are usually characterized by an abrupt, often explosive-onset, awakening of the patient from non–rapid eye movement (NREM) 2 sleep accompanied by sustained asymmetric dystonic, tonic posturing, violent hypermotor behaviors, thrashing, pedaling, and/or kicking of the lower extremities. Patients are often aware during the seizure, but say they cannot control their movements or vocalizations.

Other motor automatic movements (automatisms) that may be seen include prominent bimanual and bipedal movements, such as bicycling or kicking movements of the legs, hand clapping, and/or leg slapping. Some stand, walk, or run during the seizure, although they rarely wander far. Axial body movements, such as rocking, thrashing, running (often in an apparently agitated or distressed manner), sitting up, and head nodding are also common. Automatisms in some patients have a semipurposeful quality.[3] Sexual automatisms, such as pelvic thrusting and genital manipulation, are sometimes observed.[4]

Vocalization is common, and often consists of unintelligible screaming or moaning. Some individuals exhibit palilalia (repeating their own words) or scream obscenities; others breathe strangely but without vocalization.[3] The seizure often wakes the patient from sleep, and consciousness may be preserved during it. Some report that a brief aura wakes them, often nonspecific or sometimes an unpleasant choking sensation.[5] Although some complex partial frontal lobe seizures may include tonic postures or clonic movements, reflecting involvement of the supplementary motor area or primary motor cortex respectively, many do not and are characterized by automatisms only.

The seizures of NFLE are often characterized by paroxysmal attacks of increasing complexity and duration. Minor attacks are characterized by stereotyped limb, axial musculature, and/or head movements that typically last 2 to 4 seconds.[2] Paroxysmal arousals consist of abrupt, stereotyped arousals from sleep accompanied by trunk and head elevation often with vocalization and frightened expression that often last only 5 to 10 seconds. Major attacks (formerly called nocturnal paroxysmal dystonia) typically last 20 to 30 seconds and are characterized by stereotyped asymmetric tonic or dystonic posturing, bizarre hyperkinetic behaviors, bipedal automatisms, axial movements of the trunk and pelvis, vocalization, and tonic or dystonic posturing. Episodic nocturnal wanderings are uncommon, characterized by agitated ambulation, screaming, and sometimes semipurposeful automatisms.[6]

Patients rarely have a single type of attack. Smaller episodes are usually considered fragments of larger seizures,[2] and all events are considered to be manifestations of the same underlying epileptic process.[7] These can be difficult to distinguish from nonepileptic arousals.[8] They may occur repetitively and frequently throughout the night, and are often underreported, with some individuals being unaware of the episodes.[2]

Temporal lobe seizures

Between 50% and 80% of patients with temporal lobe epilepsy (TLE) report that some of their seizures occur during sleep,[9] although seizures in TLE more often occur when awake. Secondarily generalised tonic clonic seizures (GTC) in TLE occur most often during sleep, with partial seizures more common in wakefulness. Exclusively nocturnal TLE is uncommon.[10] Individuals with nocturnal TLE are usually woken by a typical temporal lobe aura (autonomic, experiential, or special sensory) that progresses to a complex partial seizure characterized by expressionless staring with minor oral or limb automatisms. Although TLE should be considered in the diagnosis of paroxysmal nocturnal events, in my experience, diagnostic difficulty is less common than for FLE because they usually have seizures awake, interictal epileptiform discharges (IEDs) awake and asleep, and their seizures are accompanied by ictal electroencephalogram (EEG) patterns.

Tonic seizures

Tonic seizures occur predominantly in individuals with learning disability and symptomatic generalized epilepsy, particularly Lennox-Gastaut syndrome (LGS). LGS most often appears between ages 2 and 6 years, is characterized by frequent daily seizures of multiple types, and is usually accompanied by developmental delay and psychological and/or behavioral problems. Tonic seizures are the most frequently occurring seizure type in LGS, 90% of which occur during sleep. These seizures are typically brief, lasting only seconds, and are characterized by symmetric or asymmetric posturing of the upper limbs, often with involvement of the neck, trunk, and lower limbs. They usually occur in clusters during sleep (affected individuals may have dozens of tonic seizures per night), and less often in wakefulness. Tonic seizures do not usually present diagnostic challenges, although occasionally are subtle and only recognized on video-EEG monitoring.

NONEPILEPTIC MOTOR DISORDERS OF SLEEP

Nonepileptic motor disorders of sleep are common and varied. The second edition of the International Classification of Sleep Disorders (ICSD-2), developed by the American Academy of Sleep Medicine (AASM),[11] groups such disorders into parasomnias, sleep-related movement disorders, and others (**Box 1**). A full discussion of these conditions is beyond the scope of this article, can be found elsewhere,[12] but the most commonly confused conditions are reviewed here.

Parasomnias

Parasomnias are defined in the ICSD-2 as "unpleasant or undesirable behavioral or experiential phenomena that occur predominantly or exclusively during the sleep period."[11] Parasomnias are subdivided by phenomenology into 3 subgroups: disorders of arousal (from NREM sleep), parasomnias usually associated with REM sleep, and others (see **Box 1**).

NREM arousal parasomnias

NREM arousal disorders are the most frequently encountered parasomnias and the most likely to cause diagnostic confusion with epilepsy. They are characterized by paroxysmal motor behaviors, without conscious awareness, usually occurring during stage 3 or 4 NREM sleep (rarely NREM 2). They have a broad spectrum of clinical manifestations, and are loosely subdivided into 3 main forms, albeit with significant overlap.[8] Confusional arousals are associated with sudden arousal and a period of apparent confusion, but little motor or autonomic involvement. Somnambulism (sleepwalking) is associated with motor activity, typically walking, but also other semipurposeful tasks such as moving objects, talking nonsensically, dressing, eating, and drinking,[13] but with little autonomic or affective involvement. Sleep terrors (pavor nocturnus) are dramatic events characterized by prominent autonomic and affective features; the individual suddenly arouses from deep sleep, usually with a terrified scream, appearing agitated and frightened, with tachycardia and diaphoresis.

NREM arousal parasomnias vary in duration, lasting from 1 or 2 minutes to longer than 30 minutes. They tend to begin in early childhood, and are common; an estimated 15% to 20% of

---

Box 1
The major paroxysmal motor disorders of sleep, categorized according to the second edition of the International Classification of Sleep Disorders

1. Parasomnias
   a. NREM arousal disorders
      i. Confusional arousals
      ii. Sleepwalking
      iii. Sleep terrors
   b. Parasomnias usually associated with rapid eye movement (REM) sleep
      i. REM sleep behavior disorder
      ii. Parasomnia overlap disorder
      iii. Sleep paralysis
   c. Other parasomnias
      i. Catathrenia (nocturnal groaning)
2. Sleep-related movement disorders
   a. Periodic limb movements of sleep
   b. Sleep bruxism
   c. Nocturnal leg cramps
   d. Rhythmical movement disorder (RMD; jactacio capitis nocturna)
3. Other (nonparasomnia, nonmovement disorder) paroxysmal nocturnal events
   a. Sleep starts
   b. Somniloquy
   c. Benign sleep myoclonus of infancy
   d. Nocturnal psychogenic nonepileptic seizures (PNES, or pseudoseizures)
   e. Nocturnal panic attacks
   f. Sleep-related breathing disorders
   g. Gastroesophageal reflux
   h. Newly recognized conditions
      i. Excessive fragmentary myoclonus
      ii. Propriospinal myoclonus at sleep onset
      iii. Rhythmical feet movements while falling asleep
      iv. Alternating leg muscle activation during sleep and arousals

Data from American Sleep Disorders Association. American Academy of Sleep Medicine: The International Classification of Sleep Disorders: diagnostic and coding manual. 2nd edition. Westchester (IL): American Academy of Sleep Medicine; 2005.

children[14] have at least 1 episode of sleepwalking. Although resolution in adolescence is typical, they persist in an estimated 1% to 4% of adults.[15] NREM arousal parasomnias are thought to arise through incomplete or impaired arousal from deep NREM sleep,[16] resulting in a dissociation between sleep and wake states.[17] Because of their high prevalence in otherwise normal children, they are considered to represent altered physiologic processes during brain maturation rather than true abnormality. In some cases, an underlying process causing frequent arousals (such as obstructive sleep apnea [OSA]) may precipitate parasomnias,[18] or the use of drugs that increase the intensity of slow wave sleep (gabapentin, sodium oxybate).[19]

REM sleep behavior disorder

REM sleep behavior disorder (RBD) is characterized by a loss of muscle atonia during REM sleep resulting in the acting out of dream content (oneiric behaviors). During REM sleep, patients display complex and often violent behaviors such as screaming, punching and kicking, jumping out of bed, and running.[20] These behaviors may result in injury to the patients or their bedpartners.[21] Individuals can usually be wakened from these episodes, when they may report vivid, disturbing dreams.[22] Episodes may last from a few minutes to half an hour, and although some patients have episodes several times per night, in others they are less frequent. Events occur preferentially in the second half of sleep, when the greatest proportion of REM sleep occurs.[23] Recent studies show that the motor movements in RBD are typically brief: 75% lasted less than 2 seconds, 83% were simple, 14% complex, 11% had vocalizations, and only 4% were violent. The motor behaviors of RBD tend to (1) be more severe at the end of the night when most REM sleep occurs; (2) be more in phasic (than tonic) REM sleep; (3) exhibit night-to-night variability (but not for REM sleep without atonia); (4) most often be limb jerks (most often of the arms); (5) usually not involve leaving the bed; and (6) often feature no apparent increase in the heart rate during episodes (perhaps because of loss of heart rate variability).[24–27] A strong association between chronic RBD and degenerative neurologic conditions, particularly Parkinson disease (PD) and multiple system atrophy (MSA), has been reported,[20,21] RBD often preceding parkinsonian features by several years.[28] RBD mainly affects individuals more than 50 years of age,[20] with men affected in more than 80% of large reported series.[21]

Other parasomnias

Other parasomnias, including sleep paralysis, may occasionally be considered in the differential diagnosis of epilepsy, but their presentation is so characteristic that diagnostic confusion should not occur. Sleep paralysis is characterized by episodes of absent voluntary motor activity at sleep onset or waking, usually lasting for a few minutes. Individuals are aware but paralyzed, and may experience vivid hallucinations. The episodes may subside spontaneously, and may be aborted if the individual is touched.[29] Sleep paralysis is thought to represent an intrusion of REM sleep into wakefulness. It may occur in otherwise normal individuals, particularly after a change in sleep pattern or sleep restriction,[30] but is also a feature of narcolepsy with cataplexy.

Sleep-Related Movement Disorders

Although parasomnias cause the main diagnostic confusion with seizures, some movement disorders in sleep may also occasionally cause difficulties.

Periodic limb movements during sleep

Periodic limb movements during sleep (PLMS) are characterized by repetitive and stereotyped movements of the legs (extension of the great toe and dorsiflexion of the ankle), predominantly during NREM sleep; occasionally the upper limbs may be involved. However, from a diagnostic perspective, PLMS are usually not confused with epilepsy because the interval between jerks is too long.

Rhythmic movement disorder

RMD consists of stereotyped rhythmical motor behaviors that occur primarily in drowsy wakefulness and the transition to sleep. Video-PSG studies have shown that RMD often emerges from NREM 1, NREM 2, or occasionally REM sleep.[31] RMD movements include body rocking, body rolling, head banging, and head rolling. Movements typically occur at a frequency of 0.5 to 2 movements per second for less than 15 minutes per episode. They often are accompanied by rhythmical humming or rhythmical vocalization, often in time with each rock, bang, or roll. RMD during wakefulness is associated with varying degrees of awareness; some patients acknowledge a pleasurable aspect to them, whereas others are unaware.[32] The condition is common in developmentally normal children, affecting 59% of infants at 9 months of age. It usually resolves early in childhood, with prevalence decreasing to 5% by 5 years.[33] RMD is uncommon in adults and, when present, is more likely to be associated with intellectual disability, autism, and/or anxiety, and rarely acquired following trauma or encephalitis.[34] It should not be confused with epilepsy, although the rarity of the condition in adulthood may occasionally lead to misdiagnosis in this age group.

Other Paroxysmal Nocturnal Events

Some other motor conditions also warrant consideration in the differential diagnosis of nocturnal epilepsy.

Sleep starts

Sleep starts are a common, quasiphysiologic phenomenon occurring at the transition from wakefulness to sleep. Sleep starts are characterized by sudden brief myoclonic jerks of legs, arms, or whole body at sleep onset, often associated with sensory phenomena (such as a sensation of falling, a flash of light, or other fragmentary or visual, auditory, or somesthetic hallucinations). Multiple jerks occasionally occur in succession; a sharp cry may occur. Between 60% and 70% of people have experienced these. Excessive caffeine or other stimulant use, intense work or exercise, and emotional stress can increase their intensity. Chronic severe clusters of sleep starts rarely cause sleep-onset insomnia, chronic anxiety, and fear of falling asleep. Sleep starts rarely require investigation or treatment, although, if severe, can cause sleep-onset insomnia, a condition known as excessive fragmentary hypnic myoclonus.[35]

Nocturnal psychogenic nonepileptic seizures

Psycghogenic non-epileptic attacks (PNES, or pseudoseizures) are reported from sleep in 12% to 58% of patients with PNES.[36,37] Video-EEG in this condition shows apparent sleep (so-called pseudosleep) at onset, in which the patient behaviorally appears asleep but EEG shows wakefulness. PNES restricted exclusively to pseudosleep are rare, with most patients having events both in wakefulness and apparent sleep.[36] In sleep-related panic attacks, the patient wakes with a feeling of impending doom, tachycardia, and sweating. The episodes usually last several minutes, return to sleep is difficult, and vivid recall of the events is typical.[38] They are common in panic disorder, with around half of patients with panic disorder reporting at least 1 such episode. Almost all patients with nocturnal panic attacks experience similar daytime episodes, although a small subgroup have symptoms predominantly at night.[38]

Sleep talking

Sleep talking (somniloquy) occurs predominantly during light NREM sleep or arousals from deeper sleep, although it can be a REM sleep phenomenon.[13] It is common, particularly in children, and usually consists of single words or short sentences, sometimes associated with body movement. It may be associated with NREM arousal

disorders, OSA, or RBD, but rarely causes diagnostic confusion with epilepsy.

Obstructive sleep apnea

OSA is rarely confused with epilepsy, but sometimes causes recurrent arousals from sleep that may be confused with the paroxysmal arousals pattern of NFLE. If a good witness account of snoring, choking, and apneic periods is available, diagnostic uncertainty is less likely to arise, although this distinction can be more difficult if the individual sleeps alone.

IMPORTANT FACTORS IN THE HISTORY

Taking a detailed history of the events from both the patient and witness is crucial, and is the most important part of the diagnostic workup. Obtaining the witness account is often challenging or even impossible, particularly if the patient sleeps alone. Many of the nonepileptic syndromes discussed earlier are easily distinguished from epilepsy if an adequate history is obtained. The most commonly encountered diagnostic dilemma is distinguishing parasomnias (NREM arousal parasomnias or RBD) from NFLE. Because of their similar presentations, distinguishing these conditions can be difficult, even when a good witness account is available; as a result, misdiagnosis is common and may persist for years.[39,40] There are several features in the history that may be helpful, and these aspects should be fully explored (**Table 1**).

Age of Onset

NREM parasomnias tend to appear earlier than frontal lobe seizures, with a peak prevalence between the ages of 5 and 10 years.[41,42] NFLE usually begins in middle to late childhood or adolescence. The mean age of onset of NFLE in the largest case series of 100 patients was 14 ($\pm$10) years (but the range was 1–64 years).[2] The mean age of onset was 7.5 years among 22 children with NFLE.[43] However, the range is wide within both conditions, making these population features less diagnostically useful in individual cases. In contrast, RBD appears in an older age group (predominantly men more than 50 years of age); it is rare for NFLE to appear at this age.

Frequency and Clustering of Paroxysmal Nocturnal Events

On average, individuals with NFLE report 3 to 8 events in 1 night,[2,44] and reports of greater than 20 are common. Clustering of seizures is common, with many occurring over 1 or more nights,

Table 1
Differentiating NREM arousal disorder from NFLE

	NREM Arousal Disorder (eg, Sleepwalking, Sleep Terrors)	NFLE
Age at onset	Usually <10 y	Variable; usually childhood or adolescence
Positive family history	60%–90%	Up to 40%
Attacks per night (mean)	1 or 2	3 or more
Episode frequency/mo	<1–4	20–40
Clinical course (over years)	Tends to disappear by adolescence	Often stable with increasing age
Disease duration (mean)	Approx 7 y	Approx 20 y
Episode duration	Seconds to 30 min	Seconds to 3 min (often less than 2 min)
Semiology of movements	Variable complexity; not highly stereotyped (on video)	Highly stereotyped on video monitoring, often vigorous movements
Trigger factors	Sleep deprivation, febrile illness, alcohol, stress	Often none identified
Associated conditions	Obstructive sleep apnea	Often none identified
Ictal EEG	Slow waves, no epileptiform features	Often normal, or obscured by movement. Epileptiform ictal rhythms in <10%
Time of episodes during sleep	First third of night, but usually after 90 min of sleep	Any time, but may occur in first 30–60 min
PSG sleep stages when events occur	NREM stage 3 or 4	Usually stage 2 NREM, occasionally stage 3 or 4

From Derry C, Duncan JS, Berkovic S. Paroxysmal motor disorders of sleep: the clinical spectrum and differentiation from epilepsy. Epilepsia 2006;47(11):1775–91; with permission.

followed by a period with few events. In contrast, NREM arousal disorders usually occur no more than once or twice per night, and rarely cluster.[42]

Timing

NFLE seizures characteristically occur during NREM 2 sleep, and therefore are common soon after falling asleep, or just before waking in the morning.[44] NREM parasomnias usually arise from NREM 3 or 4 sleep, and typically occur during the longest period of consolidated slow wave sleep, which is generally around 1 or 2 hours after falling asleep. Occasional daytime seizures are reported to occur in 30% of patients with NFLE; fewer than 20% report ever having a generalized convulsion.[2] Symptoms that should prompt concern for sleep-related epileptic seizures include (1) events occurring any time of the night, just after falling asleep, or shortly before awakening in the morning; (2) multiple events per night; and/or (3) occasional occurrence of these events when awake or during a brief nap.

Ictal Behaviors

There are few specific features that discriminate between the motor patterns observed during NFLE and parasomnias.[8,42] However, the prominent stiffening and dystonic posturing often seen in NFLE (reflecting involvement of the supplementary sensorimotor cortex) is unusual in parasomnias.[2,8]

Awareness, Auras, and Recollection

Patients with NFLE are often woken by their seizures and retain awareness in at least a proportion of them. In such cases, they may report a distinct aura, typically a somatic sensation or a feeling that their breath is stuck in their throats.[5,40] Although patients with parasomnias may retain vague recollections of frightening or unpleasant feelings, it is more common to have no recall.

Duration

NFLE seizures are typically brief, usually less than 1 minute and rarely lasting for more than 2 minutes.[2] Parasomnias may also be brief, but more commonly last for several minutes; some may go on for 15 minutes or longer. Events lasting for more than 2 minutes are unlikely to be frontal lobe seizures.

Stereotypy

Video studies of NFLE have revealed marked stereotypy in many patients with NFLE; in some individuals, their brief attacks are identical to the onset of their longer seizures.[2,8] Parasomnias, although often broadly similar in an individual, usually show a degree of variability.[8]

Vocalization

Vocalization is common in parasomnias and NFLE. Most commonly, this is restricted to shouts, groans, or single words, such as mum or help, when it has no discriminatory value. When more complex speech is present, this can be useful because, in NFLE, such speech often reflects retained awareness and is usually remembered, whereas the complex speech of parasomnias occurs while the individual is unaware, and is not remembered the next day.

An accurate history, taking into consideration the points discussed earlier, is often sufficient to distinguish NFLE from parasomnias,[45] although no single feature is sufficiently reliable to confirm the diagnosis. We have found the diagnostic process may be facilitated by use of the Frontal Lobe Epilepsy and Parasomnias (FLEP) scale (**Table 2**).[45] This is a short, validated clinical questionnaire, incorporating the features most useful in distinguishing NFLE and parasomnias. The scale is designed to divide patients into 1 of 3 groups: NFLE, parasomnia (nonepilepsy), and indeterminate; patients in the indeterminate group usually need further investigation (see later discussion).

The initial study using the FLEP scale reported good positive predictive values (PPV) and negative predictive values (NPV), at 0.91 and 1.00 respectively.[45] A subsequent validation study, performed by a different group, found comparable results, with a PPV of 1.00 and NPV of 0.91.[46] However, in the second study, there was a high proportion of indeterminate scores, particularly in individuals with RBD, suggesting that the scale is less useful for this condition.[46] In addition, some patients with NFLE were classified as having NREM parasomnias using the FLEP scale. Nevertheless, the statistical analyses indicate that the scale represents a reasonable screening tool for NFLE, particularly for individuals in whom further investigation may be difficult.

DIAGNOSTIC TESTING

The AASM clinical practice parameters recommend in-laboratory video-PSG (V-PSG) to evaluate parasomnias that are unusual or atypical because of the patient's age at onset; the time, duration, or frequency of occurrence of events; or the specifics of the particular motor patterns in question (eg, stereotypical, repetitive, or focal).[47] A PSG is not needed if the nocturnal events are typical, noninjurious, infrequent, and not disruptive to the child or family.[47] However, in children with sleep terrors or sleepwalking events occurring more than 2 to 3 times per week (and symptoms that suggest OSA or PLMS), a PSG should be considered. I find that prolonged inpatient video-EEG monitoring is more useful because a typical event is often not recorded in a single night (or even 2 nights) of PSG.

Because frequent unexplained paroxysmal nocturnal events are uncommon in adults, further investigation is often necessary if diagnostic uncertainty remains. An EEG with sleep is probably the first investigation if sleep-related epilepsy is suspected, but if this is normal a period of monitoring will usually be neccessary. If the patients spells occur only at night and are frequent, a V-PSG with expanded EEG may suffice, especially if concomitant OSA or RBD is suspected. If the first (or second with 24-hours of sleep deprivation) routine EEG with sleep is normal, inpatient video-EEG monitoring for 2 to 5 days is probably the next best step. Prolonged video-EEG monitoring is often a better choice when (1) the events do not occur nightly or every other night, (2) a primary sleep disorder (eg, OSA) is unlikely, (3) there is a history of postictal agitation or wandering, and/or (4) cooperation of the patient is questionable.

Other standard investigations are often unhelpful. In NFLE, neuroimaging (magnetic resonance imaging [MRI]) and interictal EEG are usually normal,[2] as they are in NREM parasomnias. Although these investigations should be performed in most cases, in practice they often add little to the diagnosis. In those individuals in whom events occur only infrequently, home video of events (on mobile phones or cameras) may be helpful, although it is often difficult to record an attack in its entirety using this method.

Even when an individual has events recorded on video-EEG or PSG with expanded EEG monitoring, difficulties remain. Ictal scalp-recorded EEG in individuals with NFLE often shows no ictal EEG changes, and is often marred by artefact. Only around half of NFLE seizures are associated with an ictal rhythm or other epileptiform EEG changes,[2] and there are no specific EEG features in NREM arousal parasomnias. The stage of sleep

Table 2
The FLEP scale

Clinical Feature		Score
Age at onset		
At what age did the patient have the first clinical event (y)?	<55	0
	≥55	−1
Duration		
What is the duration of a typical event (min)?	<2	+1
	2–10	0
	>10	−2
Clustering		
What is the typical number of events to occur in a single night?	1 or 2	0
	3–5	+1
	>5	+2
Timing		
At what time of night do the events most commonly occur?	Within 30 min of sleep onset	+1
	Other times (including if no clear pattern is identified)	0
Symptoms		
Are the events associated with a definite aura?	Yes	+2
	No	0
Does the patient ever wander outside the bedroom during the events?	Yes	−2
	No (or uncertain)	0
Does the patient perform complex, directed behaviors (eg, picking up objects, dressing) during events?	Yes	−2
	No (or uncertain)	0
Is there a history of prominent dystonic posturing, tonic limb extension, or cramping during events?	Yes	+1
	No (or uncertain)	0
Stereotypy		
Are the events highly stereotyped or variable in nature?	Highly stereotyped	+1
	Some variability/uncertain	0
	Highly variable	−1
Recall		
Does the patient recall the events?	Yes; lucid recall	+1
	No or vague recollection only	0
Vocalization		
Does the patient speak during the events and, if so, is there subsequent recollection of this speech?	No	0
	Yes; sounds only or single words	0
	Yes; coherent speech with incomplete or no recall	−2
	Yes; coherent speech with recall	+2
Total score		

From Derry C, Davey M, Johns M, et al. Distinguishing sleep disorders from seizures: diagnosing bumps in the night. Arch Neurol 2006;63(7):1037; with permission.

from which events arise is an important clue; most NFLE seizures occur from NREM 2 sleep (often with multiple minor events being seen),[2] whereas NREM arousal parasomnias are usually isolated events arising from NREM 3 or 4.[8]

Thus, analysis of ictal semiology is the critical step. The ictal semiological features of NFLE, although varied, are well described.[2,7] In particular,

the recording of asymmetric tonic posturing typical of supplementary sensorimotor area involvement, or agitated axial or bipedal bicycling automatisms, may enable a confident diagnosis of NFLE, even if the EEG is unhelpful or obscured by artifact.[8] Likewise, various semiological features have been identified that favor a diagnosis of parasomnias.[8] A waxing and waning pattern of behaviors, verbal

Table 3
Important quantitative and qualitative features which can be used in the positive identification of parasomnias.[8]

Features Strongly Favouring Parasomnias	Features Moderately Favouring Parasomnias	Features Which do not Discriminate Between Parasomnias and NFLE
Yawning	Tremor/trembling	Brevity
Scratching and prominent nose-rubbing	Myoclonic jerks Coughing	Sitting
Rolling over in bed	Semipurposeful behaviours, fumbling, manipulation of nearby objects	Standing or walking
Internal or external trigger (noise, cough, snore)	Variability/absence of stereotypy	Preceding 'normal' arousal
Waxing and waning pattern	No events recorded on first night of monitoring	Brief arousals (up to 10 seconds) without definite semiological features of epilepsy
Physical or verbal interaction	Few events recorded in total (less than 3)	Fearful emotional behaviour
Sobbing, sad emotional behaviour		
Indistinct offset		
Failure to fully arouse after event with complex behaviour		
Prolonged duration (>2 minutes)		
Discordance between severity and duration of *reported* event and *recorded* event		

interaction, failure to rouse to full wakefulness after prominent motor activity, and an indistinct offset to episodes (in which the end of the attack cannot be clearly demarcated) all favor an NREM arousal parasomnia rather than NFLE. A summary of important semiological features, including those that have been shown to have no discriminatory value, are shown in **Table 3**. A simple algorithm (**Fig. 1**) is available for analyzing events,[8] although independent validation is still required.

In some patients, despite recording events on video-EEG monitoring, diagnostic doubt may remain because many of the behavior patterns seen in NFLE and parasomnias are similar and, in some cases, indistinguishable. These similarities may be caused by the same neuronal networks (central pattern generators [CPGs]) being involved in both conditions.[48] CPGs are neural networks that endogenously (ie, without sensory or cortical input) produce patterns of behavior.[49,50]

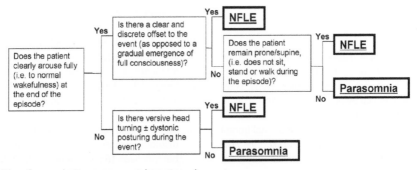

Fig. 1. Algorithm for analysing paroxysmal nocturnal events.

Bibliography

Although some are continuously active (eg, those involved in respiration), others (eg, those involved in locomotion) can be turned on and off; in mammals the latter are largely under neocortical control.[48,51] It has been hypothesized that CPGs may play a role in oral automatisms in TLE (feeding-related CPGs), and bipedal automatisms in FLE (locomotor CPGs).[48,52] Tassinari and colleagues[48] advanced this concept, suggesting that parasomnias may also reflect activation of CPGs, providing a possible explanation for why parasomnias are sometimes difficult to distinguish from NFLE. CPGs are discussed in detail elsewhere in this issue.

SUMMARY

Differentiating seizures from other paroxysmal events in sleep poses challenges for the clinician. An appreciation of the range and characteristic features of sleep disorders and sleep-related epileptic seizures is critical; in practice, the most common diagnostic dilemma is between parasomnias and epileptic seizures, particularly NFLE. The most important diagnostic information is obtained from the history, and obtaining adequate descriptions from witnesses, whenever possible, is paramount. Use of the FLEP scale may be a helpful guide in this context, although its limitations should be recognized. Routine investigations including MRI brain and EEG may sometimes be helpful but are often normal in nonepileptic parasomnias and NFLE. When events are sufficiently frequent, comprehensive video-EEG monitoring may be diagnostic. For situations in which this is not practicable, home video recordings of events may be helpful. In most cases, it is possible to make a confident diagnosis using a combination of these modalities.

ACKNOWLEDGMENTS

I would like to thank Dr Richard Davenport and Dr Susan Duncan for their comments on the manuscript.

REFERENCES

1. Rodin EA. Differential diagnosis of epileptic versus psychogenic seizures. In: Dam M, Gram L, Penry JK, editors. Advances in epileptology: XIIth Epilepsy International Symposium. New York: Raven Press; 1981. p. 337–41.
2. Provini F, Plazzi G, Tinuper P, et al. Nocturnal frontal lobe epilepsy. A clinical and polygraphic overview of 100 consecutive cases. Brain 1999;122(Pt 6): 1017–31.
3. Chauvel P, Kliemann F, Vignal JP, et al. The clinical signs and symptoms of frontal lobe seizures: phenomenology and classification. Adv Neurol 1995;1995(66): 115–26.
4. Spencer SS, Spencer DD, Williamson PD, et al. Sexual automatisms in complex partial seizures. Neurology 1983;33(5):527–33.
5. Scheffer IE, Bhatia KP, Lopes-Cendes I, et al. Autosomal dominant nocturnal frontal lobe epilepsy. A distinctive clinical disorder. Brain 1995;118(Pt 1): 61–73.
6. Plazzi G, Tinuper P, Montagna P, et al. Epileptic nocturnal wanderings. Sleep 1995;18(9):749–56.
7. Provini F, Plazzi G, Lugaresi E. From nocturnal paroxysmal dystonia to nocturnal frontal lobe epilepsy. Clin Neurophysiol 2000;111(Suppl 2):S2–8.
8. Derry C, Harvey A, Walker M, et al. NREM arousal parasomnias and their distinction from nocturnal frontal lobe epilepsy: a video EEG analysis. Sleep 2009;32(12):1637–44.
9. Chokroverty S, Quinto C. Sleep and epilepsy. In: Chokroverty S, editor. Sleep disorders medicine. Boston: Butterworth-Heinemann; 1999. p. 697–727.
10. Bernasconi A, Andermann F, Cendes F, et al. Nocturnal temporal lobe epilepsy. Neurology 1998; 50(6):1772–7.
11. American Sleep Disorders Association. American Academy of Sleep Medicine: The International Classification of Sleep Disorders: diagnostic and coding manual. 2nd edition. Westchester (IL): American Academy of Sleep Medicine; 2005.
12. Derry C, Duncan JS, Berkovic S. Paroxysmal motor disorders of sleep: the clinical spectrum and differentiation from epilepsy. Epilepsia 2006;47(11):1775–91.
13. Aldrich M. Parasomnias. In: Aldrich M, editor. Sleep medicine. Oxford (United Kingdom): Oxford University Press; 1999.
14. Laberge L, Tremblay RE, Vitaro F, et al. Development of parasomnias from childhood to early adolescence. Pediatrics 2000;106(1 Pt 1):67–74.
15. Hublin C, Kaprio J, Partinen M, et al. Prevalence and genetics of sleepwalking: a population-based twin study. Neurology 1997;48(1):177–81.
16. Broughton RJ. Sleep disorders: disorders of arousal? Science 1968;159(3819):1070–8.
17. Bassetti C, Vella S, Donati F, et al. SPECT during sleepwalking. Lancet 2000;356(9228):484–5.
18. Espa F, Dauvilliers Y, Ondze B, et al. Arousal reactions in sleepwalking and night terrors in adults: the role of respiratory events. Sleep 2002;25(8):871–5.
19. Lange CL. Medication-associated somnambulism. J Am Acad Child Adolesc Psychiatry 2005;44(3): 211–2.
20. Schenck CH, Mahowald MW. REM sleep behavior disorder: clinical, developmental, and neuroscience perspectives 16 years after its formal identification in SLEEP. Sleep 2002;25(2):120–38.

21. Olsen EJ, Boeve BF, Silber MH. Rapid eye movement sleep behaviour disorder: demographic, clinical and laboratory findings in 93 cases. Brain 2002;123:331–9.

22. Fantini ML, Ferini-Strambi L, Montplaisir J. Idiopathic REM sleep behavior disorder: toward a better nosologic definition. Neurology 2005;64(5):780–6.

23. Schenck CH, Bundlie SR, Ettinger MG, et al. Chronic behavioural disorders of REM sleep: a new category of parasomnia. Sleep 1986;9:293–308.

24. Iranzo A, Ratti PL, Casanova-Molla J, et al. Excessive muscle activity increases over time in idiopathic REM sleep behavior disorder. Sleep 2009;32(9): 1149–53.

25. Frauscher B, Gschliesser V, Brandauer E, et al. Video analysis of motor events in REM sleep behavior disorder. Mov Disord 2007;22(10):1464–70.

26. Frauscher B, Iranzo A, Hogl B, et al. Quantification of electromyographic activity during REM sleep in multiple muscles in REM sleep behavior disorder. Sleep 2008;31(5):724–31.

27. Oudiette D, De Cock VC, Lavault S, et al. Nonviolent elaborate behaviors may also occur in REM sleep behavior disorder. Neurology 2009;72(6):551–7.

28. Schenck CH, Bundlie SR, Mahowald MW. Delayed emergence of a parkinsonian disorder in 38% of older men initially diagnosed with idiopathic rapid eye movement behaviour disorder. Neurology 1996;46:388–93.

29. Sheldon SH. Disorders of development and maturation of sleep, and sleep disorders of infancy, childhood and cerebral palsy. In: Culebras A, editor. Sleep disorders and neurological disease. New York: Marcel Dekker; 2000.

30. Takeuchi T, Miyasita A, Sasaki Y, et al. Isolated sleep paralysis elicited by sleep interruption. Sleep 1992; 15(3):217–25.

31. Dyken ME, Rodnitzky RL. Diagnosing rhythmic movement disorder with video-polysomnography. Pediatr Neurol 1992;16:37–41.

32. Zaiwalla Z. Parasomnias. Clin Med 2005;5(2):109–12.

33. Klackenberg G. A prospective longitudinal study of children. Data on psychic health and development up to 8 years of age. Acta Paediatr Scand Suppl 1971;224:1–239.

34. Chisholm T, Morehouse RL. Adult headbanging: sleep studies and treatment. Sleep 1996;19:343–6.

35. Vetrugno R, Plazzi G, Provini F, et al. Excessive fragmentary hypnic myoclonus: clinical and neurophysiological findings. Sleep Med 2002;3(1):73–6.

36. Duncan R, Oto M, Russell AJ, et al. Pseudosleep events in patients with psychogenic non-epileptic seizures: prevalence and associations. J Neurol Neurosurg Psychiatry 2004;75(7):1009–12.

37. Thacker K, Devinsky O, Perrine K, et al. Nonepileptic seizures during apparent sleep. Ann Neurol 1993; 33:414–8.

38. Craske MG, Tsao JC. Assessment and treatment of nocturnal panic attacks. Sleep Med Rev 2005;9(3): 173–84.

39. Lombroso CT. Pavor nocturnus of proven epileptic origin. Epilepsia 2000;41(9):1221–6.

40. Scheffer IE, Bhatia KP, Lopes-Cendes I, et al. Autosomal dominant frontal epilepsy misdiagnosed as sleep disorder. Lancet 1994;343(8896):515–7.

41. Kales JD, Kales A, Soldatos CR, et al. Night terrors. Clinical characteristics and personality patterns. Arch Gen Psychiatry 1980;37(12):1413–7.

42. Zucconi M, Ferini-Strambi L. NREM parasomnias: arousal disorders and differentiation from nocturnal frontal lobe epilepsy. Clin Neurophysiol 2000; 111(Suppl 2):S129–35.

43. Sinclair DB, Wheatley M, Snyder T. Frontal lobe epilepsy in childhood. Pediatr Neurol 2004;30(3): 169–76.

44. Berkovic SF, Scheffer IS. Autosomal dominant nocturnal frontal lobe epilepsy. In: Bazil CW, Malow BA, Samaritno MR, editors. Sleep and epilepsy: the clinical spectrum. Amsterdam: Elsevier Science; 2002. p. 217–22.

45. Derry C, Davey M, Johns M, et al. Distinguishing sleep disorders from seizures: diagnosing bumps in the night. Arch Neurol 2006;63(7):1037.

46. Manni R, Terzaghi M, Repetto A. The FLEP scale in diagnosing nocturnal frontal lobe epilepsy: data from a tertiary sleep and epilepsy unit. Epilepsia 2008;49(9):1581–5.

47. Kushida CA, Littner MR, Morgenthaler T, et al. Practice parameters for the indications for polysomnography and related procedures: an update for 2005. Sleep 2005;28(4):499–521.

48. Tassinari CA, Rubboli G, Gardella E, et al. Central pattern generators for a common semiology in fronto-limbic seizures and in parasomnias. A neuroethologic approach. Neurol Sci 2005;26(Suppl 3): s225–32.

49. Hooper SL. Central pattern generators. Curr Biol 2000;10(5):R176.

50. Grillner S, Wallen P. Central pattern generators for locomotion, with special reference to vertebrates. Annu Rev Neurosci 1985;8:233–61.

51. Grillner S. The motor infrastructure: from ion channels to neuronal networks. Nat Rev Neurosci 2003; 4(7):573–86.

52. Meletti S, Cantalupo G, Volpi L, et al. Rhythmic teeth grinding induced by temporal lobe seizures. Neurology 2004;62(12):2306–9.

Relationship of Central Pattern Generators with Parasomnias and Sleep-Related Epileptic Seizures

Carlo Alberto Tassinari, MD[a], Elena Gardella, MD, PhD[b,c],
Gaetano Cantalupo, MD[d], Guido Rubboli, MD[b,e],*

KEYWORDS

- Central pattern generators • Parasomnias
- Sleep-related epileptic seizures • Arousal

In 1911, Graham Brown[1] was the first to show the existence of neuronal networks within the thoracic spinal cord capable of producing repetitive rhythmic hind limb movements resembling locomotion. He reported that rhythmic alternating locomotorlike motor movements were observed in antagonistic muscles in each hind limb for a short time after experimental thoracic spinal cord transection in an animal model that had previously had its dorsal sensory roots sectioned.[1] These experiments unequivocally showed that neuronal aggregates in the spinal cord (deprived from sensory inputs and supraspinal influences) can generate a coordinated rhythmic motor movement.

Since then, a wealth of molecular, genetic, and neuroimaging studies have confirmed that such autonomous motor neural networks (now called central pattern generators [CPGs]) are present in all animals. CPGs are located in the midbrain, pons, and vertebrate spinal cord. They are genetically determined neural networks (circuits) that are capable of producing self-sustained patterns of innate motor behaviors critical for survival (eg, feeding, locomotion, reproduction, respiration, fleeing from danger) without sensory or motor feedback.[2–4] Although they are present in all organisms (from worms to humans), CPGs display species-specific features.[5]

Recently, we proposed that certain motor behaviors observed in parasomnias and epileptic seizures have similar features and resemble the output of particular CPGs. A temporary loss of cerebral cortical control can occur in both sleep and certain sleep-related seizures; an arousal can then permit the emergence of stereotyped, inborn, fixed-action motor patterns that are independent of the nature of the trigger (seizure or parasomnia) and reflect activation of the same CPGs.[6–9]

In this review, the motor expressions of events related to epileptic seizures and parasomnias are discussed, and other important, albeit relevant, components, such as subjective feelings, impairments of consciousness or memory, variations of vegetative functions, and site of origin of the epileptic seizure, are disregarded. We argue that these motor fragments, regardless of whether they are

All the authors report no conflicts of interest or financial disclosures related to this paper.
[a] Neuroscience Department, University of Parma, via Volturno 39, 43125 Parma, Italy
[b] Danish Epilepsy Center, Epilepsihospitalet, Dianalund, Denmark
[c] Epilepsy Center, San Paolo Hospital, University of Milan, 20142 Milan, Italy
[d] Child Neuropsychiatry Unit, University of Parma, via Gramsci 14, 43126 Parma, Italy
[e] Neurology Unit, Bellaria Hospital, IRCCS Institute of Neurological Sciences, via Altura 3, 40139 Bologna, Italy
* Corresponding author. Doctor Sells Vej 22, 4293 Dianalund, Denmark.
E-mail address: grubboli@libero.it

Sleep Med Clin 7 (2012) 125–134
doi:10.1016/j.jsmc.2012.01.003
1556-407X/12/$ – see front matter © 2012 Elsevier Inc. All rights reserved.

a product of an epileptic seizure or a parasomnia, induce remarkably similar repetitive stereotyped motor sequences, which represent inborn motor patterns that are, from an ethological perspective, crucial to the survival of our species. In this respect, these behavioral motor activities represent genetically determined inborn motor patterns, resulting from genes that code for neuronal networks subserving instinctive motor behaviors, as well as for hormones, peptides, enzymes, and other factors responsible for such behavioral manifestations. Our argument is that a motor fragment that occurs during a particular epileptic seizure has identical features to motor activities that characterize some parasomnias because they represent the activation of the same CPGs during sleep.

OROMOTOR CPG BEHAVIORS

Brainstem masticatory CPGs are essential to generate motor patterns in cranial motoneurons of the tongue, facial, and masticatory muscles involved in swallowing, chewing, respiration, self-defense, and predatory functions.[10] Masticatory CPGs can produce rhythmic licking, lapping, and chewing movements, which can be refined by sensory feedbacks from the peripheral nervous system to the brainstem, showing that CPGs are adaptable and capable of responding to different environmental situations.[11–13] The basic jaw movement rhythm can be modified by proprioceptive information coming mainly from muscle spindles of masticatory muscles, which accounts for the sensory feedback and feedforward information that modulates the CPG.[14–16]

Masticatory brainstem CPGs can be subdivided into 2 neuronal aggregates: (1) a central timing network (CTN), which provides the timing signal for rhythmic alternation of jaw opening and closing, and (2) the CPG neuronal group, which orchestrates jaw, tongue, and facial muscle activity patterns, organizes the intracycle motor pattern, and executes the movement.[17,18] Each oscillation of the CTN drives the CPG to produce the motor output for 1 movement cycle. Other brainstem masticatory CPGs (such as chewing, licking, and lapping motor movements) probably share the same CTN but the CPGs producing the motor movements may differ.[17–19]

Sleep bruxism (SB) is a sleep disorder that is characterized by recurring episodes of rhythmic masticatory activity of the masseter and temporalis muscles accompanied by the noise of grinding or clenching teeth.[20] SB usually follows an arousal, and sometimes concludes with a swallow, and can occur in any stage of sleep but most often non-rapid eye movement (NREM) stage 1 or NREM

stage 2. SB is probably an extreme audible expression of another brainstem masticatory CPG, rhythmic masticatory muscle activity.[21]

Sleep-related faciomandibular myoclonus (FM) is another primary sleep-related movement disorder that at first glance resembles SB but is characterized on polysomnography by spontaneous myoclonic jerks of the facial, masticatory, and sometimes sternocleidomastoid muscles during NREM sleep without the tonic electromyographic masticatory activity typical of SB.[22] Sleep-related FM can cause repetitive tongue biting and bleeding, and has been mistaken for sleep-related epilepsy.[23] Biting often accompanying aggression has rarely been observed to occur during epileptic seizures.[24,25] Repetitive fly-biting or jaw-snapping is a frequent and characteristic feature of epileptic seizures in dogs.[26] Jaw-snapping, which can lead to biting, has also been observed during both epileptic and nonepileptic events in humans and dogs.

Periodic limb movements in sleep (PLMS) are more common in patients with SB. Repetitive leg movements sometimes accompany episodes of SB.[21] PLMS are believed to reflect disinhibition of the locomotor CPG.[27] Studies in humans have shown that PLMS are associated with increased spinal cord excitability with lower thresholds and greater spatial spread of the spinal flexor reflexes.[28] Rhythmic teeth grinding and leg movements have been observed in patients with anterior and mesial temporal lobe seizures (**Fig. 1**A).[29] Seizure-related oroalimentary automatisms in focal seizures are believed to indicate involvement of the amygdalohippocampal structures by the epileptic discharge.[20,21,30,31] Mild masticatory movements also occur in prolonged absence seizures (lasting >20 seconds or longer), even triggered by merely inserting something chewable in the mouth of the patient during an absence seizure.[32] Rhythmic orofacial contractions and perioral myoclonia seen in some absence seizures may also represent a release of normally inhibited brainstem masticatory CPGs.[33] These data suggest that the same masticatory CPGs can be activated in etiologically different pathologic conditions (SB, PLMS) and seizure types (absence and temporal lobe complex partial seizures) (see **Fig. 1**).

Oroalimentary activity during sleep may be particularly prominent in individuals with sleep-related eating disorders (SRED). SRED is defined as a parasomnia with recurrent episodes of eating after arousal from nighttime sleep that have adverse consequences. Episodes are described as compulsive, involuntary, and most often patients cannot be easily awakened during them. Epidemiologic studies suggest that nocturnal eating and

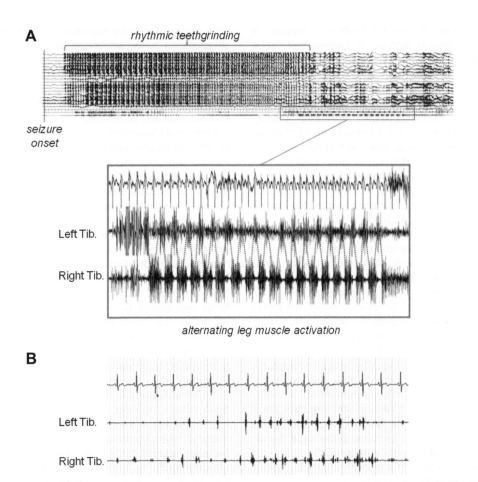

Fig. 1. (*A*) Polygraphic recording of a sleep-related focal epileptic seizure in a patient with left mesial temporal lobe epilepsy, characterized by prolonged rhythmic teeth grinding (note the muscular artifacts masquerading the electroencephalographic traces in the first part of the seizure) (see also Ref.[29]). As the seizure evolves and ends, teeth grinding progressively fades away to be followed by rhythmic alternating leg movements (magnified in the lower insert showing electromyographic activity in the left and right tibialis anterior), which persist also in the postictal phase. (*B*) In a different patient, detail of a polygraphic recording showing sleep-related nonepileptic rhythmic alternating leg movements (see also Ref.[91]). The rhythmic alternating pattern of electromyographic contractions shown in (*A*) and (*B*) is similar, suggesting activation of the same CPG. (*Courtesy of* Lino Nobili, Centre of Sleep Medicine, Niguarda Hospital, Milan.)

SRED are particularly common in patients with restless legs syndrome (RLS) and PLMS. A recent case-control study found 33% of 100 adults with RLS self-reported SRED compared with 1% of 100 matched controls randomly selected from the general population.[34]

Masticatory automatisms have been described during episodes of postural hypotension in a patient with multiple system atrophy,[35] and in normal individuals during reflex-induced vasovagal syncope,[36] further supporting the hypothesis that the same CPG can be activated in a variety of pathophysiologically and etiologically different conditions.

EMOTIONAL CPG BEHAVIORS

The expression of emotions is a universal behavior in both animals[37] and humans.[38] The facial expression for each emotion results from selective and distinctive inborn motor patterns, elegantly codified in humans by Ekman and Friesen.[39] The ability to accurately interpret facial expressions is of primary importance for humans to interact socially with one another. Facial expressions communicate information from which one can quickly infer the state of mind of one's peers, and adjust one's behavior accordingly. From this point of view, the human face can be viewed as a transmitter of expression signals and the brain as a decoder of these expression signals. It follows that facial expressions and the underlying motor circuitry (regulated by brainstem CPGs that orchestrate the facial nerves and musculature) have evolved to optimize the transmission of these signals.[39,40]

Humans during epileptic seizures display a coherent pattern of activation of facial muscles comparable with that observed in genuine universal facial emotions in normal individuals (in addition to several nonemotional facial displays).[7,41] Coherent patterns of facial emotions are particularly observed during seizures involving the medial temporal, cingulate, and orbitofrontal cortex. Using a facial action coding system (FACS), we documented that both fear and sadness are facially expressed during epileptic seizures and use the same physiologic patterns of facial muscle activation that normal individuals use to express the same emotions (**Fig. 2**).[7,41] In another study, we found a few frontotemporal epileptic seizures that were also associated with displays of emotions and the corresponding complex behavior, suggesting the involvement of a wide physiologic network including prefrontal, frontomesial, and temporal limbic structures.[42] Ictal discharges for all emotions showed a right hemisphere predominance (except for happiness, which is associated with left-sided seizures), confirming the right hemispheric specialization for emotion.

A recent retrospective study[43] reported a gender dimorphism in the ictal facial expression of emotions, which reproduces a physiologic dimorphism of human expression of emotion, reflecting either inborn or sociobehavioral differences. These investigators found no gender difference for ictal fear in children. However, more adult women reported ictal fear than adult men, and more men than women had ictal fear during childhood that disappeared during adulthood. Studies of human behavioral psychology document the prevalence of expression of rage in males and of happiness/sadness in females, relating this dimorphism to different gender social roles: competitive in males and more joining in females.

Emotional parasomnias such as sleep terrors and nightmares clearly indicate a high level of emotional arousal. In rapid eye movement sleep behavior disorder (RBD), facial expressions of emotions, mainly of negative valence, are frequently observed.[44] Are facial expressions of basic emotions the same whether related to an epileptic event (limbic-hypothalamic network) or nonepileptic emotional parasomnias? Are sleep terrors and nightmares expressed by the same encoded muscle activation pattern in epilepsy as in physiologic conditions? To our knowledge, no study of facial expression during these sleep terrors or nightmares has been performed. It is relevant that decoding recognition of facial emotions is significantly impaired in epileptic patients with damage to the medial temporal lobe network occurring early in infancy.[45,46]

Aggressive behaviors related to epilepsy have been widely reported,[47,48] and can occur in the ictal, postictal, and interictal periods.[49,50] Investigation of biting behavior as a model of aggressive behavior related to epileptic seizures has been shown to occur as a reflexive behavior in the context of strong emotional arousal, fear, or anger. Biting acts were evoked (both during and after seizures) by external stimuli such as actions of people in close contact with the patient. Using stereoelectroencephalography with intracranial recording, we demonstrated that the amygdala/hippocampal region and orbitomedial prefrontal

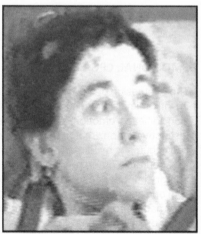 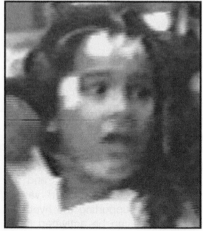

Fig. 2. Facial emotion expressing surprise during a temporal lobe seizure (*left*) and fear during a nocturnal frontal lobe seizure (*right*).

cortex were both involved when ictal biting behaviors were observed.[25] These data suggest that seizure-related biting behavior could result from a loss of inhibitory control of higher centers on CPGs modulating instinctive behaviors (ie, aggressive behavior),[25,51] findings that are in agreement with the views of Jasper[52] on epileptic automatisms representing a paretic phenomenon (ie, the expression of loss of control).

Violent and aggressive behaviors during sleep are observed in patients with a variety of sleep disorders including NREM arousal disorders, RBD, and sleep-related epilepsies (especially nocturnal frontal lobe epilepsy [NFLE]).[53] One study found a high prevalence of NREM arousal parasomnias and SB in the personal and family histories of patients with NFLE compared with normal age-matched healthy controls.[54] Single-photon emission tomography studies have shown similar patterns of cingulate and cerebellar hyperperfusion during episodes of sleepwalking and epileptic paroxysmal arousals.[55,56] Current evidence showing that sleepwalking, sleep terrors, and some epileptic seizures display similar ictal semiology and can be similarly provoked by sleep deprivation and arousal are in keeping with our hypothesis that both arousal disorders and NFLE share the same final common pathway (ie, activation of the same CPGs in the brainstem and spinal cord).[8,9,53]

LOCOMOTOR CPG BEHAVIORS

Experimental studies in animals have shown that electrical stimulation of the spinal cord and supraspinal structures, such as brainstem (the so-called mesencephalic locomotor region)[3,57,58] and cerebellum,[59] can initiate locomotion. We also know that the basal ganglia are responsible for selecting the appropriate locomotory CPGs by the inhibitory action of striatal neurons on the globus pallidus, which in turn exert a tonic inhibitory drive on CPG networks. Striatal neurons can in turn be activated by the neocortex.[60,61] Some data in humans have shown that electrical stimuli delivered to the lumbar spinal cord can evoke locomotorlike activity in spinal cord–transected paraplegic patients.[62,63] Involuntary rhythmic stepping leg movements were described in a patient whose spinal cord was transected.[64] Therefore, based on this evidence, we and others assume that locomotory CPGs exist in the spinal cord in humans.[61,65] There is likely to be a shared interphyletic basis for motor actions such as swaying, creeping, swimming, climbing, walking, crawling, trotting, and galloping.

Rhythmic leg activity during epileptic seizure has also been described by Wada[66] (who called it bipedal activity).[67] Epileptic seizures manifested by alternating leg flexion and extension at the hip, or pedaling, suggest a frontal involvement, but the origin of the seizure may be from mesiofrontal[68] or extrafrontal networks.[66,69–71] Crawling progression can be observed during a seizure when a patient is in a prone position. In some instances, the prone position is assumed from other initial body postures (need to pronate). Semipurposeful and prolonged ambulatory activity (sometimes called episodic or paroxysmal nocturnal wandering) can occur during sleep-related partial epileptic seizures as a part of complex motor manifestations,[72,73] resembling the features of sleepwalking.[74]

Gardella and colleagues[75] reported a patient with long-standing drug-resistant focal epilepsy who took a few steps forward when standing after they performed high-frequency electrical stimulation of his right frontodorsolateral cortex, which provoked a paroxysmal afterdischarge that spread into the frontomesial region (**Fig. 3**). Because these

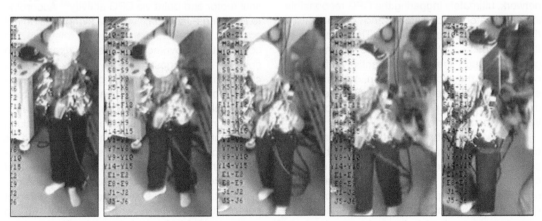

Fig. 3. Locomotor activity in a standing patient suffering from drug-resistant focal epilepsy induced by intracerebral (stereoelectroencephalographic) high-frequency electrical stimulation of the right frontodorsolateral cortex, which was accompanied by a paroxysmal discharge spreading into the frontomesial region (see also Ref.[75]).

motor movements were seen only when associated with an afterdischarge involving a wide frontomesial and lateral region, the investigators postulated that the relationship between dorsofrontal electrical stimulation and the appearance of a locomotor behavior was mediated by a relatively widespread cortical dysfunction involving mesial frontal regions, which led ultimately via a release mechanism to the activation of spinal locomotor CPGs. Similar alternating leg movements during sleep of nonepileptic nature, mimicking locomotor activity and consistent with the activation of spinal locomotor CPGs, characterize RLS in augmentation.[9,76]

In individuals with NFLE, highly stereotyped minor motor events (MMEs) in the form of short-lasting stereotyped movements involving the limbs, the axial musculature, or the head have been described in either the presence or absence of an epileptic ictal discharge (ED). In addition, the occurrence of both EDs and MMEs was associated with higher levels of arousal.[77] These findings support the hypothesis that because recurrence of EDs can in itself increase the arousal level, the occurrence of MMEs would not depend on a direct effect of EDs, but rather originate from an indirect effect related to loss of cortical inhibition, secondary to arousal. Accordingly, MMEs associated or not with EDs may result from a specific disinhibition triggered by internal epileptic stimuli of innate motor patterns generated by CPGs.[77]

PHYSIOPATHOGENIC SPECULATIONS

Seizure-induced cortical dysfunction (related to excessive epileptic discharges or the postictal phase) might result in the activation of the basal ganglia, thereby impinging on the locomotor network, ultimately triggering the CPG responsible for masticatory, copulatory, and deambulatory rhythmic CPG motor activity.[75] The selection of the appropriate CPG is mediated by the basal ganglia through the inhibitory activity of striatal neurons on the globus pallidum, which in turn exerts an inhibitory effect on other CPG networks. In addition, striatal neurons can be directly activated by the neocortex.[61,78]

Rhythmic oral motor and ambulatory sequences can be observed in acute hypoxic cerebral episodes. Hypoxia reduces the firing of cerebral cortical neurons, a condition that is exactly the opposite of an epileptic seizure.[73,79] Sleep-related disorders, such as bruxism and RLS, do not share any common physiopathogenic mechanisms with epileptic seizures or hypoxic episodes, yet they show the same oral motor and ambulatory behavior-related CPG activity. Sleep per se is a condition characterized by cyclic functional rearrangement of the corticosubcortical-spinal network, favoring profound modifications of motor functions such as axial muscle atonia, hypnic myoclonus, areflexia, and eye movements. Furthermore, the Babinski sign can be evoked during physiologic sleep,[80] as well as in relation to various parasomnias.[81]

In the triune brain concept proposed by MacLean,[82] when neomammalian function is disrupted, the paleomammalian and reptilian brains take over, expressing their old functional networks. In the ontogenesis of premature and newborn babies, it is possible to trace a variety of oromotor (alimentary) and ambulatory (automatic creeping, alternating progression) behaviors and motor reflexes (grasping and the Babinski sign), which indicates that the neomammalian cortical networks are anatomically and functionally unable to interact with the subcortical-spinal CPG (Fig. 4).

Progressive maturation of the neocortex leads to a parallel functional modification; as the infant acquires the ability to voluntarily control different behaviors, natatory and automatic quadrupedal progression disappears along with other primitive reflexes (including the spontaneous Babinski sign). Grasping also subsides for selected finger grips, although grasping can reappear during frontal seizures (Fig. 5).[83,84] However, the CPG and various reflex networks persist as a sort of carillon,[8] ready to act in their own rhythmic way to play their unchanging rhythmic motor symphony: the kinetic melody of Luria.[85] The CPG expressed is independent of its cause, whether a seizure, an anoxic event, or a parasomnia.

We believe that the general mechanism of release might explain how these different causes can set a cascade in motion, terminating with the final motor end point via CPG activity[86] According to Hughlings-Jackson,[87] "These symptoms do not occur in, but after, the paroxysm; they are too coordinated movements to result directly from epileptic discharges; there is, I think, a duplex condition: (1) negatively, loss of control; (2) positively, increased activity of healthy lower centers. Nevertheless, the association, or sequence, is very significant". Furthermore, Jasper,[52] along with Penfield, referred to some automatisms as "psychoparetic rather than psychomotor", suggesting that the motor event is a consequence of an inhibitory ictal event or a postictal depression.

Lorenz,[88] coming from a completely different perspective, similarly wrote "from worm to man... the central automatic motor sequences... would be continuous; when not necessary they are 'braked' by the central inhibition." The

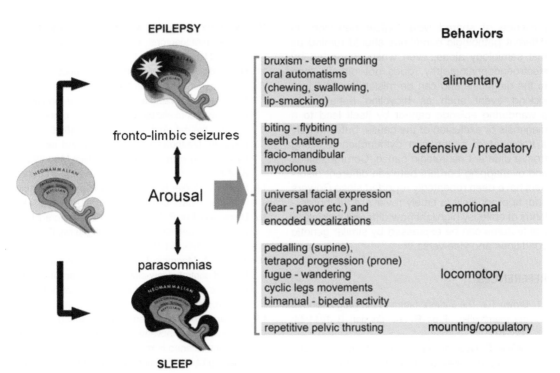

EPILEPSY

Behaviors

fronto-limbic seizures

Arousal

parasomnias

bruxism - teeth grinding oral automatisms (chewing, swallowing, lip-smacking)	alimentary
biting - flybiting teeth chattering facio-mandibular myoclonus	defensive / predatory
universal facial expression (fear - pavor etc.) and encoded vocalizations	emotional
pedalling (supine), tetrapod progression (prone) fugue - wandering cyclic legs movements bimanual - bipedal activity	locomotory
repetitive pelvic thrusting	mounting/copulatory

SLEEP

Fig. 4. The triune brain by MacLean (see also Ref.[82]), who proposed that the human brain is composed of 3 super-imposed brains (neomammalian, paleomammalian, and reptilian), each one representing a distinct evolutionary stage and formed on the preceding older layer (*left*). Both epilepsy and sleep can lead to a temporary loss of control of neomammalian cortex on lower layers favoring, through a common platform (arousal), the emergence of motor phenomena (*middle*), which can be referred to stereotyped, inborn, fixed-action patterns subserving innate motor behaviors critical for survival (behaviors, *right*). (*Modified from* Tassinari CA, Rubboli G, Gardella E, et al. Central pattern generators for a common semiology in fronto-limbic seizures and in parasomnias. A neuro-ethologic approach. Neurol Sci 2005;26(Suppl 3):s227; with permission.)

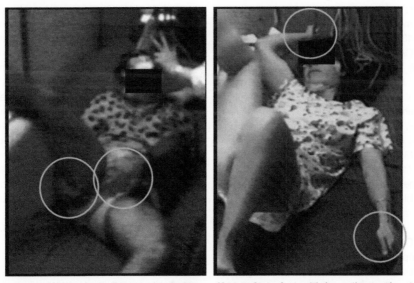

Fig. 5. Seizure-related repetitive grasping in 2 patients suffering from frontal lobe epilepsy. The circle indicates the hand grasping of the genitals and thigh (*left*) and of the headboard and mattress (*right*) (see also Refs.[83,84]).

presence of shared semiological behaviors in different pathologic conditions should remind us that semiology alone, even when supported by electroencephalography, does not directly lead to the diagnosis and can be misleading.[89] A leg-kicking event such as bicycling behavior or a wandering episode cannot by itself lead to a diagnosis or exclusion of the cause, but is merely a fragment of a common dysfunction resulting from a different neurologic cause. Commonalities and overlapping borders between different disorders have been repeatedly reported since Gowers and, appropriately, a timely review of the borderlands of epilepsy highlight how different semiological features can be expressed by similar genetic conditions and vice versa.[90]

REFERENCES

1. Brown TG. The intrinsic factor in the progression of the mammalian. Proc R Soc London B 1911;44:308–19.
2. Grillner S. Neurobiological basis of rhythmic motor acts in vertebrates. Science 1985;228:143–9.
3. Grillner S, Georgopoulos AP, Jordan LM. Selection and initiation of motor behavior. In: Stein PS, Grillner S, Seleverston AI, et al, editors. Neurons, networks and motor behavior. Cambridge (United Kingdom): MIT Press; 1997. p. 3–19.
4. Rossignol S, Dubuc R, Gossard J. Dynamic sensorimotor interactions in locomotion. Physiol Rev 2006;86:89–154.
5. Grillner S, Wallen P. Central pattern generators for locomotion, with special reference to vertebrates. Annu Rev Neurosci 1985;8:233–61.
6. Tassinari CA. A neuroethological approach to "motor behaviours" related to epileptic seizures–characterization of motor behaviour events in epilepsy. Epilepsia 2002;43(Suppl 8):35.
7. Tassinari CA, Gardella E, Meletti S, et al. The neuroethological interpretation of motor behaviours in "nocturnal-hyperkineticfrontal seizures": emergence of "innate" motor behaviours and role of central pattern generators. In: Beaumanoir A, Andermann F, Chauvel P, et al, editors. Frontal lobe seizures and epilepsies in children. Paris: John Libbey Eurotext; 2003. p. 43–8.
8. Tassinari CA, Rubboli G, Gardella E, et al. Central pattern generators for a common semiology in fronto-limbic seizures and in parasomnias. A neuroethologic approach. Neurol Sci 2005;26(Suppl 3):S225–32.
9. Tassinari CA, Cantalupo G, Hogl B, et al. Neuroethological approach to frontolimbic epileptic seizures and parasomnias: the same central pattern generators for the same behaviours. Rev Neurol 2009;165:762–8.
10. Yamada Y, Yamamura K, Makoto I. Coordination of cranial motoneurons during mastication. Respir Physiol Neurobiol 2005;147:177–89.
11. Hess WR, Akert K, McDonald DA. Functions of the orbital gyri in cats. Brain 1952;75:244–58.
12. Morimoto T, Kawamura Y. Properties of tongue and jaw movements elicited by stimulation of the orbital gyrus in the cat. Arch Oral Biol 1973;18:361–72.
13. Lund JP, Matthews B. Mastication and its control by the brain stem. Crit Rev Oral Biol Med 1991;2:33–64.
14. Scutter S, Turker K. The role of the muscle spindles in human masseter. Hum Mov Sci 2001;20:489–97.
15. Dessem D, Luo P. Jaw-muscle spindle afferent feedback to the cervical spinal cord in the rat. Exp Brain Res 1999;128:451–9.
16. Komuro A, Morimoto T, Iwata K, et al. Putative feedforward control of jaw-closing muscle activity during rhythmic jaw movements in the anesthetized rabbit. J Neurophysiol 2001;86:2834–44.
17. Lennard PR. Afferent perturbations during "monopodal" swimming movements in the turtle: phase-dependent cutaneous modulation and proprioceptive resetting of the locomotor rhythm. J Neurosci 1985;5:1434–45.
18. Nakamura Y, Katakura N. Generation of masticatory rhythm in the brainstem. Neurosci Res 1995;23:1–19.
19. Juch PJ, van Willigen JD, Broekhuijsen ML, et al. Peripheral influences on the central pattern-rhythm generator for tongue movements in the rat. Arch Oral Biol 1985;30:415–21.
20. Macaluso GM, Guerra P, Di Giovanni G, et al. Sleep bruxism is a disorder related to periodic arousals during sleep. J Dent Res 1998;77:565–73.
21. Lavigne GJ, Kato T, Kolta A, et al. Neurobiological mechanisms involved in sleep bruxism. Crit Rev Oral Biol Med 2003;14:30–46.
22. Loi D, Provini F, Vetrugno R, et al. Sleep-related faciomandibular myoclonus: a sleep-related movement disorder different from bruxism. Mov Disord 2007;22(12):1819–22.
23. Vetrugno R, Provini F, Plazzi G, et al. Familial nocturnal faciomandibular myoclonus mimicking sleep bruxism. Neurology 2002;58:644–7.
24. van Rijckevorsel K, Abu Serieh B, de Tourtchaninoff M, et al. Deep EEG recordings of the mammillary body in epilepsy patients. Epilepsia 2005;46:781–5.
25. Tassinari CA, Tassi L, Calandra-Buonaura G, et al. Biting behavior, aggression and seizures. Epilepsia 2005;46:654–63.
26. Heynold Y, Faissler D, Steffen F, et al. Clinical, epidemiological and treatment results of idiopathic epilepsy in 54 Labrador retrievers: a long-term study. J Small Anim Pract 1997;38:7–14.
27. Trenkwalder C, Paulus W. Why do restless legs occur at rest?–pathophysiology of neuronal structures in

RLS. Neurophysiology of RLS (part 2). Clin Neurophysiol 2004;115:1975–88.

28. Bara-Jimenez W, Aksu M, Graham B, et al. Periodic limb movements in sleep: state-dependent excitability of the spinal flexor reflex. Neurology 2000; 54(8):1609–16.

29. Meletti S, Cantalupo G, Volpi L, et al. Rhythmic teeth grinding induce by temporal lobe seizures. Neurology 2004;62:2306–9.

30. Munari C, Bancaud J, Bonis A, et al. Role du noyau amygdalien dans la survenue de manifestations oro-alimentaires au cours des crises épileptiques chez l'homme. Rev Electroencephalogr Neurophysiol Clin 1979;9:236–40 [in French].

31. Beauvais K, Biraben A, Vérin M, et al. Mouvements buccaux complexes critiques explorés en stéréo-EEG. Epilepsies 2002;14:171–6 [in French].

32. Penry JK, Porter RJ, Dreifuss RE. Automatisms associated with the absence of petit mal epilepsy. Arch Neurol 1969;21:142–9.

33. D'Orsi G, Demaio V, Trivisano M, et al. Ictal video-polygraphic features of perioral myoclonia with absences. Epil Behav 2011;21:314–7.

34. Provini F, Antelmi E, Vignatelli L, et al. Association of restless legs syndrome with nocturnal eating: a case-control study. Mov Disord 2009;30:871–7.

35. Iani C, Attanasio A, Manfredi M. Paroxysmal staring and masticatory automatisms during postural hypotension in s232, a patient with multiple system atrophy. Epilepsia 1996;37:690–3.

36. Lempert T, Bauer M, Schmidt D. Syncope: a videometric analysis of 56 episodes of transient cerebral hypoxia. Ann Neurol 1994;36:233–7.

37. Darwin CR. The expression of the emotions in man and animals. London: John Murray; 1872.

38. Eibl-Eibesfeldt I. Die Biologie des menschlichen Verhaltens. Grundriss der Humanethologie. München (Germany): R. Piper; 1984 [in German].

39. Ekman P, Friesen WV. Pictures of facial affect. Palo Alto (CA): Consulting Psychologist Press; 1976.

40. Smith ML, Cottrell GW, Gosselin F, et al. Transmitting and decoding facial expressions. Psychol Sci 2005; 16:184–9.

41. Tassinari CA, Gardella E, Rubboli G, et al. The expression of facial emotion in temporal and frontal lobe epileptic seizures. In: Ekman P, Campos JJ, Davidson RJ, et al, editors. Emotions inside out: 130 years after Darwin's, 'The expression of the emotions in man and animals', vol. 1000. New York: Ann NY Acad Sci; 2003. p. 393–4.

42. Gardella E, Rondelli F, Stanzani Maserati M, et al. Facial display of emotions during epileptic seizures. Epilepsia 2006;(Suppl 3):2.

43. Chiesa V, Gardella E, Tassi L, et al. Age-related gender differences in reporting ictal fear: analysis of case histories and review of the literature. Epilepsia 2007;48:2361–4.

44. Frauscher B, Gschliesser V, Brandauer E, et al. Video analysis of motor events in REM sleep behavior disorder. Mov Disord 2007;22:1464–70.

45. Meletti S, Benuzzi F, Rubboli G, et al. Impaired facial emotion recognition in early onset right mesial temporal lobe epilepsy. Neurology 2003;60:426–31.

46. Benuzzi F, Meletti S, Zamboni G, et al. Impaired fear processing in right mesial temporal sclerosis: a fMRI study. Brain Res Bull 2004;63:269–81.

47. Schachter ST. Aggressive behaviour in epilepsy. In: Kanner AM, editor. Psychiatric issues in epilepsy. Philadelphia: Lippincott Williams & Wilkins; 2001. p. 201–13.

48. Marsh L, Krauss GL. Aggression and violence in patients with epilepsy. Epilepsy Behav 2000;1:160–8.

49. Delgado-Escueta AV, Mattson RH, King L, et al. Special report: the nature of aggression during epileptic seizures. N Engl J Med 1981;305:711–6.

50. Treiman DM. Psychobiology of ictal aggression. Adv Neurol 1991;55:341–56.

51. Stanzani Maserati M, Meletti S, Cantalupo G, et al. Biting behavior as a model of aggression associated with seizures. In: Schacthter SC, Holmes GL, Kasteleijn-Nolst Trenitè DG, editors. Behavioral aspects of epilepsy, principles and practice. New York: Demos; 2008. p. 227–34.

52. Jasper HH. Some physiological mechanisms involved in epileptic automatisms. Epilepsia 1964;23:1–20.

53. Siclari F, Khatami R, Urbaniok F, et al. Violence in sleep. Brain 2010;133:3494–509.

54. Bisulli F, Vignatelli L, Naldi I, et al. Increased frequency of arousal parasomnias in families with nocturnal frontal lobe epilepsy: a common mechanism. Epilesia 2010;51(9):1852–60.

55. Bassetti C, Vella S, Donati F, et al. SPECT during sleep-walking. Lancet 2000;356:484–5.

56. Vetrugno R, Mascalchi M, Vella A, et al. Paroxysmal arousal in epilepsy associated with cingulate hyperperfusion. Neurology 2005;64:356–8.

57. Shik ML, Severin FV, Orlovsky GN. Control of walking and running by means of electrical stimulation of the mid-brain. Biophysics 1966;11:756–65.

58. Jordan LM. Brainstem and spinal cord mechanisms for the initiation of locomotion. In: Shimamura M, Grillner S, Edgerton VR, editors. Neurobiological basis of human locomotion. Tokyo: Japan Scientific Societies Press, Springer Verlag; 1991. p. 3–20.

59. Mori S, Matsui T, Kuze B, et al. Cerebellar-induced locomotion: reticulospinal control of spinal rhythm generating mechanism in cats. In: Kiehn O, Harris-Warrick R, Jordan LM, et al, editors. Neuronal mechanisms for generating locomotor activity. Annals of the New York Academy of Sciences, vol. 860. New York: Blackwell Synergy; 1998. p. 94–105.

60. Grillner S. The motor infrastructure: from ion channels to neuronal networks. Nat Rev Neurosci 2003; 4:573–86.

61. Grillner S. Biological pattern generation: the cellular and computational logic of networks in motion. Neuron 2006;52:751–66.

62. Dimitrijevic MR, Gerasimenko Y, Pinter MM. Evidence for a spinal central pattern generator in humans. In: Kiehn O, Harris-Warrick R, Jordan LM, et al, editors. Neuronal mechanisms for generating locomotor activity. Annals of the New York Academy of Sciences, vol. 860. New York: Blackwell Synergy; 1998. p. 360–76.

63. Shapkova EI. Spinal locomotor capability revealed by electrical stimulation of the lumbar enlargement in paraplegic patients. In: Latash M, Levin M, editors. Progress in motor control, vol. 3. Human Kinetic Publishers; 2004. p. 253–89.

64. Calancie B, Needham-Shropshire B, Jacobs P, et al. Involuntary stepping after chronic spinal cord injury. Evidence for a central rhythm generator for locomotion in man. Brain 1994;117:1143–59.

65. Hultborn H, Nielsen JB. Spinal control of locomotion–from cat to man. Acta Physiol 2007;189:111–21.

66. Wada JA. Predominantly nocturnal recurrence of intensively affective vocal and facial expression associated with powerful bimanual, bipedal and axial activity as ictal manifestations of mesial frontal lobe epilepsy. Adv Epileptol 1989;17:261–7.

67. Swartz BE. Electrophysiology of bimanual-bipedal automatisms. Epilepsia 1994;35:264–74.

68. Williamson PD. Frontal lobe epilepsy: some clinical characteristics. In: Jasper HH, Riggio S, Goldman-Rakic PS, editors. Epilepsy and the functional anatomy of the frontal lobe. New York: Raven Press; 1995. p. 127–52.

69. Biraben A, Taussig D, Beillard S, et al. Motor automatisms in limbic seizures. In: Avanzini G, Beumanoir A, Mira L, editors. Limbic seizures in children. Montrouge (France): John Libbey Eurotext; 2001. p. 89–103.

70. Nobili L, Cossu M, Mai R, et al. Sleep-related hyperkinetic seizures of temporal lobe origin. Neurology 2004;62:482–5.

71. Vaugier L, Aubert S, McGonigal A, et al. Neural networks underlying hyperkinetic seizures of "temporal lobe" origin. Epilepsy Res 2009;86:200–8.

72. Pedley TA, Guilleminault C. Episodic nocturnal wanderings responsive to anticonvulsant drug therapy. Ann Neurol 1977;2:30–5.

73. Plazzi G, Tinuper P, Provini F, et al. Epileptic nocturnal wanderings. Sleep 1995;18:749–56.

74. Gastaut H, Broughton R. A clinical and polygraphic study of episodic phenomena during sleep. In: Wortis J, editor. Recent advances in biology and psychiatry, vol. 7. New York: Plenum Press; 1965. p. 197–222.

75. Gardella E, Rubboli G, Francione S, et al. Seizure-related automatic locomotion triggered by intracerebral electrical stimulation. Epileptic Disord 2008;10: 247–52.

76. Hogl B, Zucconi M, Provini F. RLS, PLM, and their differential diagnosis–a video guide. Mov Disord 2007;22(Suppl 18):S414–9.

77. Terzaghi M, Sartori I, Mai R, et al. Coupling of minor motor events and epileptiform discharges with arousal fluctuations in NFLE. Epilepsia 2008;49:670–6.

78. Grillner S. On the central generation of locomotion in the low spinal cat. Exp Brain Res 1979;34:241–61.

79. Gastaut H, Meyers JS. Cerebral anoxia and the electroencephalogram. Boston: Charles C Thomas; 1961.

80. Bickel A. Der Babinski'sche Zehnenreflex unter physiologischen und pathologischen Bedingungen. Dsche Z Nervenheilk 1902;22:163–5 [in German].

81. Martinelli P, Coccagna G, Lugaresi E. Nocturnal myoclonus, restless legs syndrome, and abnormal electrophysiological findings. Ann Neurol 1987;21:515.

82. MacLean PD. The triune brain in evolution: role in paleocerebral functions. New York: Plenum Press; 1990.

83. Gardella E, Rubboli G, Tassinari CA. Video-EEG analysis of ictal repetitive grasping in "frontal-hyperkinetic" seizures. Epileptic Disord 2006;8:267–73.

84. Gardella E, Rubboli G, Tassinari CA. Ictal grasping: prevalence and characteristics in seizures with different semiology. Epilepsia 2006;47(Suppl 5):59–63.

85. Luria AR. The working brain. New York: Basic Books; 1973.

86. Parrino L, Halasz P, Tassinari CA, et al. CAP, epilepsy and motor events during sleep: the unifying role of arousal. Sleep Med Rev 2006;10:267–85.

87. Hughlings-Jackson J. On temporary mental disorders after epileptic paroxysms. West Riding Lunatic Asylum Medical Reports (WRLAMR) 1875;5: 105–29.

88. Lorenz K. Die Ruckseite des spiegels. Versuch einer Naturgeschichte des menschlichen Erkennens. Munchen: R. Piper; 1973 [in German].

89. Scheffer IE, Bhatia KP, Lopes-Cendes I, et al. Autosomal dominant frontal epilepsy misdiagnosed as sleep disorder. Lancet 1994;343:515–7.

90. Crompton DE, Berkovic SF. The borderland of epilepsy: clinical and molecular features of phenomena that mimic epileptic seizures. Lancet Neurol 2009;8:370–81.

91. Chervin RD, Consens FB, Kutluay E. Alternating leg muscle activation during sleep and arousals: a new sleep-related motor phenomenon? Mov Disord 2003;18:551–9.

Benign Rolandic and Occipital Epilepsies of Childhood

Oliviero Bruni, MD[a],*, Luana Novelli, PhD[a,b],
Alice Mallucci, MD[c], Martina della Corte, MD[c],
Antonino Romeo, MD[d], Raffaele Ferri, MD[e]

KEYWORDS

- Rolandic epilepsy • Occipital epilepsy
- Panayiotopoulos syndrome • Sleep

Benign childhood focal seizures represent the most common epileptic manifestations in childhood and affect approximately 22% of children. Three identifiable electro clinical syndromes are coded by the International League against Epilepsy (ILAE)[1]: benign epilepsy with centrotemporal spikes (BECTS), Panayiotopoulos syndrome (PS), and the idiopathic childhood occipital epilepsy of Gastaut (ICOE-G).

The term "benign" refers to the positive prognosis of these disorders in regard to the EEG pattern and the seizures. However, a significant number of children with BECTS present various cognitive deficits affecting language and memory functions the severity of which associated with the intensity and the duration of interictal epileptic discharges (IED) and resolve with EEG normalization.[2–6]

Since the publication of the ILAE classification of epileptic syndromes,[7] the group of focal idiopathic epilepsies has been enlarged to a subgroup of epileptic encephalopathies (EE) with continuous spike-and-waves during slow-wave sleep (CSWS) in which the appearance and persistence of IED are associated with cognitive regression. BECTS and EE with CSWS represents opposite ends of a spectrum, behavioral and cognitive deficits are often milder in BECTS and severe in the CSWS epileptic encephalopathy.[8–14]

BENIGN CHILDHOOD EPILEPSY WITH CENTRO-TEMPORAL SPIKES

BECTS, also known as *Rolandic Epilepsy*, is the most common among the benign focal epilepsies of childhood, occurring in 15–25% of pediatric epilepsy patients.[15–18] The age at onset is between 2 and 14 years, with a peak of incidence (80% of the cases) at 5 to 10 years. Absence seizures develop in approximately 2% of cases.[19,20]

Loiseau and Duché[21] specified 5 criteria for the diagnosis of BECTS: (1) age at onset between 2 and 13 years; (2) lack of neurologic/intellectual deficit at the time of the onset; (3) partial seizures with motor signs, often associated with somatosensory symptoms or precipitated by sleep; (4) a spike focus located in the centrotemporal area with normal background activity on the interictal

The authors have nothing to disclose.

[a] Department of Developmental Neurology and Psychiatry, Centre for Paediatric Sleep Disorders, Sapienza University, via dei Sabelli 108, Rome 00185, Italy
[b] Department of Neuroscience, AFaR-Fatebenefratelli Hospital, Isola Tiberina, Rome, Italy
[c] Faculty of Medicine and Psychology, S. Andrea Hospital, via di Grottarossa 1035, Rome 00189, Italy
[d] Department of Neurosciences, Epilepsy Center, Fatebenefratelli e Oftalmico Hospital, Corso di Porta Nuova 23, Milano 20121, Italy
[e] Department of Neurology, I.C., Sleep Research Centre, Oasi Institute for Research on Mental Retardation and Brain Aging (IRCCS), via Conte Ruggero 73, Troina 94018 (EN), Italy
* Corresponding author.
E-mail address: oliviero.bruni@uniroma1.it

sleep.theclinics.com

EEG; and (5) spontaneous remission (generally during adolescence).

Seizure Manifestations

Seizures are usually brief, lasting for 1 to 3 minutes, and their clinical manifestations include (see Video 1):

- Unilateral facial motor symptoms (30% of cases), in the form of clonic contractions, mostly localized in the lower lip that may extend to the ipsilateral hand. Symptoms can include numbness in the corner of the mouth.[19,22]
- Oro-pharyngo-laryngeal symptoms (53%), consisting of unilateral sensorimotor symptoms or paresthesias inside the mouth, associated with vocalizations.[19,22]
- Speech arrest in 40% of patients, who are unable to utter intelligible words and can communicate only with gestures.[19,22]
- Hypersalivation (30%), often associated with hemifacial seizures.[19,22]

Generalized convulsive status epilepticus is rare. Opercular status epilepticus occurs in atypical evolutions of BECTS or, exceptionally, it may be induced by carbamazepine.[23] This status may last for hours to months and consists of continuous unilateral or bilateral contractions of the mouth, tongue, or eyelids, positive or negative subtle perioral or other myoclonia, dysarthria, anarthria, or speech arrest, buccofacial apraxia and hypersalivation.[24]

EEG Features

The interictal EEG is distinctive in BECTS, showing centrotemporal spike-and-wave discharges which have a tangential dipole that is negative in the centrotemporal area and positive frontally. Centrotemporal spikes (CTS) are the hallmark of the BECTS syndrome and are mainly localized in the left central (C3) and right central (C4) or the supra-sylvian electrodes (C5, C6 using the International 10-10 system of electrode placement) and not in the temporal ones.[25] CTS are markedly activated by drowsiness, occur independently over both hemispheres at frequencies of 4 to 20 discharges per minute, and usually occur in clusters (**Fig. 1**). Recent studies show that the main negative spike component is modeled by a stable tangential dipole source, with the positive pole was maximum in the frontal region, while the negative pole was maximum in the central region.[26] The main spike (sharp wave) component is diphasic with a maximum surface, negative, rounded peak that is followed by a smaller positive peak. The amplitude of the main spike component often exceeds 200 µV, though it may be much smaller or much higher. The negative phase is larger than the positive phase of the spike, as well as the preceding or following components of the spike–slow wave complex. About 4% of patients with rolandic epilepsy also show brief bursts of 3-5 Hz slow waves with internalized small spikes lasting 1-3 seconds, without overt clinical symptoms.[27] The frequency, location and persistence of CTS are not specific for BECTS.[27,28] In fact,

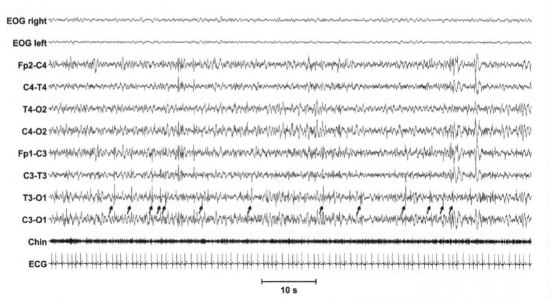

Fig. 1. Example of EEG tracing of a patient with rolandic epilepsy with typical spikes in the left fronto-centrotemporal area with spreading in the right corresponding area (*arrows*).

they occur in 2-3% of normal school-aged children, of whom less than 10% develop rolandic seizures.[16] They are also seen in children with other organic brain diseases with or without seizures[27–29] as well as in non-epileptic children with symptoms such as headaches, and speech, behavioral, or learning difficulties.

Somatosensory stimulation activates CTS in 10% to 20% of cases and evokes giant somatosensory evoked spikes (GSES) that, like spontaneous CTS, appear in children with or without seizures and disappear with age.[27,30,31] Generalized tonic-clonic seizures (GTCS), in BECTS are preceded by focal clinical and EEG features.[27,32]

Etiology and Pathophysiology

Twin studies[33] suggest the existence of a genetic basis for BECTS. Specifically, there is a proven linkage with chromosome 15q14.[34] Even if there was an early hypothesis of an autosomal inheritance pattern, later studies suggested a multifactorial inheritance; more recent work has shown that noninherited factors are more important than once believed.[35]

The seizures occur during sleep, mostly night sleep but also during daytime sleep, in approximately 75% of the affected children, and usually appear after the child falls asleep or close to the wake-up time. Although the rolandic seizures occur mainly during sleep, studies on sleep in patients with BECTS are rare. One of the first studies on this topic[36] showed that no specific or clear-cut pathologic alterations of sleep were found. The authors concluded that epileptic malfunctioning of neuronal aggregates does not affect sleep organization and that the lack of detrimental interactions between epilepsy and sleep in this group may be related to the benign course of BECTS. The same authors showed a clear increase in spike activity in the first cycle of sleep and another increase near the end of night sleep. These periods of sleep correspond to the periods favored by seizures in BECTS. The level of spike activation (ie, spike density) decreased across the night: peak of activation in the first sleep cycle, followed by a marked decrease in the second cycle, especially during NREM 3 sleep and an increase in the third sleep cycle mostly related to NREM 1 and 2.[37]

Nobili and colleagues[38] found a highly significant correlation between IED and sigma (12-16 Hz) activity; the IED in BECTS patients during sleep are sensitive to the IED-promoting action of the spindle-generating mechanism, while delta activity does not seem to play a facilitating role or is even inversely correlated with IED distribution.[38–40]

Recently, Bruni and colleagues[41] studied sleep architecture in children with BECTS, analyzing conventional sleep parameters and microstructure using cyclic alternating pattern (CAP). In agreement with previous studies,[37,38] they confirmed that sleep architecture is not significantly altered in patients with BECTS with only mild decreases in total sleep time, sleep efficiency, and REM sleep percentage and the presence of the IEDs does not seem to alter sleep structure. However, CAP analysis of sleep microstructure in the subjects with BECTS compared with normal age-matched controls showed a reduced total NREM 2 CAP rate and reduced EEG slow oscillations during stages NREM 1 and 2 sleep. In BECTS there might be a reduction of CAP rate and a decrease of the CAP A phases, with special effect on the slow-wave containing A1 subtypes. This microstructural analysis reveals, therefore, a decrease of NREM instability, mainly in sleep stage 2.

In order to better understand these findings, one has to take into account the results of the EEG spectral analysis carried out in different types of benign epilepsies.[38,42] Data derived from spectral analysis highlight a strong correlation between the temporal distribution of CTS and that of the sigma activity, the frequency band to which spindles contribute most. The facilitating influence of sigma activity on the activation of spike activity during sleep has been found in many epilepsies of childhood that seem to be characterized by a strong NREM sleep spike activation. Spindle-related spike activation is present in functional partial epilepsies, such as BECTS,[43] benign epilepsy with occipital paroxysms,[39] lesional and cryptogenetic partial epilepsies with strong activation of epileptic discharges during sleep,[38] the Landau-Kleffner syndrome,[40] and the fragile-X syndrome.[44] Nobili and colleagues[43] also stated that, taking into account that sigma activity reflects the intra-night dynamics of sleep spindles, the neural mechanisms involved in the generation of sleep spindles might also facilitate the production of CTS. Sleep spindles are associated with sleep-protecting mechanisms and are considered to be microstates gating the sensory input toward the cortex in an inhibitory way[45] and, therefore, inhibiting slow oscillations and arousals.[46]

Therefore, since CTS and spindles are strictly interdependent, and taking into account the inhibitory action of spindle activity on arousals, it can be supposed that the decrease of oscillations and of arousal-related transient events (reduction of A1 and A2 index in NREM 2), might be related to the CTS typically present in BECTS. Although this remains speculative, based on previous studies and to better clarify the relationships between sleep microstructure and spike activity, it has been shown that CAP rate decrease in NREM 2 was more evident in patients with BECTS who also showed an increase of spike density in NREM 2 versus NREM 3. This decrease was mainly related to the A1 component of CAP rate, as the A1 index was significantly lower during NREM 2. To summarize, there is a spindle-related spike activation in BECTS, and the decrease of CAP rate, EEG slow oscillations and arousals may be linked with the inhibitory action of sleep spindle activity and spikes on arousals.

An increase of the age-related, area-specific cortical excitability has been hypothesized to be at the basis of the origin of BECTS.[31,47,48] This increased excitability of the cortex is able to transform the thalamic volley that normally induces sleep spindles in a mechanism inducing epileptic discharges, as shown in animals[49,50] and in humans.[51] Due to the age-related regional hyperexcitability, the cortex could react with spikes to the thalamocortical volleys that generate spindles, even in physiologic conditions in predisposed children. This hypothetical transformation of spindles into spike activity might explain the strict relationships between sigma activity and CTS but might also account for the particular sleep microstructure with spike activity independent from CAP phase A and the increase of CTS during non-CAP (NCAP).

Prognosis

Remission in BECTS usually occurs 2–4 years after the onset and typically before the age of 16 years. Most patients have less than a total of 10 lifetime seizures, 10–20% have just a single seizure, and about 10–20% may have frequent seizures that also remit with age.

In the past 10 years, several studies have indicated that patients with BECTS have a variety of cognitive disturbances, including language impairment, memory dysfunction, and auditory processing difficulties; this indicates that BECTS is not benign with respect to cognitive consequences.

During the active phase of the BECTS syndrome, the children may develop mild linguistic, cognitive, and behavioral abnormalities[52–55] which may be worse in those in whom the epilepsy syndrome begins at 8 years of age and/or in those with a high rate of seizure and multifocal EEG spikes.[56,57] Deonna and colleagues[2] showed that children with BECTS presented mild, varied, and transient cognitive difficulties during the course of their epilepsy, and in most cases this probably had a direct relation with the paroxysmal EEG activity.

A case-control study of families affected by BECTS indicates that family members of the proband who have not had seizures, demonstrate reading disabilities and speech sound disorders.[58] The families of the probands were not studied with EEG so it is unclear whether the spike-wave discharges were present in the 55% who manifested the disabilities. Assuming that BECTS is a autosomal dominant trait and would be expected to be present in 50% of family members, this study suggests that most or all of the individuals with the trait may express the disabilities.

Recently, Sarco and colleagues[59] revealed an association between mood disorder (anxiety, depression, aggression, and conduct problems) and spike frequency in BECTS: increased epileptic activity in children with BECTS may predict higher rates of mood and behavioral problems.

BENIGN OCCIPITAL EPILEPSIES OF CHILDHOOD
Panayiotopoulos Syndrome

Panayiotopoulos syndrome (PS), otherwise defined as susceptibility to early-onset benign childhood seizures with mainly autonomic symptoms, is a common childhood epileptic syndrome with benign age-related focal seizures occurring in early and mid-childhood. After BECTS, this is the most frequent epilepsy syndrome of childhood with a mild female preponderance.

The prevalence of PS may be high, probably affecting approximately13% of children 3-6 years old with one or more nonfebrile seizures and 6% of the age group from 1 to 15 years.[60]

Seizure manifestations
PS seizures mainly occurring during sleep, are infrequent, often single, with a constellation of autonomic, mainly emetic symptoms, behavioral changes, and other more conventional ictal clinical manifestations, such as unilateral deviation of the eyes and convulsions.[60] Other autonomic manifestations include pallor, flushing or cyanosis, mydriasis or miosis, cardiorespiratory and thermoregulatory alterations, urinary and/fecal incontinence, hypersalivation, cephalic auras, and altered gastrointestinal motility.[61,62] Emesis is usually the first apparent ictal symptom, but it may occur long after the other manifestations that include pallor, enuresis and encopresis, hypersalivation, cyanosis, mydriasis and less often miosis, coughing, and abnormalities of intestinal motility.[63,64] Cardiorespiratory arrest due to a PS seizure is rare, probably occurring in 1 per 200 individuals with the syndrome. Headache or migraine symptoms are often reported with other

autonomic symptoms at seizure onset. Syncopal-like manifestations occur in at least one-fifth of seizures.[65–67] Parents are always frightened by the manifestations of seizures because the child is completely unresponsive and flaccid like a rag doll, before or after the other seizure symptoms. Restlessness, agitation, terror, or quietness may occur at the onset of seizures.

Autonomic manifestations can be missed by the parents, who are more likely to report the more obvious seizure symptoms, including uni-lateral deviation of the eyes or eyes opening, speech arrest, hemifacial convulsions, visual hallu-cinations, unilateral drooping of the mouth, and rarely eyelid or limb jerks, nystagmus, or automa-tisms. PS seizures can evolve to hemiconvulsive or generalized. Visual auras are rarely reported (1%) and not present in recurrent seizures.[60,68] Duration of PS vary from few minutes to hours leading to autonomic status epilepticus.[60,67] which occurs in 10% of patients. Two-thirds of seizures start in sleep. Long-lasting seizures are equally common in sleep and wakefulness. Even after the most severe seizures and autonomic status, the child is back to normal after a few hours of sleep.

EEG features
Although the semiology of these events may resemble panic attacks, sleep terrors, and other parasomnias, routine EEG will usually confirm the diagnosis of benign epilepsy of childhood with occipital paroxysms.[69,70] The interictal EEG in PS shows multifocal, high-amplitude, continuous occipital sharp slow-wave complexes (occipital paroxysms), often shifting from one region to another in the same or the contralateral hemi-sphere in sequential EEGs of the same child. Occipital spikes predominate but they do not occur in one-third of patients. The main focus is often posterior, and secondarily other spikes appear in secondary foci in different hemispheric sides[60,63,71–74] and rarely they are generalized as discharges of slow waves, intermixed with small spikes.

The IEDs in PS are typically enhanced by sleep, and not activated by photic stimulation. As in BECTS, the frequency, location, and persistence of spikes do not influence the clinical manifesta-tions, duration, severity, and frequency of seizures or their prognosis.

The ictal discharge in PS is characterized by rhythmic monomorphic decelerating theta or delta activity, while in Gastaut-type late-onset idiopathic childhood occipital epilepsy, the ictal pattern of visual seizures is represented by an episodic fast activity.[75–77] The onset of the ictal discharge is usually from the posterior brain regions, but frontal onset has also been documented.[77] In the few re-ported ictal EEGs, the discharges consist mainly of posterior unilateral rhythmic slow activity, usually in-termixed with fast rhythms and small spikes.[64,65]

Etiology
PS has probably a genetic background but usually there is no family history of similar seizures, although siblings with PS and/or BECTS have been reported.[61,63,68,71,72] There is a high preva-lence of febrile seizures (about 17%).[60] SCN1A gene mutations have been recently reported in a child[78] and two siblings[79] with relatively early onset of seizures, a prolonged time over which many seizures have occurred and strong associa-tion with febrile precipitants, even after the age of 5 years.

Prognosis
One-third of PS patients have a single seizure, and another half have 2-5 lifetime seizures. Only 5% of patients have more than 10 lifetime seizures. Even after the most severe seizures and status, the patient recovers within a few hours.[63] Remission of seizures and the EEG patterns are the norm and usually occurs within 1 to 2 years from onset; the prognosis is in general very good with no risk of developing epilepsy in adult life.[60,63,68,71,77,80,81] However, autonomic seizures are of concern since four cases of cardiorespiratory arrest have been reported, even if all of them were successfully resuscitated and recovered completely.[60,66,67,82] Approximately 10% of patients may have more pro-tracted active seizure periods. Twenty percent develop other benign forms of epilepsies, including BECTS rolandic and less often ICOE-G.[60] Atypical evolution of PS to CSWS syndrome is rare and the risk of epilepsy in adult life appears to be no higher than in the general population.[60,66,68] Prognosis is also good for cognitive functioning, although subtle neuropsychological deficits during the active phase have been described.[68,83]

Differential diagnosis
The difficulty making a diagnosis of PS is related to the challenge of recognizing the ictal vomiting and other autonomic manifestations as epileptic seizures. Autonomic symptoms in these children are too often initially misdiagnosed as signs of encephalitis, migraine, syncope or gastroenter-itis.[60,80,84] When these are excluded, the diagnosis is easy because of the characteristic clinical semi-ology and interictal EEG findings.

PS is significantly different from BECTS and the ICOE-G, despite some overlapping clinical and/or EEG features. Differentiating PS and other epileptic syndromes and seizures is typically straightforward, as (1) PS and Gastaut-type childhood occipital epilepsy have entirely different clinical manifestations despite common interictal EEG when occipital paroxysms occur; (2) photosensitive occipital seizures may show autonomic disturbances and ictal vomiting, but manifestations of visual seizures usually precede them[81]; and (3) rolandic seizures have different clinical manifestations, and emesis is not commonly reported.[71]

Idiopathic Childhood Occipital Epilepsy of Gastaut

The third benign childhood epilepsy syndrome is the idiopathic childhood occipital epilepsy of Gastaut (ICOE-G) also known as late-onset childhood occipital epilepsy. It is relatively rare, accounting for 2–7% of benign focal epilepsies of childhood. It manifests with frequent and brief elementary visual hallucinations, blindness or both. Onset is between ages 3 to 15 years (most often around age 8) of both sexes. ICOE-G is rare, of uncertain prognosis, and markedly different from PS, despite sharing some common interictal EEG finding of occipital spikes.

Seizure manifestations
Seizures in ICOE-G are typically simple partial elementary visual hallucinations which appear as colored circular patterns commonly in the periphery of the visual field which enlarge and multiply during the course of the seizure. They are frequently the first and often the only seizure symptom. As opposed to PS, seizures in ICOE-G most often occur awake. ICOE-G seizures usually last a few seconds to 1–3 minutes unless they spread to the contralateral occipital or extra-occipital regions.

Ictal blindness with total loss of vision is the second most common symptom and usually begins at the onset of the seizure, lasts 3–5 minutes, can be the only ictal manifestation in patients who at other times have seizures characterized by visual hallucinations. Other non-visual occipital symptoms which usually appear after the elementary visual hallucinations include: forced sustained deviation of eyes seen in approximately 70% of cases; it is often accompanied by ipsilateral turning of the head.[85–89]

Consciousness is preserved during the visual symptoms but may be altered or lost in the course of the seizure, usually before or during eye deviation or convulsions. Forced eye closure and eyelid blinking occur in 10% of patients usually when consciousness becomes impaired and warns of an impending GTCS.

Progression from elementary visual hallucination to complex focal seizures occurs in 14%, hemiconvulsions in 43%, and GTCS in 13% of cases.[90] Postictal headache (severe, unilateral, pulsating) develops in half of the patients, and in 10% of the cases it is associated with nausea and vomiting.[86,89,90]

EEG features
The interictal EEG shows occipital discharges which occur as long as fixation and central vision are eliminated by eye closure, absolute darkness or +10 spherical lenses.[85,90] Some patients only have random occipital spikes, others occipital spikes only in sleep.[86,91] The reported presence of the classical fixation-off occipital spikes ranges from 100%[90] to 88%[89] and 19%,[86] varying because this distinctive EEG feature is not always formally tested. Centrotemporal, frontal, and giant somatosensory evoked potentials occur together with occipital spikes in about 20% of patients, less often than in patients with PS.[90,92] Occipital spikes are not specific for this syndrome, also occur in children with congenital or early onset visual and ocular deficits. Moreover, occipital spikes occur in 0.8–1.0% of normal preschool children. The ictal EEG in ICOE-G is characterized by the sudden appearance of fast spikes or rhythmic activity and seen when the patient reports the elementary visual hallucinations. Ictal blindness is characterized by semi-periodic spike-slow waves. Post-ictal EEG abnormalities are usually absent.

Etiology and differential diagnosis
The seizures originate in the occipital lobes. Elementary visual hallucinations originate from the primary visual cortex, complex visual hallucinations from the junction of the occipital with the parietal and temporal lobes, formed visual illusions from the lateral occipital-posterior temporal junction, and tonic deviation of the eyes from the medial occipital cortex, above or below the calcarine sulcus. Ictal blindness may reflect bi-occipital seizure spreading but this may not explain its sudden onset, without any other preceding manifestation. A family history of epilepsy (21%–37%) or migraine (9%–16%) is common,[85–89] but familial ICOE-G is rare.[72] Occipital epilepsies due to structural lesions can imitate ICOE-G so a thorough neuro-ophthalmological examination and a high-resolution brain MRI is warranted to exclude subtle structural occipital lesions. Occipital seizures are common in children with mitochondrial disorders, coeliac or Lafora disease.

Prognosis and treatment strategies
ICOE-G remits in 50–60% of children within 2–4 years from onset.[86,89,90] Unfortunately, 40–50% continue having visual seizures and infrequent

secondarily GTCS. On rare occasion, children with ICOE-G may evolve to CSWS syndrome.[93] I-COE-G may develop typical absence seizures which usually appear after the onset of occipital seizures.[93]

Children with ICOE-G had lower performance scores for attention, memory, and intellectual functioning compared with control subjects.[94] As opposed to the other benign focal epilepsies, children with ICOE-G most often have frequent seizures and require medication. Seizures show a dramatically good response to carbamazepine in 90% of patients.

INFLUENCE OF SLEEP ON INTERICTAL DISCHARGES IN ROLANDIC AND OCCIPITAL EPILEPSIES

It is known that, generally, NREM sleep activates and REM sleep inhibits IED but the type of epilepsy influences the expression of IED. In benign epilepsies of childhood, early studies demonstrated an activation of IED during sleep,[95] particularly NREM sleep. Some studies showed that IED progressively increase with deeper stages of NREM sleep,[96–98] while others have found greater activation during NREM 1 and 2 sleep, not NREM 3.[99,100]

NREM 1 and 2 sleep facilitates the spread of epileptic discharges in the form of clinical or subclinical seizures; whereas in deep sleep stages, irritative neuronal discharges increase, but the spreading capacity is reduced. On the other hand, REM sleep inhibits both phenomena.

Both interictal and ictal discharges occur most often during NREM sleep and show a strict association with K-complexes or spindles.[101] Steriade and Amzica[102] showed that generalized epileptic spike-and-waves are driven by conversion of slow cortical oscillation (<1 Hz) into recurrent paroxysmal discharges.

Cyclic alternating pattern (CAP) represents a modulating factor of IEDs and epileptic seizures.[103–107] However, all the benign forms of epilepsy in childhood, focal spike discharges seem to show no significant relationship with CAP.[107,108] The first study on CAP in children with BECTS was conducted more than 15 years ago, evaluating how the CAP and non-CAP conditions affected CTS distribution during sleep[107]: no significant differences in spike distribution throughout CAP and NCAP modalities were found, demonstrating that, despite the high burst frequency during NREM sleep, IEDs of CTS are not modulated by the arousal-related mechanisms of CAP.

The finding that the IEDs in BECTS coincide with the peaks of the sigma band (sleep spindles)

activation,[43] suggested a relationship between CTS and the spindle-generating mechanism, while slow-wave activity does not seem to play a facilitating role or is even inversely correlated with CTS distribution.[40,43]

The strict relationship of CTS with spindles might explain the relative independence of CTS from the CAP A phase modulation since during the entire duration of phase A there is a sustained depression of the sigma spectral band activities[109,110] and, therefore, the neurophysiological substrate for the occurrence of CTS is lacking.

Sleep stage architecture in patients with BECTS is not altered,[37,41,43] and the presence of CTS does not seem to alter sleep structure. However, sleep microstructure in these patients shows mainly a reduction of A1 index in NREM 2 but not in NREM 3 sleep associated with an increase in the percentage of A2 and A3 indexes.

The results of the EEG spectral analysis in different types of benign epilepsies[38,43] highlight a strong correlation between the temporal distribution of CTS and that of the sigma activity. Spindle-related spike activation is present in functional partial epilepsies such as BECTS,[43] benign epilepsy with occipital paroxysms,[39] lesional and cryptogenetic partial epilepsies with strong activation of epileptiform discharges during sleep,[38] the fragile-X syndrome,[29] and the Landau-Kleffner syndrome.[40] Since CTS and spindles are strictly interdependent and spindling activity has an inhibitory action on arousals, Bruni and colleagues[41] hypothesized that the decrease of EEG slow oscillations and of arousal-related transient events (reduction of A1 and A2 index in sleep stage 2) might be related to CTS typically present in BECTS. Theoretically, these CAP alterations in BECTS patients might be in some way related to the transitory cognitive impairment reported during the active phase of the disease.[3,111]

SUMMARY

Despite significant progress, the pathophysiology of IED-induced cognitive deficits in patients with focal idiopathic epilepsy is not completely understood. The potential role of IED on sleep-related memory consolidation was evaluated in two patients with CSWS; they found that memory consolidation was restored in that patient whose EEG normalized after treatment with corticosteroids but not in the other patient whose EEG was improved but not normalized.[112] Since similar memory impairment has been observed in four children with focal idiopathic epilepsy, IEDs in these patients may disrupt the brain processes underlying sleep-related memory consolidation.[112] As interictal spiking is most intense and diffuse during NREM sleep, this might interfere with the NREM-dependent physiological processes of neuronal plasticity supporting memory consolidation in children. More research is needed to unravel the pathophysiology of these benign, but probably not so innocent benign focal epilepsies of childhood.

SUPPLEMENTARY DATA

Supplementary data related to this article can be found online at doi:10.1016/j.jsmc.2011.12.004.

REFERENCES

1. Engel J Jr. Report of the ILAE classification core group. Epilepsia 2006;47:1558–68.
2. Deonna T, Zesiger P, Davidoff V, et al. Benign partial epilepsy of childhood: a longitudinal neuropsychological and EEG study of cognitive function. Dev Med Child Neurol 2000;42:595–603.
3. Baglietto MG, Battaglia FM, Nobili L, et al. Neuropsychological disorders related to interictal epileptic discharges during sleep in benign epilepsy of childhood with centrotemporal or Rolandic spikes. Dev Med Child Neurol 2001;43:407–12.
4. Metz-Lutz MN, Kleitz C, de Saint Martin A, et al. Cognitive development in benign focal epilepsies of childhood. Dev Neurosci 1999;21:182–90.
5. Massa R, de Saint-Martin A, Carcangiu R, et al. EEG criteria predictive of complicated evolution in idiopathic rolandic epilepsy. Neurology 2001;57: 1071–9.
6. Nicolai J, van der Linden I, Arends JB, et al. EEG characteristics related to educational impairments in children with benign childhood epilepsy with centrotemporal spikes. Epilepsia 2007;48: 2093–100.
7. Proposal for revised classification of epilepsies and epileptic syndromes. Commission on Classification and Terminology of the International League Against Epilepsy. Epilepsia 1989;30:389–99.
8. Fejerman N. Atypical rolandic epilepsy. Epilepsia 2009;50(Suppl 7):9–12.
9. Kramer U. Atypical presentations of benign childhood epilepsy with centrotemporal spikes: a review. J Child Neurol 2008;23:785–90.
10. Parisi P, Bruni O, Villa MP, et al. The relationship between sleep and epilepsy: the effect on cognitive functioning in children. Dev Med Child Neurol 2010;52:805–10.
11. Saltik S, Uluduz D, Cokar O, et al. A clinical and EEG study on idiopathic partial epilepsies with evolution into ESES spectrum disorders. Epilepsia 2005;46:524–33.
12. Stephani U, Carlsson G. The spectrum from BCECTS to LKS: the rolandic EEG trait impact on cognition. Epilepsia 2006;47(Suppl 2):67–70.
13. Tassinari CA, Rubboli G, Volpi L, et al. Encephalopathy with electrical status epilepticus during slow sleep or ESES syndrome including the acquired aphasia. Clin Neurophysiol 2000;111(Suppl 2): S94–102.
14. Van Bogaert P, Aeby A, De Borchgrave V, et al. The epileptic syndromes with continuous spikes and waves during slow sleep: definition and management guidelines. Acta Neurol Belg 2006; 106:52–60.
15. Aicardi J. Benign epilepsy of childhood with Rolandic spikes (BECRS). Brain Dev 1979;1:71–3.
16. Cavazzuti GB. Epidemiology of different types of epilepsy in school age children of Modena, Italy. Epilepsia 1980;2:57–62.
17. Holmes GL. Benign focal epilepsies of childhood. Epilepsia 1993;34(Suppl. 3):S49–61.
18. Shields D, Snead OC. Benign epilepsy with centrotemporal spikes. Epilepsia 2009;50(Suppl 8):10–5.
19. Panayiotopoulos CP, Michael M, Sanders S, et al. Benign childhood focal epilepsies: assessment of established and newly recognized syndromes. Brain 2008;131:2264–86.
20. Caraballo RH, Cersosimo RO, Medina CS, et al. Panayiotopoulos-type benign childhood occipital epilepsy. A prospective study. Neurology 2000; 55:1096–100.
21. Loiseau P, Duché B. Benign childhood epilepsy with centrotemporal spikes. Cleve Clin J Med 1989;56(Suppl Pt 1):S17–22.
22. Fejerman N, Caraballo R, Tenembaum SN. Atypical evolutions of benign partial epilepsy of infancy with centro-temporal spikes. Rev Neurol 2000;31: 389–96.
23. Parmeggiani L, Seri S, Bonanni P, et al. Electrophysiological characterization of spontaneous and carbamazepine-induced epileptic negative myoclonus in benign childhood epilepsy with centrotemporal spikes. Clin Neurophysiol 2004;115:50–8.
24. Panayiotopoulos CP. The epilepsies: seizures, syndromes and management. Oxfordshire (UK): Bladon Medical Publishing; 2005.
25. Panayiotopoulos CP. Benign childhood partial seizures and related epileptic syndromes. London: John Libbey and Company Ltd; 1999.
26. Boor R, Jacobs J, Hinzmann A, et al. Combined spike-related functional MRI and multiple source analysis in the non-invasive spike localization of benign rolandic epilepsy. Clin Neurophysiol 2007; 118:901–9.
27. Panayiotopoulos CP. Extra-occipital benign childhood seizures with ictal vomiting and excellent prognosis. J Neurol Neurosurg Psychiatry 1999; 66:82–5.

28. Lerman P, Kivity S. Benign focal epilepsy of child-hood. A follow-up study of 100 recovered patients. Arch Neurol 1975;32:261–4.

29. Musumeci SA, Colognola RM, Ferri R, et al. Fragile-X syndrome: a particular epileptogenic EEG pattern. Epilepsia 1988;29:41–7.

30. De Marco P, Tassinari CA. Extreme somatosensory evoked potential (ESEP): an EEG sign forecasting the possible occurrence of seizures in children. Epilepsia 1981;22:569–75.

31. Ferri R, Del Gracco S, Elia M, et al. Age-related changes of cortical excitability in subjects with sleep-enhanced centrotemporal spikes: a somato-sensory evoked potential study. Clin Neurophysiol 2000;111:591–9.

32. Watanabe K. Recent advances and some prob-lems in the delineation of epileptic syndromes in children. Brain Dev 1996;18:423–37.

33. Eeg-Olofsson O, Safwenberg J, Wigertz A. HLA and epilepsy: an investigation of different types of epilepsy in children and their families. Epilepsia 1982;23:27–34.

34. Neubauer BA, Fiedler B, Himmelein B, et al. Centro-temporal spikes in families with rolandic epilepsy: linkage to chromosome 15q14. Neurology 1998; 51:1608–12.

35. Vadlamudi L, Kjeldsen MJ, Corey LA, et al. Analyzing the etiology of benign rolandic epilepsy: a multicenter twin collaboration. Epilepsia 2006;47: 550–5.

36. Clemens B, Oláh R. Sleep studies in benign epilepsy of childhood with rolandic spikes. I. Sleep pathology. Epilepsia 1987;28:20–3.

37. Clemens B, Majoros E. Sleep studies in benign epilepsy of childhood with rolandic spikes. II. Anal-ysis of discharge frequency and its relation to sleep dynamics. Epilepsia 1987;28:24–7.

38. Nobili L, Baglietto MG, Beelke M, et al. Modulation of sleep interictal epileptiform discharges in partial epilepsy of childhood. Clin Neurophysiol 1999;110: 839–45.

39. Beelke M, Nobili L, Baglietto MG, et al. Relationship of sigma activity to sleep interictal epileptic discharges: a study in children affected by benign epilepsy with occipital paroxysms. Epilepsy Res 2000;40:179–86.

40. Nobili L, Baglietto MG, Beelke M, et al. Spindles-inducing mechanism modulates sleep activation of interictal epileptiform discharges in the Landau-Kleffner syndrome. Epilepsia 2000;41:201–6.

41. Bruni O, Novelli L, Luchetti A, et al. Reduced NREM sleep instability in benign childhood epilepsy with centro-temporal spikes. Clin Neurophysiol 2010; 121:665–71.

42. Nobili L, Baglietto MG, Beelke M, et al. Temporal relationship of generalized epileptiform discharges to spindle frequency activity in childhood absence epilepsy. Clin Neurophysiol 2001;112:1912–6.

43. Nobili L, Ferrillo F, Baglietto MG, et al. Relationship of sleep interictal epileptiform discharges to sigma activity (12–16 Hz) in benign epilepsy of childhood with rolandic spikes. Clin Neurophysiol 1999;110: 39–46.

44. Ferri R, Bergonzi P, Elia M, et al. Modulation of the interictal epileptiform EEG activity during sleep: from oscillations to complex dynamics. Neurophy-siol Clin 1991;21:1–14.

45. Steriade M, McCormick DA, Sejnowski TJ. Thala-mocortical oscillations in the sleeping and aroused brain. Science 1993;262:679–85.

46. Naitoh P, Antony-Baas V, Muzet A, et al. Dynamic relation of sleep spindles and K-complexes to spontaneous phasic arousal in sleeping human subjects. Sleep 1982;5:58–72.

47. Guerrini R, Belmonte A, Veggiotti P, et al. Delayed appearance of interictal EEG abnormalities in early onset childhood epilepsy with occipital paroxysms. Brain Dev 1997;19:343–6.

48. Tassinari CA, De Marco P, Plasmati R, et al. Extreme somatosensory evoked potentials (ESEPs) elicited by tapping of hands or feet in children: a somatosensory cerebral evoked potentials study. Neurophysiol Clin 1988;18:123–8.

49. Kostopoulos G, Avoli M, Pellegrini A, et al. Laminar analysis of spindles and of spikes of the spike and wave discharge of feline generalized penicillin epilepsy. Electroencephalogr Clin Neurophysiol 1982;53:1–13.

50. Steriade M, Amzica F. Dynamic coupling among neocortical neurons during evoked and sponta-neous spike-wave seizure activity. J Neurophysiol 1994;72:2051–69.

51. Kellaway P, Frost JD Jr, Crawley JW. Time modula-tion of spike-and-wave activity in generalized epilepsy. Ann Neurol 1980;8:491–500.

52. Giordani B, Caveney AF, Laughrin D, et al. Cogni-tion and behavior in children with benign epilepsy with centrotemporal spikes (BECTS). Epilepsy Res 2006;70:89–94.

53. Nicolai J, Aldenkamp AP, Arends J, et al. Cognitive and behavioral effects of nocturnal epileptiform discharges in children with benign childhood epilepsy with centrotemporal spikes. Epilepsy Be-hav 2006;8:56–70.

54. Riva D, Vago C, Franceschetti S, et al. Intellectual and language findings and their relationship to EEG characteristics in benign childhood epilepsy with centrotemporal spikes. Epilepsy Behav 2007; 10:278–85.

55. Byars AW, Byars KC, Johnson CS, et al. The relation-ship between sleep problems and neuropsycholog-ical functioning in children with first recognized seizures. Epilepsy Behav 2008;13:607–13.

56. Bulgheroni S, Franceschetti S, Vago C, et al. Verbal dichotic listening performance and its relationship

with EEG features in benign childhood epilepsy with centrotemporal spikes. Epilepsy Res 2008; 79:31–8.

57. Piccinelli P, Borgatti R, Aldini A, et al. Academic performance in children with rolandic epilepsy. Dev Med Child Neurol 2008;50:353–6.

58. Clarke T, Strug LJ, Murphy PL, et al. High risk of reading disability and speech sound disorder in rolandic epilepsy families: case-control study. Epilepsia 2007;48:2258–65.

59. Sarco DP, Boyer K, Lundy-Krigbaum SM, et al. Benign rolandic epileptiform discharges are associated with mood and behavior problems. Epilepsy Behav 2011;22:298–303.

60. Panayiotopoulos CP. Panayiotopoulos syndrome: a common and benign childhood epileptic syndrome. London: John Libbey and Company; 2002.

61. Ferrie CD, Beaumanoir A, Guerrini R, et al. Early-onset benign occipital seizure susceptibility syndrome. Epilepsia 1997;38:285–93.

62. Vigevano F, Lispi ML, Ricci S. Early onset benign occipital susceptibility syndrome: video-EEG documentation of an illustrative case. Clin Neurophysiol 2000;111(Suppl 2):S81–6.

63. Lada C, Skiadas K, Theodorou V, et al. A study of 43 patients with Panayiotopoulos syndrome: a common and benign childhood seizure susceptibility. Epilepsia 2003;44:81–8.

64. Koutroumanidis M, Rowlinson S, Sanders S. Recurrent autonomic status epilepticus in Panayiotopoulos syndrome: video/EEG studies. Epilepsy Behav 2005;7:543–7.

65. Parisi P, Ferri R, Pagani J, et al. Ictal video-polysomnography and EEG spectral analysis in a child with severe Panayiotopoulos syndrome. Epileptic Disord 2005;7:333–9.

66. Ferrie C, Caraballo R, Covanis A, et al. Panayiotopoulos syndrome: a consensus view. Dev Med Child Neurol 2006;48:236–40.

67. Ferrie CD, Caraballo R, Covanis A, et al. Autonomic status epilepticus in Panayiotopoulos syndrome and other childhood and adult epilepsies: a consensus view. Epilepsia 2007;48:1165–72.

68. Caraballo R, Cersósimo R, Fejerman N. Panayiotopoulos syndrome: a prospective study of 192 patients. Epilepsia 2007;48:1054–61.

69. Capovilla G, Striano P, Beccaria F. Changes in Panayiotopoulos syndrome over time. Epilepsia 2009; 50(Suppl 5):45–8.

70. Michael M, Tsatsou K, Ferrie CD. Panayiotopoulos syndrome: an important childhood autonomic epilepsy to be differentiated from occipital epilepsy and acute non-epileptic disorders. Brain Dev 2010; 32:4–9.

71. Covanis A, Lada C, Skiadas K. Children with Rolandic spikes and ictal vomiting: Rolandic epilepsy or Panayiotopoulos syndrome? Epileptic Disord 2003; 5:139–43.

72. Taylor I, Berkovic SF, Kivity S, et al. Benign occipital epilepsies of childhood: clinical features and genetics. Brain 2008;13:2287–94.

73. Leal AJ, Ferreira JC, Dias AI, et al. Origin of frontal lobe spikes in the early onset benign occipital lobe epilepsy (Panayiotopoulos syndrome). Clin Neurophysiol 2008;119:1985–91.

74. Ohtsu M, Oguni H, Hayashi K, et al. EEG in children with early-onset benign occipital seizure susceptibility syndrome: Panayiotopoulos syndrome. Epilepsia 2003;44:435–42.

75. Beaumanoir A. Semiology of occipital seizures in infants and children. In: Andermann F, Beaumanoir A, Mira L, et al, editors. Occipital seizures and epilepsies in children. London: John Libbey and Company Ltd; 1993. p. 71–86.

76. Vigevano F, Ricci S. Benign occipital epilepsy of childhood with prolonged seizures and autonomic symptoms. In: Andermann F, Beaumanoir A, Mira L, et al, editors. Occipital seizures and epilepsies in children. London: John Libbey and Company Ltd; 1993. p. 133–40.

77. Oguni H, Hayashi K, Imai K, et al. Study on the early-onset variant of benign childhood epilepsy with occipital paroxysms otherwise described as early-onset benign occipital seizure susceptibility syndrome. Epilepsia 1999;40:1020–30.

78. Grosso S, Orrico A, Galli L, et al. SCN1A mutation associated with atypical Panayiotopoulos syndrome. Neurology 2007;69:609–11.

79. Livingston JH, Cross JH, Mclellan A, et al. A novel inherited mutation in the voltage sensor region of SCN1A is associated with Panayiotopoulos syndrome in siblings and generalized epilepsy with febrile seizures plus. J Child Neurol 2009;24: 503–8.

80. Panayiotopoulos CP. Vomiting as an ictal manifestation of epileptic seizures and syndromes. J Neurol Neurosurg Psychiatry 1988;51:1448–51.

81. Guerrini R, Dravet C, Genton P, et al. Idiopathic photosensitive occipital lobe epilepsy. Epilepsia 1995;36:883–91.

82. Verrotti A, Salladini C, Trotta D, et al. Ictal cardiorespiratory arrest in Panayiotopoulos syndrome. Neurology 2005;64:1816–7.

83. Germanò E, Gagliano A, Magazù A, et al. Benign childhood epilepsy with occipital paroxysms: neuropsychological findings. Epilepsy Res 2005;64: 137–50.

84. Covanis A. Panayiotopoulos syndrome: a benign childhood autonomic epilepsy frequently imitating encephalitis, syncope, migraine, sleep disorder, or gastroenteritis. Pediatrics 2006;118: e1237–43.

85. Gastaut H. A new type of epilepsy: benign partial epilepsy of childhood with occipital spike-waves. Clin Electroencephalogr 1982;13:13–22.

86. Panayiotopoulos CP. Benign childhood epilepsy with occipital paroxysms: a 15-year prospective study. Ann Neurol 1989;26:51–6.

87. Covanis A. Photosensitivity in idiopathic generalized epilepsies. Epilepsia 2005;46(Suppl 9):67–72.

88. Gobbi G, Boni A, Filippini M. The spectrum of idiopathic Rolandic epilepsy syndromes and idiopathic occipital epilepsies: from the benign to the disabling. Epilepsia 2006;47(Suppl 2):62–6.

89. Caraballo RH, Cersósimo RO, Fejerman N. Childhood occipital epilepsy of Gastaut: a study of 33 patients. Epilepsia 2008;49:288–97.

90. Gastaut H, Zifkin BG. The risk of automobile accidents with seizures occurring while driving: relation to seizure type. Neurology 1987;37:1613–6.

91. Panayiotopoulos CP. Inhibitory effect of central vision on occipital lobe seizures. Neurology 1981; 31:330–3.

92. Herranz Tanarro FJ, Saénz Lope E, Cristobal Sassot S. Occipital spike-wave with and without benign epilepsy in the child. Rev Electroencephalogr Neurophysiol Clin 1984;14:1–7 [in French].

93. Caraballo RH, Cersósimo RO, Fejerman N. Late-onset, "Gastaut type," childhood occipital epilepsy: an unusual evolution. Epileptic Disord 2005;7:341–6.

94. Gülgönen S, Demirbilek V, Korkmaz B, et al. Neuropsychological functions in idiopathic occipital lobe epilepsy. Epilepsia 2000;41:405–11.

95. Niedermeyer E, Rocca U. The diagnostic significance of sleep electroencephalograms in temporal lobe epilepsy. A comparison of scalp and depth tracings. Eur Neurol 1972;7:119–29.

96. Malow BA. Sleep and epilepsy. Neurol Clin 1996; 14:765–89.

97. Malow BA, Lin X, Kushwaha R, et al. Interictal spiking increases with sleep depth in temporal lobe epilepsy. Epilepsia 1998;39:1309–16.

98. Sammaritano M, Gigli GL, Gotman J. Interictal spiking during wakefulness and sleep and the localization of foci in temporal lobe epilepsy. Neurology 1991;41:290–7.

99. Ferrillo F, Beelke M, De Carli F, et al. Sleep-EEG modulation of interictal epileptiform discharges in adult partial epilepsy: a spectral analysis study. Clin Neurophysiol 2000;111:916–23.

100. Montplaisir J, Laverdière M, Saint-Hilaire JM, et al. Sleep and temporal lobe epilepsy: a case study with depth electrodes. Neurology 1981;31:1352–6.

101. Sinha SR. Basic mechanisms of sleep and epilepsy. J Clin Neurophysiol 2011;28:103–10.

102. Steriade M, Amzica F. Slow sleep oscillation, rhythmic K-complexes, and their paroxysmal developments. J Sleep Res 1998;7(Suppl 1):30–5.

103. Eisensehr I, Parrino L, Noachtar S, et al. Sleep in Lennox-Gastaut syndrome: the role of the cyclic alternating pattern (CAP) in the gate control of clinical seizures and generalized polyspikes. Epilepsy Res 2001;46:241–50.

104. Manni R, Zambrelli E, Bellazzi R, et al. The relationship between focal seizures and sleep: an analysis of the cyclic alternating pattern. Epilepsy Res 2005;67:73–80.

105. Parrino L, Halasz P, Tassinari CA, et al. CAP, epilepsy and motor events during sleep: the unifying role of arousal. Sleep Med Rev 2006;10: 267–85.

106. Terzaghi M, Sartori I, Tassi L, et al. Evidence of dissociated arousal states during NREM parasomnia from an intracerebral neurophysiological study. Sleep 2009;32:409–12.

107. Terzano MG, Parrino L, Spaggiari MC, et al. Discriminatory effect of cyclic alternating pattern in focal lesional and benign rolandic interictal spikes during sleep. Epilepsia 1991b;32:616–28.

108. Terzano MG, Parrino L, Garofalo PG, et al. Activation of partial seizures with motor signs during cyclic alternating pattern in human sleep. Epilepsy Res 1991a;10:166–73.

109. Bruni O, Novelli L, Finotti E, et al. All-night EEG power spectral analysis of the cyclic alternating pattern at different ages. Clin Neurophysiol 2009; 120:248–56.

110. Ferri R, Bruni O, Miano S, et al. All-night EEG power spectral analysis of the cyclic alternating pattern components in young adult subjects. Clin Neurophysiol 2005;116:2429–40.

111. Holmes GL, Lenck-Santini PP. Role of interictal epileptiform abnormalities in cognitive impairment. Epilepsy Behav 2006;8:504–15.

112. Urbain C, Di Vincenzo T, Peigneux P, et al. Is sleep-related consolidation impaired in focal idiopathic epilepsies of childhood? A pilot study. Epilepsy Behav 2011;22:380–4.

Electrical Status Epilepticus in Sleep

Elina Liukkonen, MD, PhD[a],[*],
Madeleine M. Grigg-Damberger, MD[b]

KEYWORDS

- Epilepsy • Children • ESES • CSWS • Clinical • Outcome

Electrographic status epilepticus in slow-wave sleep (ESES) is an electroencephalographic pattern characterized by continuous (or near-continuous) spike-wave discharges during non–rapid eye movement (NREM) sleep. ESES is most often associated with an encephalopathy (ESES syndrome) characterized by epileptic seizures; continuous spike-wave discharges in NREM sleep; global or selective regression of cognitive functions; and motor impairments, such as ataxia, dyspraxia, and unilateral dysfunction. The importance of this electrophysiological phenomenon lies in the detrimental effects it has on the neurologic and neuropsychological development of affected children.

ESES (the electroencephalogram [EEG] pattern alone) and the ESES syndrome may occur in children with no previous neurologic problems (idiopathic type) as well as in children with preexisting neurodevelopmental impairment or marked structural changes in the central nervous system (symptomatic form). The pathophysiological basis of the disorder is not fully understood. The EEG pattern and seizures of ESES are thought to be self-limited in that they usually disappear by puberty, but the neuropsychological outcome of the patients is often poor even if ESES was eradicated early by medications or epilepsy surgery.

This review provides an overview of the clinical features, treatment options, outcome, and suggested mechanisms of neuropsychological deterioration of encephalopathy with ESES. In this review, the term ESES will refer to the EEG pattern and ESES syndrome to the EEG pattern associated with clinical symptoms and signs.

HISTORY AND DEFINITIONS

In 1971, Patry and colleagues[1] first reported the EEG pattern of continuous spike and waves during slow-wave sleep in 6 children. They called the EEG pattern electrical or subclinical status epilepticus because it was not associated with any clinical signs when it occurred during sleep. All of these children had moderate to severe cognitive impairment, and 5 had epileptic seizures when the ESES pattern was first observed.

As other cases were reported, it became clear that ESES was an epileptic encephalopathy; the onset of it was most often associated with or followed by neurologic regression and seizures. Epileptic encephalopathies are conditions in which the epileptiform EEG abnormalities themselves are thought to contribute to a progressive disturbance in cerebral function.[2] In 1977, Tassinari and colleagues[3] proposed that the abbreviation, ESES, should stand for encephalopathy with status epilepticus during sleep. More recent classifications by the International League Against Epilepsy (ILAE) call it "epileptic encephalopathy with continuous spike and wave during sleep (CSWS)."[4,5]

The ILAE classification defines the ESES syndrome as an age-related and self-limited disorder characterized by 1) epilepsy with focal and apparently generalized seizures (unilateral or bilateral clonic seizures, tonic-clonic seizures, absences,

Elina Liukkonen has received lecture honoraria from Eisai.

[a] Epilepsy Unit, Department of Pediatric Neurology, Helsinki University Central Hospital, Stenbäckinkatu 28 F, 00250 Helsinki, Finland

[b] Department of Neurology, University of New Mexico School of Medicine, MSC10 5620, One University of NM, Albuquerque, NM 87131-0001, USA

* Corresponding author.

E-mail addresses: elina.liukkonen@hus.fi; elina.liukkonen@fimnet.fi

Sleep Med Clin 7 (2012) 147–156
doi:10.1016/j.jsmc.2011.12.003
1556-407X/12/$ – see front matter © 2012 Elsevier Inc. All rights reserved.

partial motor seizures, complex partial seizures, or epileptic falls); 2) neuropsychological impairment in the form of global or selective regression of cognitive functions; 3) motor impairment in the form of ataxia, dyspraxia, dystonia, or unilateral deficit; and 4) typical EEG findings with a pattern of diffuse spike wave (or more or less unilateral or focal occurring up to 85% of slow-wave sleep and persisting on 3 or more recordings over a period of at least 1 month).[2] The percentage of NREM sleep occupied by spike-wave discharges varies in the literature from greater than 25% to greater than 85%.[6-8] **Fig. 1** shows an example of ESES during NREM sleep.

CLINICAL PRESENTATION

ESES syndrome is a rare age-related condition occurring only in childhood, with a suggested incidence of 0.2% to 0.5% of childhood epilepsies.[9] The first clinical symptoms usually emerge between 5 and 9 years of age.[10] In most cases, the clinical course can be divided into 3 stages.[9,11-13] The first stage of ESES syndrome is usually heralded by the onset of seizures between 1 and 10 years of age (peak 4–5 years). The first seizure occurs in sleep in half of the cases, and in 40% it consists of unilateral convulsions that can last more than 30 minutes (hemiclonic status epilepticus).[13] Other seizure types observed include focal motor, myoclonic, atypical absence, and generalized tonic-clonic. Seizures during the first stage tend to be infrequent and occur primarily in sleep.[13] Tonic seizures are never seen in patients with ESES at any stage in the disease and when present warrant consideration of another diagnosis.

The second stage is often observed 1 to 2 years after epilepsy onset with the development of ESES with specific or global neuropsychological deterioration or behavioral problems. Habitual seizures become more frequent; and new seizure types are often observed, such as hemifacial, hemiconvulsive, atypical absences, and negative myoclonus (an interruption of tonic muscular activity time locked to a spike on the EEG without evidence of an antecedent myoclonus). Convulsive seizures continue to occur primarily during sleep. The neuropsychological regression tends to be gradual and progressive. Other neurologic deficits that occur in the second phase include ataxia, hemiparesis, or dyspraxia. Some develop an acquired epileptiform opercular syndrome characterized by dysarthria, drooling, face/tongue weakness, or speech arrest. The third stage of ESES syndrome is residual stage with alleviation of epilepsy and ESES by puberty, but permanent neuropsychological sequelae remain in half of the patients.[9,10]

In the prospective longitudinal study of 32 children with ESES syndrome, 53% (17) had a symptomatic cause, 6 (19%) had atypical rolandic epilepsy, and 9 (28%) had Landau-Kleffner syndrome (LKS).[14] Eleven children had congenital hemiplegia, 8 had unilateral thalamic injury on magnetic resonance imaging (MRI), and 5 had obstructive hydrocephalus. The mean age of epilepsy onset was 3.1 years, which was earlier in the symptomatic group than in the idiopathic group. Twenty (63%) of the children were cognitively normal before the development of ESES. Clinical symptoms of ESES syndrome (motor, language, behavioral, or cognitive deterioration) emerged at a mean age of 4.4 years. Symptoms

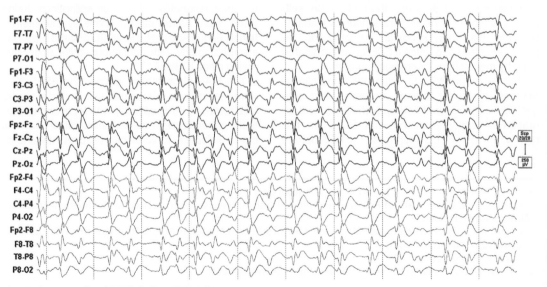

Fig. 1. An example of ESES during NREM sleep.

of encephalopathy most often observed were deterioration of motor functions, including oral motor problems, combined with marked cognitive and behavioral problems in the symptomatic group. Mean delay from symptom onset to diagnosis of ESES was 1.0 year (0.1–4.8 years). In 7 children with a symptomatic cause and previous neuropsychological evaluation, the mean drop of the IQ by the time of the diagnosis of ESES syndrome was 29 points. Within the whole group of 32 children, the mean subsequent reduction of the IQ score during ESES, despite active treatment, was 23 points.

Others report at least one-third of the patients with ESES syndrome have symptomatic focal epilepsy with prenatal and perinatal problems or deviations in early development or structural abnormalities on brain imaging.[10,15] MRI abnormalities reported in children with ESES include unilateral or diffuse cortical atrophy, focal porencephaly, and cortical malformations. Cases of ESES in children with congenital hemiplegia either with prenatal/perinatal vascular or dysgenetic cause,[14–19] obstructive hydrocephalus,[16,17] or thalamic injury[14,20] have been reported. However, epidemiologic data on ESES syndrome in children with these conditions are not available.

ESES syndrome may occur in children with normal previous development and with normal brain structure in MRI. Some cases of ESES syndrome seem to evolve from idiopathic focal epilepsies of childhood, such as benign epilepsy of childhood with centrotemporal spikes[16,21,22] and the benign occipital epilepsy of childhood.[23] The risk of atypical evolution in idiopathic focal epilepsies seems to be low, less than 1%.[21] Other idiopathic epilepsies that may be associated with ESES include the opercular syndrome with oral motor dysfunction, drooling, and epileptic negative myoclonus[24] and atypical benign partial epilepsy with frequent atypical absences.[25,26] The ESES syndrome needs to be distinguished from the acquired epileptic aphasia syndrome of LKS defined primarily by a gradually acquired aphasia combined with marked activation of primarily temporal epileptiform activity in sleep.[27–31] The clinical features of these syndromes are discussed in greater detail in this issue in the article authored by Bruni and colleagues.

EEG FINDINGS

The EEG pattern that defines the ESES syndrome is characterized by continuous spike-wave discharges during NREM sleep that are usually generalized and symmetric repeating at frequencies varying from 1.5 to 2.0 Hz, the pattern appearing as soon as the child falls asleep. The discharges

may be asymmetrical, lateralized, or relatively focal, often frontally or centrally maximum, and sometimes consisting of sharp, spike discharges.[9,32] Discharges in wakefulness are infrequent, focal, or multifocal spikes or spike waves. In some, atypical absences are seen in wakefulness. During REM sleep, spike waves are far less frequent, occupying less than 25% of the REM sleep times. Discharges during REM sleep are often focal and similar to those in the wake EEG.[9] Focal or multifocal spikes or spike waves occur infrequently.

The typical EEG finding in these patients *before* ESES develops are focal spikes or spike waves predominantly in centrotemporal or frontotemporal regions, sometimes with generalized spike waves that occur mainly in sleep.[9] Some investigators suggest EEG features that increase the risk a child with benign idiopathic epilepsy could evolve to ESES include (1) focal spike-wave activity that spreads to adjacent regions or to the contralateral hemisphere and (2) focal slowing in the region of major epileptiform activity.[33] As the ESES pattern begins to resolve, the spike-wave discharges in sleep become shorter, less frequent, and more fragmented. The EEG typically normalizes, often 3 to 5 years after the onset of the syndrome. Rare focal discharges may persist in a few.

SPIKE-WAVE INDEX

Investigators have used the spike-wave index (SWI) to quantify the percentage of NREM sleep occupied by spike-wave discharges. The SWI is usually defined by total minutes of spike waves multiplied by 100 and divided by the total minutes of NREM sleep without spike waves.[15] The SWI is usually greater than 85% of the total duration of NREM sleep. Other investigators have defined ESES with lower SWI of greater than 25% to greater than 60%, justifying this by as the discharges are markedly activated by sleep. The duration of the sleep recording period needed to define the SWI varies from whole night sleep, first sleep cycle, and daytime nap.[7,8] Computerized digital EEG techniques allow semiautomated calculation of the SWI,[34] making analysis of it far less laborious. In 2009, Scheltens-deBoer[35] proposed quantitative and qualitative methods for classifying the EEG in patients with ESES that could make the comparison and interpretation of the published studies easier and possibly facilitate multicenter studies for this rare condition.

SLEEP ARCHITECTURE

Sleep spindles, K-complexes, or vertex waves are seldom recognizable during ESES. The SWI often lessens across the night, and later NREM cycles contain lower percentages of spike-wave discharges (such that the average SWI for all NREM sleep is greater than 85%, with much higher percentages in earlier NREM sleep periods). The onset of REM sleep is often recognized by the disappearance of ESES. It is fairly easy to score REM sleep then because discharges are much less frequent. When the ESES pattern is fragmented, sleep architecture seems to be preserved with approximately 80% of the sleep time spent in NREM sleep and the remaining 20% in REM sleep.[13,15] Sleep organization and sleep stages are normal after the ESES pattern disappears.

LOCALIZATION OF THE EPILEPTIFORM ACTIVITY AND CLINICAL PICTURE

At first glance, the ESES pattern is typically generalized and focal features are often evident. Initially, the ILAE classified the epilepsy associated with ESES as "undetermined as to whether it is focal or generalized."[36] In 1994, Kobayashi and colleagues[37] argued that ESES has a focal cortical origin that is secondarily generalized in NREM sleep. The synchronizing nature of NREM sleep leads to focal discharges that seem widespread (a term called secondary bilateral synchrony).[38] ESES is now regarded as a focal epilepsy; the discharges generalized during NREM sleep are focal (or multifocal) during wake and REM sleep.

Some investigators argue that the neuropsychological deficits in ESES syndrome reflect the localization of the spikes. Cognitive dysfunction in children with frontal or prefrontal ESES often results in frontal lobe dysfunction with hyperkinesia, disinhibition, inattention, aggression, psychosis, or dementia, whereas temporal lobe ESES tends to produce prominent language deficits, especially for the expression of it (as compared with comprehension).

TREATMENT STRATEGIES

Treatment choices for ESES syndrome are based primarily on case reports and small cases series; no randomized controlled studies to treat it exist. Various antiepileptic drugs (AEDs), such as valproate (VPA), ethosuximide (ESM), benzodiazepines, sulthiame, and levetiracetam and intravenous immunoglobulin (IV-IG) or corticosteroids have been reported to abolish the ESES pattern from the EEG.[7,8,16,39–48] Carbamazepine, oxcarbazepine, and phenobarbital may aggravate seizures and ESES and should be avoided.[7,49] Carbamazepine may provoke generalization of the spike-wave discharges.[11,13,49]

Kramer and colleagues[16] (2009) reported treatment responses in 30 children with ESES syndrome treated between 1994 and 2007 in 4 pediatric neurology outpatient clinics. The antiepileptic drugs that were found to be efficacious were levetiracetam (41%), clobazam (31%), and sulthiame (17%). In this case series, VPA, lamotrigine, topiramate, and ESM showed no efficacy. Corticosteroids were effective in 65%, and immunoglobulins were efficacious in a third. A third of the patients responded to high-dose diazepam, but this effect was only temporary.

The author (EL) prospectively evaluated the efficacy of VPA in all 32 children and a combination of VPA and ESM in children with bilaterally synchronous ESES or atypical absences.[14] The primary treatment response was defined by total abolition of ESES, although permitting possible residual focal spiking. No response to VPA as the sole AED therapy (monotherapy) was observed, whereas ESES disappeared in 3 (18%) of the 17 children treated with the combination of VPA and ESM. In all, ESES disappeared with drug treatment in 16 children (50%) using different combinations of antiepileptic drugs and prednisone.

Treatment with oral corticosteroids, adrenocorticotropic hormone, or IV-IG is tried most often in patients who do not respond to AEDs. Some patients have clinical and EEG improvement. One case series treated 44 children with ESES with hydrocortisone (5 mg/kg/d during the first month, 4 mg/kg/d the second, 3 mg/kg/d the third, 2 mg/kg/d during months 4 to 12, then slowly tapering over a total treatment period of 21 months.[42] Seizures or neuropsychological deficits improved in 34 patients (77%). Seizures were completely controlled in 77%, EEG normalized in 21 (47%), and the long-term remission rate was 45%. Only a few case reports of immunoglobulin therapy improving ESES syndrome have been reported.[48,50,51]

Several small case series have recently been published reporting the benefits of epilepsy surgeries on ESES refractory to medical treatment.[52–56] The author's (EL) group recently reported the benefits of epilepsy surgery in 13 children with medically refractory ESES syndrome.[52] The group found that after surgery (1) the ESES EEG pattern terminated in 2 patients, restricted to 1 region in 1 patient, and lessened after surgery in 4 patients; (2) cognitive deterioration was halted in 12 patients; and (3) cognitive catch-up of greater than 10 IQ points was seen in 3 patients (all of whom had shown a first measured IQ of >75).[52] Loddenkemper and colleagues (2009)[53] reported a beneficial outcome of epilepsy surgery on 8 children with ESES. Symptomatic causes for ESES were a perinatal infarction in 7 patients and a cortical malformation in 1 patient. Six patients became seizure free after resection, and 2 patients continued to have rare seizures. The postoperative EEG demonstrated resolution of generalized interictal epileptic discharges (IEDs) and ESES in all. Formal preoperative and postoperative neuropsychological testing showed overall improvement of age-equivalent scores.

Epilepsy surgery should be considered in patients with a unilateral brain lesion, even when the EEG activity shows no localizing features. Successful treatment of epilepsy and ESES by hemispherectomy or functional hemispherectomy and resective surgery report overall improvements in one-half of the patients undergo them.[52,53,55,57] The frequency of atypical absences was markedly reduced in the case series of children with ESES syndrome who had anterior or total corpus callosotomy.[52]

PROGNOSIS

The studies on the outcome of children with ESES syndrome are often difficult to interpret and compare with other studies because patients with idiopathic focal epilepsy and a symptomatic cause are presented and discussed together. Moreover, in many studies the subjects are grouped by the extent of the epileptiform discharge (SWI), which makes the evaluation of the impact of the underlying clinical/neurologic and etiologic factors on the outcome difficult.[6,15,58–60] Clinical seizures and the ESES EEG pattern tend to resolve by adolescence.[9,61] It is not clear whether this finding is spontaneous or the result of drug treatment. Seizures generally stop before the ESES pattern disappears.[9,14,33,61] Complete neuropsychological and cognitive recovery is possible but rarely observed.[14,59,60,62]

Rousselle and Revol[63] reviewed 44 articles published from 1974 to 1992 of 209 children who had continuous or near-continuous spikes during non-REM 3 (slow wave sleep). They divided the children into groups based on their premorbid neurologic condition and subsequent neuropsychological deterioration. They also divided them into 4 groups: (1) 35 children with atypical idiopathic epilepsy; (2) 33 children with language problems (the majority consistent with LKS); (3) 99 children who had normal development before; and (4) 42 children who had focal of diffuse brain lesions and preexistent global cognitive problems.

They found that the long-term cognitive prognosis was favorable in most of the first group (atypical idiopathic epilepsy), only one-fourth of the children in the third group (idiopathic form), and less than 20% of the fourth group regained their previous level. The SWI and duration of CSWS increased successively from group 1 to group 4, and these were considered to be one of the determinant factors of the prognosis. Duration of the ESES EEG pattern for longer than 2 years was associated with poor cognitive outcome.

In the studies that included more than 15 patients, the neuropsychological and psychosocial prognosis has been reported to be poor in at least half.[6,15,16,33,58,62,64] **Table 1** presents the studies in which data on cognitive outcome could be extracted. Generally, neuropsychological evaluations were not detailed, and the degree of permanent deterioration was not clearly defined.

Our study on the long-term cognitive outcome of 32 children was the first prospective longitudinal study of ESESS.[14] The mean follow-up was 5.4 years, and some were followed up to 13 years after the diagnosis. The effects of drug treatment for ESES syndrome included the following: (1) ESES was abolished with drug treatment in 50% (n = 16) of the children (including 6 of 17 patients with symptomatic, 4 of 6 patients with atypical rolandic epilepsy, and 6 of 9 patients with LKS) who had ESES for 1.2 to 6.9 years; (2) cognitive catch-up to a pre-ESES cognitive level (levels: IQ >85, IQ 70–85, IQ 50–69, IQ 30–49 and IQ <30) occurred in 28% (n = 9, all treatment responders), including 2 of 6 patients with symptomatic, 4 of 4 patients with atypical rolandic, and 3 of 6 patients with LKS; and (3) a permanent cognitive decline by 2 or 3 IQ levels persisted in 44% (14), including 9 of 16 patients with symptomatic forms of ESES syndrome, 1 of 6 patients with atypical rolandic, and 4 of 9 patient with LKS.

Earlier age of onset of the ESES was associated with a poor outcome, which may reflect more extensive disturbance during the developmentally important early years. Children who had a higher IQ at the time of the ESES diagnosis had better cognitive outcomes (mean IQ 90 vs 72), suggesting more extensive brain abnormality or more severe epilepsy to begin with in the latter group. Cognitive catch-up only occurred in the drug responders.[14]

Fig. 2 shows the cognitive course of the 16 children with a symptomatic cause. The patients who showed no response to drug treatments showed steady cognitive decline. **Fig. 3** shows how their cognitive deterioration was halted in those who went to epilepsy surgery. The patients who showed no response to drug treatment and were not candidates for epilepsy surgery were those with the lowest pre-ESES cognitive level. Features that predicted a favorable response to epilepsy surgery among 13 children with medically refractory symptomatic ESES syndrome were (1) a unilateral brain abnormality; (2) interhemispheric propagation pattern on the EEG; and (3) normal or nearly normal initial cognitive development before was associated with cognitive catch-up of +10 or more IQ points 2 years postoperatively.[52]

Table 1
Clinical characteristics and course of ESES syndrome in published studies with at least 15 patients

Author, Year of Publication (Retrospective/Prospective)	Number of Patients (Patient Groups)	Previous Development	Definition of CSWS/ESES (N If Varying)	Age at dx of ESES, Mean (Range)	Duration of ESES, Mean (Range)	Definition of ESES Disappearance	Follow-up, Mean (Range)	Cognitive Outcome	Prognostic Factors
Tassinari et al,[15] 1992 (Retrospective)	29 (15 symptomatic)	18 normal, 11 deficit	SWI >85%	8 y (3–15 y)	3 y	EEG normal/focal	7 y	50% permanent deficit, not defined	Better if previously normal; Poor if ESES >2 y; No correlation with age of epilepsy onset epilepsy severity symptomatic cause
Veggiotti et al,[62] 1999 (Retrospective)	32 (13 cryptogenic, 19 symptomatic)	18 normal or mild delay, 4 moderate delay, 10 severe delay	SWI >85%	5.8 y	(0.5–5.0 y) cryptogenic mean 2 y, symptomatic mean 1.5 y	Not defined (SWI <85%)	Not reported	11 lost at least one IQ level	
Robinson et al,[64] 2001 (Prospective)	17 (Landau-Kleffner syndrome)	13 normal, 4 delay	SWI >70%	4.7 y (2–7 y)	3.7 y (1–8 y)	Not defined (SWI <85%)	5.5 y (1–15 y)	3 regained normal language, 4 less than 50% of age level	Normal outcome possible if ESES <3 y
Saltik et al,[33] 2005 (Prospective)	16 (idiopathic)	All normal	SWI >85%, symmetric or mildly asymmetric	7.8 y (4.5–13.0 y)	1.2 y (3 mo to 3 y)	SWI 50%–85%, hemi CSWS, focal, normal	5.8 y (4–11 y)	3 previous level, 9 not previous level (3 severe impairment)	No correlation with ESES duration
Kramer et al,[16] 2009 (Retrospective)	30 (12 symptomatic, 11 idiopathic, 7 unknown)	20 normal, 10 mental retardation	SWI >85% (24), 50%–85% (5), 30%–50% (1)	6.7 y	9 mo (2 mo to 5 y)	Normal, >75%, >50%, >25% improvement of SWI, or focal	6.6 y (2–14 y)	14 permanent cognitive deficit; Also 3/6 with SWI 40%–85% and 3/7 of focal ESES	No one with ESES duration >1.5 y regained previous level; Cause did not predict outcome
Liukkonen et al,[14] 2010 (Prospective)	32 (17 symptomatic, 6 idiopathic, 9 Landau-Kleffner syndrome)	18 normal, 8 nearly normal, 4 mild II, 2 moderate or severe II	SWI >85%	5.4 y (2.7–9.2 y)	3.5 y (1.2–6.9 y) in treatment responders	Normal or focal spiking	5.4 y (0.2–13.4 y) 8 surgical patients excluded	16 ESES abolished, 10 regained previous level, 14 lost 2 IQ levels (see text)	No correlation of ESES duration and outcome, but definition of ESES disappearance very strict; Better outcome with idiopathic cause

Abbreviations: dx, diagnosis; II, intellectual impairment.

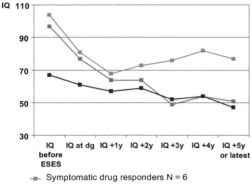

Fig. 2. The cognitive course of the 16 children with symptomatic cause.

PATHOPHYSIOLOGICAL MECHANISMS

We do not know what causes ESES or its syndrome. Some suggest that the ESES pattern represents pathologic hyperexcitable neuronal firing of the corticothalamic neuronal network, which generates sleep spindles in NREM sleep.[65,66] More research evaluating the role of the thalamus in the development of ESES is needed. It may explain why focal discharges become generalized in NREM sleep in patients with ESES (so-called secondary bilateral synchrony)[37] and the observations of thalamic injury in children with ESES syndrome.[14,20]

Even a single IED can transiently interfere with cognitive processes (via membrane hyperpolarization). IEDs in ESES, if particularly frequent and widespread, may impair daytime cognitive abilities by interfering with synaptic plasticity and memory consolidation of learning and memories, which seem to normally occur preferentially during sleep.[61,67–69] Functional neuroimaging studies in children with ESES syndrome suggest that surround

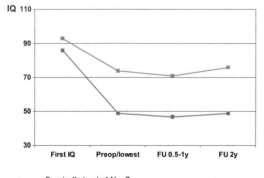

Fig. 3. Effect on cognitive deterioration in those who were suitable candidates for epilepsy surgery.

and remote inhibition may represent one possible mechanism for how the neurophysiological effects of ESES activity spread to connected brain areas.[70–72] De Tiege and colleagues have published a series of studies examining evaluating positron emission tomography[70,72] or functional MRI[71] in children with ESES. In the first, they found 3 different types of metabolic patterns in 18 children with ESES: 55% had focal hypermetabolism with distant hypometabolism primarily involving the frontal, parietal, or temporal associative cortical areas; 28% of the children had focal hypometabolism; and 17% did not have any significant metabolic abnormality.[72] In 2008, De Tiege and colleagues[70] performed PET studies using FDG in 9 children during acute and recovery phases of ESES. They found altered effective neuronal network connectivity between areas of focal hypermetabolism in the centroparietal regions and right fusiform gyrus and widespread hypometabolism (prefrontal and orbitofrontal cortices, temporal lobes, left parietal cortex, precuneus, and cerebellum) during the acute phase of ESES. Recovery from ESES was characterized by a complete or near complete regression of these abnormalities. The investigators argued that these results show that the neurophysiological effects of CSWS activity are not restricted to the epileptic foci but spread via the inhibition of remote neurons within connected brain areas. They suggested that these reversible remote effects seen in children with ESES syndrome contribute to the cognitive dysfunction seen in children with ESES syndrome. They also reported on an EEG–functional MRI (fMRI) study[71] on a girl with CSWS and marked problems in executive functions and memory. During interictal secondarily generalized spike-wave discharges, EEG-fMRI demonstrated deactivations in the lateral and medial frontoparietal cortices, posterior cingulate gyrus, and cerebellum, with focal relative activations in the right frontal, parietal, and temporal cortices. These findings suggest that the neuropsychological dysfunctions could be related to secondary cortical dysfunction spreading from localized epileptic foci.

Despite etiologic heterogeneity and different epileptic foci, Siniatchkin and colleagues[73] (2010) found that spike-wave discharges in NREM 3 sleep in 12 children with ESES syndrome produced a similar pattern of neuronal network activation in the perisylvian region, insula, and cingulate gyrus using EEG- fMRI. Simultaneously, other brain regions (precuneus, parietal cortex, and medial frontal cortex in all and the caudate nucleus in 4) showed deactivation time locked to the spike-wave activity. The investigators argued that these findings demonstrate how the spiking of ESES in sleep could impact on normal brain function by causing repetitive interruptions of neurophysiological function. These networks seem important in neuropsychological processes, and consolidations of memories in sleep and disturbance in the function of these networks could explain neuropsychological deficits in ESES syndrome.[61] Sleep seems to play a critical role in brain synaptic plasticity, which is the basis for consolidation of memories and learning.[67,68] Continuous spiking in NREM sleep in children with ESES may interfere with these crucial processes and, if occurring at a crucial developmental age, leave permanent cognitive deficits that linger long after the ESES pattern has remitted.

SUMMARY

ESES syndrome is a devastating childhood epileptic encephalopathy that may permanently and considerably disturb the developmental potential of a child with either idiopathic or symptomatic epilepsy. The original SWI criteria of at least 85% only reveals the tip of the iceberg, and total abolishment of ESES may be needed for a complete catch-up of neuropsychological impairment. Results of drug treatment are variable, and surgical treatment should be offered as early as possible to potential candidates, such as children with congenital hemiplegia. Complete cognitive recovery is possible but rarely observed, and at least half of the children have permanent cognitive impairments. Patients with idiopathic epilepsy generally have better cognitive outcome than those with a symptomatic cause. To make the diagnosis as early as possible, sleep EEG is recommended whenever any new epileptic, developmental, or behavioral concern in a child aged less than 10 years arises. The exact pathophysiological mechanisms of ESES and cognitive deterioration are still unclear.

REFERENCES

1. Patry G, Lyagoubi S, Tassinari CA. Subclinical "electrical status epilepticus" induced by sleep in children. A clinical and electroencephalographic study of six cases. Arch Neurol 1971;24(3):242–52.
2. Engel J Jr. A proposed diagnostic scheme for people with epileptic seizures and with epilepsy: report of the ILAE Task Force on Classification and Terminology. Epilepsia 2001;42(6):796–803.
3. Tassinari C, Dravet C, Roger JS. ESES: encephalopathy related to electrical status during slow wave sleep. Proceedings of the ninth congress of the International Federation of EEG and clinical neurophysiology. Amsterdam: Elsevier; 1977. p. 529–30.
4. Engel J Jr. Report of the ILAE classification core group. Epilepsia 2006;47(9):1558–68.
5. Berg AT, Berkovic SF, Brodie MJ, et al. Revised terminology and concepts for organization of seizures and epilepsies: report of the ILAE Commission on Classification and Terminology, 2005-2009. Epilepsia 2010; 51(4):676–85.
6. Beaumanoir A, Bureau M, Mira L. Identification of the syndrome. In: Beaumanoir A, Bureau M, Deonna T, et al, editors. Continuous spikes and waves during slow wave sleep. London: John Libbey; 1995. p. 243–9.
7. Inutsuka M, Kobayashi K, Oka M, et al. Treatment of epilepsy with electrical status epilepticus during slow sleep and its related disorders. Brain Dev 2006;28(5):281–6.
8. Aeby A, Poznanski N, Verheulpen D, et al. Levetiracetam efficacy in epileptic syndromes with continuous spikes and waves during slow sleep: experience in 12 cases. Epilepsia 2005;46(12):1937–42.
9. Tassinari CA, Rubboli G, Volpi L, et al. Encephalopathy with electrical status epilepticus during slow sleep or ESES syndrome including the acquired aphasia. Clin Neurophysiol 2000;111(Suppl 2): S94–102.
10. Bureau M. Outstanding cases of CSWS and LKS: analysis of the data provided by the participants. In: Beaumanoir A, Bureau M, Deonna T, et al, editors. Continuous spikes and waves during slow sleep. London: John Libbey; 1995. p. 213–6.
11. Loddenkemper T, Fernandez IS, Peters JM. Continuous spike and waves during sleep and electrical status epilepticus in sleep. J Clin Neurophysiol 2011; 28(2):154–64.
12. Hughes JR. A review of the relationships between Landau-Kleffner syndrome, electrical status epilepticus during sleep, and continuous spike-waves during sleep. Epilepsy Behav 2011;20(2):247–53.
13. Panayiotopoulos CP. Epileptic encephalopathy with continuous spike-and-wave in sleep. A clinical guide to epileptic syndromes and their treatment. Revised 2nd edition. London (United Kingdom): Springer; 2010. p. 309–15.
14. Liukkonen E, Kantola-Sorsa E, Paetau R, et al. Long-term outcome of 32 children with encephalopathy with status epilepticus during sleep, or ESES syndrome. Epilepsia 2010;51(10):2023–32.
15. Tassinari CA, Michelucci R, Forti A, et al. The electrical status epilepticus syndrome. Epilepsy Res Suppl 1992;6:111–5.
16. Kramer U, Sagi L, Goldberg-Stern H, et al. Clinical spectrum and medical treatment of children with electrical status epilepticus in sleep (ESES). Epilepsia 2009;50(6):1517–24.
17. Veggiotti P, Beccaria F, Papalia G, et al. Continuous spikes and waves during sleep in children with shunted hydrocephalus. Childs Nerv Syst 1998; 14(4–5):188–94.
18. Guerrini R, Genton P, Bureau M, et al. Multilobar polymicrogyria, intractable drop attack seizures, and

sleep-related electrical status epilepticus. Neurology 1998;51(2):504–12.

19. Ohtsuka Y, Tanaka A, Kobayashi K, et al. Childhood-onset epilepsy associated with polymicrogyria. Brain Dev 2002;24(8):758–65.

20. Guzzetta F, Battaglia D, Veredice C, et al. Early thalamic injury associated with epilepsy and continuous spike-wave during slow sleep. Epilepsia 2005; 46(6):889–900.

21. Fejerman N, Caraballo R, Tenembaum SN. Atypical evolutions of benign localization-related epilepsies in children: are they predictable? Epilepsia 2000; 41(4):380–90.

22. Fejerman N. Atypical rolandic epilepsy. Epilepsia 2009;50(Suppl 7):9–12.

23. Caraballo RH, Astorino F, Cersosimo R, et al. Atypical evolution in childhood epilepsy with occipital paroxysms (panayiotopoulos type). Epileptic Disord 2001;3(3):157–62.

24. de Saint-Martin A, Petiau C, Massa R, et al. Idiopathic rolandic epilepsy with "interictal" facial myoclonia and oromotor deficit: a longitudinal EEG and PET study. Epilepsia 1999;40(5):614–20.

25. Aicardi J. Atypical semiology of rolandic epilepsy in some related syndromes. Epileptic Disord 2000; 2(Suppl 1):S5–9.

26. Aicardi J, Chevrie JJ. Atypical benign partial epilepsy of childhood. Dev Med Child Neurol 1982; 24(3):281–92.

27. Landau WM, Kleffner FR. Syndrome of acquired aphasia with convulsive disorder in children. Neurology 1957;7(8):523–30.

28. Beaumanoir A, Hillion C, Mira L. Clinical differential diagnosis between benign and malignant epileptic syndromes with generalized seizures in early childhood. Epilepsy Res Suppl 1992;6:169–74.

29. Stefanatos G. Changing perspectives on Landau-Kleffner syndrome. Clin Neuropsychol 2011;25(6): 963–88.

30. Fandino M, Connolly M, Usher L, et al. Landau-Kleffner syndrome: a rare auditory processing disorder series of cases and review of the literature. Int J Pediatr Otorhinolaryngol 2011;75(1):33–8.

31. Rudolf G, Valenti MP, Hirsch E, et al. From rolandic epilepsy to continuous spike-and-waves during sleep and Landau-Kleffner syndromes: insights into possible genetic factors. Epilepsia 2009;50(Suppl 7):25–8.

32. Tassinari CA, Rubboli G, Volpi L, et al. Electrical status epilepticus during slow sleep (ESES or CSWS) including acquired epileptic aplasia (Landau-Kleffner syndrome). In: Roger J, Bureau M, Dravet C, et al, editors. Epileptic syndromes in infancy, childhood and adolescence. 4th edition (with video). Montrouge (France): John Libbey Eurotext; 2005. p. 295–314.

33. Saltik S, Uluduz D, Cokar O, et al. A clinical and EEG study on idiopathic partial epilepsies with evolution into ESES spectrum disorders. Epilepsia 2005; 46(4):524–33.

34. Larsson PG, Wilson J, Eeg-Olofsson O. A new method for quantification and assessment of epileptiform activity in EEG with special reference to focal nocturnal epileptiform activity. Brain Topogr 2009; 22(1):52–9.

35. Scheltens-de Boer M. Guidelines for EEG in encephalopathy related to ESES/CSWS in children. Epilepsia 2009;50(Suppl 7):13–7.

36. Proposal for revised classification of epilepsies and epileptic syndromes. Commission on Classification and Terminology of the International League Against Epilepsy. Epilepsia 1989;30(4):389–99.

37. Kobayashi K, Nishibayashi N, Ohtsuka Y, et al. Epilepsy with electrical status epilepticus during slow sleep and secondary bilateral synchrony. Epilepsia 1994;35(5): 1097–103.

38. Lombroso CT, Erba G. Primary and secondary bilateral synchrony in epilepsy; a clinical and electroencephalographic study. Arch Neurol 1970;22(4): 321–34.

39. Hoppen T, Sandrieser T, Rister M. Successful treatment of pharmacoresistant continuous spike wave activity during slow sleep with levetiracetam. Eur J Pediatr 2003;162(1):59–61.

40. Wang SB, Weng WC, Fan PC, et al. Levetiracetam in continuous spike waves during slow-wave sleep syndrome. Pediatr Neurol 2008;39(2):85–90.

41. Chhun S, Troude P, Villeneuve N, et al. A prospective open-labeled trial with levetiracetam in pediatric epilepsy syndromes: continuous spikes and waves during sleep is definitely a target. Seizure 2011; 20(4):320–5.

42. Buzatu M, Bulteau C, Altuzarra C, et al. Corticosteroids as treatment of epileptic syndromes with continuous spike-waves during slow-wave sleep. Epilepsia 2009;50(Suppl 7):68–72.

43. Yasuhara A, Yoshida H, Hatanaka T, et al. Epilepsy with continuous spike-waves during slow sleep and its treatment. Epilepsia 1991;32(1):59–62.

44. Roulet Perez E, Davidoff V, Despland PA, et al. Mental and behavioural deterioration of children with epilepsy and CSWS: acquired epileptic frontal syndrome. Dev Med Child Neurol 1993;35(8):661–74.

45. De Negri M, Baglietto MG, Battaglia FM, et al. Treatment of electrical status epilepticus by short diazepam (DZP) cycles after DZP rectal bolus test. Brain Dev 1995;17(5):330–3.

46. Sinclair DB, Snyder TJ. Corticosteroids for the treatment of Landau-Kleffner syndrome and continuous spike-wave discharge during sleep. Pediatr Neurol 2005;32(5):300–6.

47. von Stulpnagel C, Kluger G, Leiz S, et al. Levetiracetam as add-on therapy in different subgroups of "benign" idiopathic focal epilepsies in childhood. Epilepsy Behav 2010;17(2):193–8.

48. Mikati MA, Saab R, Fayad MN, et al. Efficacy of intravenous immunoglobulin in Landau-Kleffner syndrome. Pediatr Neurol 2002;26(4):298–300.

49. Lerman P. Seizures induced or aggravated by anticonvulsants. Epilepsia 1986;27(6):706–10.

50. Mikati MA, Saab R. Successful use of intravenous immunoglobulin as initial monotherapy in Landau-Kleffner syndrome. Epilepsia 2000;41(7):880–6.

51. Mikati MA, Shamseddine AN. Management of Landau-Kleffner syndrome. Paediatr Drugs 2005; 7(6):377–89.

52. Peltola ME, Liukkonen E, Granstrom ML, et al. The effect of surgery in encephalopathy with electrical status epilepticus during sleep. Epilepsia 2011; 52(3):602–9.

53. Loddenkemper T, Cosmo G, Kotagal P, et al. Epilepsy surgery in children with electrical status epilepticus in sleep. Neurosurgery 2009;64(2):328–37 [discussion: 337].

54. Cross JH, Neville BG. The surgical treatment of Landau-Kleffner syndrome. Epilepsia 2009;50(Suppl 7): 63–7.

55. Battaglia D, Veggiotti P, Lettori D, et al. Functional hemispherectomy in children with epilepsy and CSWS due to unilateral early brain injury including thalamus: sudden recovery of CSWS. Epilepsy Res 2009;87(2–3):290–8.

56. Moseley BD, Dhamija R, Wirrell EC. The cessation of continuous spike wave in slow-wave sleep following a temporal lobectomy. J Child Neurol 2011. [Epub ahead of print].

57. Kallay C, Mayor-Dubois C, Maeder-Ingvar M, et al. Reversible acquired epileptic frontal syndrome and CSWS suppression in a child with congenital hemiparesis treated by hemispherectomy. Eur J Paediatr Neurol 2009;13(5):430–8.

58. Van Hirtum-Das M, Licht EA, Koh S, et al. Children with ESES: variability in the syndrome. Epilepsy Res 2006;70(Suppl 1):S248–58.

59. Praline J, Hommet C, Barthez MA, et al. Outcome at adulthood of the continuous spike-waves during slow sleep and Landau-Kleffner syndromes. Epilepsia 2003;44(11):1434–40.

60. Scholtes FB, Hendriks MP, Renier WO. Cognitive deterioration and electrical status epilepticus during slow sleep. Epilepsy Behav 2005;6(2):167–73.

61. Tassinari CA, Rubboli G. Cognition and paroxysmal EEG activities: from a single spike to electrical status epilepticus during sleep. Epilepsia 2006;47(Suppl 2): 40–3.

62. Veggiotti P, Beccaria F, Guerrini R, et al. Continuous spike-and-wave activity during slow-wave sleep: syndrome or EEG pattern? Epilepsia 1999;40(11): 1593–601.

63. Rousselle C, Revol M. Relations between cognitive functions and continuous spikes and waves during slow sleep. In: Beaumanoir A, Bureau M, Deonna T, editors. Continuous spikes and waves during slow sleep. London: John Libbey; 1995. p. 123–33.

64. Robinson RO, Baird G, Robinson G, et al. Landau-Kleffner syndrome: course and correlates with outcome. Dev Med Child Neurol 2001;43(4):243–7.

65. Steriade M, Amzica F. Sleep oscillations developing into seizures in corticothalamic systems. Epilepsia 2003;44(Suppl 12):9–20.

66. Steriade M. Sleep, epilepsy and thalamic reticular inhibitory neurons. Trends Neurosci 2005;28(6):317–24.

67. Dang-Vu TT, Desseilles M, Peigneux P, et al. A role for sleep in brain plasticity. Pediatr Rehabil 2006; 9(2):98–118.

68. Holmes GL, Lenck-Santini PP. Role of interictal epileptiform abnormalities in cognitive impairment. Epilepsy Behav 2006;8(3):504–15.

69. Seri S, Thai JN, Brazzo D, et al. Neurophysiology of CSWS-associated cognitive dysfunction. Epilepsia 2009;50(Suppl 7):33–6.

70. De Tiege X, Ligot N, Goldman S, et al. Metabolic evidence for remote inhibition in epilepsies with continuous spike-waves during sleep. Neuroimage 2008;40(2):802–10.

71. De Tiege X, Harrison S, Laufs H, et al. Impact of interictal epileptic activity on normal brain function in epileptic encephalopathy: an electroencephalography-functional magnetic resonance imaging study. Epilepsy Behav 2007;11(3):460–5.

72. De Tiege X, Goldman S, Laureys S, et al. Regional cerebral glucose metabolism in epilepsies with continuous spikes and waves during sleep. Neurology 2004; 63(5):853–7.

73. Siniatchkin M, Groening K, Moehring J, et al. Neuronal networks in children with continuous spikes and waves during slow sleep. Brain 2010;133(9):2798–813.

Sudden Unexpected Death in Epilepsy: What Does Sleep Have to Do With It?

Madeleine M. Grigg-Damberger, MD

KEYWORDS

- Sudden unexpected death in epilepsy
- Sleep-related hypoventilation • Cerebral shutdown
- Prolonged generalized EEG suppression
- Sudden death in sleep

Sudden unexpected death in epilepsy (SUDEP) refers to the sudden unexpected death of a seemingly healthy individual with epilepsy. A recently published article recommending a unified definition and classification for SUDEP defines it as a "sudden, unexpected, witnessed or unwitnessed, nontraumatic and nondrowning death, occurring in benign circumstances, in an individual with epilepsy, with or without evidence for a seizure and excluding documented status epilepticus (seizure duration ≥30 minutes or seizures without recovery in between) in which postmortem examination does not reveal a cause of death."[1] SUDEP is the commonest cause of death directly attributable to epilepsy, and most often occurs at or around the time of a seizure and during sleep. This article reviews the current medical literature on the epidemiology, risk factors, and preventive measures for SUDEP in people with epilepsy, and also discusses the roles of sleep, respiration, impaired autonomic functioning, and nocturnal seizures in SUDEP.

EPIDEMIOLOGY OF DEATH IN PEOPLE WITH EPILEPSY

Sudden death is 20 to 40 times more common in people with epilepsy compared with the general population.[2–5] Between 8% and 17% of deaths in people with epilepsy are SUDEP (most often in people aged 20–40 years).[6] The incidence of SUDEP increases 100-fold from 0.09 per 1000 patient-years in prospective-based community samples, 1.2 to 5.9 per 1000 patient-years in tertiary care epilepsy centers, up to 6.0 to 9.3 per 1000 patient-years among patients with medically refractory epilepsies being evaluated for epilepsy surgery.[5–7]

A recently published longitudinal population-based cohort study prospectively followed 245 Finnish children with epilepsy for more than 40 years and found that 24% (n = 60) had died, a rate 3 times higher than for the general population.[8] Of the 60 deaths, 33 (55%) were related to epilepsy, including sudden unexplained death in 18 subjects (30%), definite or probable seizure in 9 (15%), and accidental drowning in 6 (10%). Epilepsy was not in remission in 48% of the cohort. The cumulative risk of sudden unexplained death was 7% at 40 years overall and 12% in subjects whose epilepsy was not controlled. Most of the deaths occurred in adulthood.

SUDEP MOST OFTEN OCCURS IN BED DURING THE NIGHT

SUDEP most often occurs in bed during the night, presumably during sleep, and following a generalized tonic-clonic seizure (GTCS) or complex partial seizure (CPS).[9–11] Circumstantial evidence of a recent seizure (tongue laceration, urinary incontinence, disheveled bedroom) was present in 67%

Conflicts of interest and financial disclosures: None related to this paper.
Department of Neurology, University of New Mexico School of Medicine, MSC10 5620, One University of NM, Albuquerque, NM 87131-0001, USA
E-mail address: MGriggD@salud.unm.edu

Sleep Med Clin 7 (2012) 157–170
doi:10.1016/j.jsmc.2012.01.004
1556-407X/12/$ – see front matter © 2012 Elsevier Inc. All rights reserved.

of 42 SUDEP deaths, 60% were sleep-related, and 71% of subjects were found lying prone.[11] Most of 50 SUDEP deaths occurred in sleep and evidence suggests that a seizure preceded death in 22%.[12] A prospective case-control study of 50 cases of SUDEP and 50 subjects with epilepsy who died of other causes found that the SUDEP group were more likely to be found dead in bed with evidence of a terminal seizure.[13]

Only 11% to 14% of cases of SUDEP are witnessed.[14–16] In one study, a GTCS preceded 12 of 15 witnessed SUDEP deaths, 70% were in a prone position, and respiratory difficulties were noted in 80%.[14] Half of witnessed cases of SUDEP were preceded by a GTCS, the rest by a sudden loss of consciousness.[16] SUDEP occurred in sleep in at least 40% of a case series in which sufficient clinical data are available, which is greater than could be expected by chance.[17]

A case-control study found that patients with predominantly nocturnal seizures had a greater risk of SUDEP.[15] They compared seizure patterns in a cohort of 154 cases of SUDEP and 616 controls living with epilepsy who had either exclusively diurnal or nocturnal seizures.[15] They found that (1) 86% of SUDEP deaths were unwitnessed and 58% occurred in sleep, (2) SUDEP was 4.4 times more likely to be unwitnessed if it occurred in sleep, and (3) those who died of SUDEP were 3.9 times more likely to have a history of primarily nocturnal seizures compared with the living controls with epilepsy.[15] After correcting for other SUDEP risk factors,[18] nocturnal seizures increased the risk of SUDEP 2.6 times. The investigators argued that nocturnal seizures should be considered an independent risk factor for SUDEP.

SUDEP occurs less often in children than adults.[19,20] A retrospective cohort from the United Kingdom General Practice Database found that the incidence of SUDEP was 3.3 per 10,000 person-years (9/6190).[21] Most of those who died had severe symptomatic epilepsies. A recently published prospective longitudinal study following 1012 children for approximately 10 years reported that 1.1% (11) had died of SUDEP.[19] Another study by the same group found that nearly all cases of SUDEP occurred in children who had poorly controlled epilepsy.[19]

CASES OF SUDEP OCCURRING DURING LONG-TERM VIDEO-ELECTROENCEPHALOGRAPHIC MONITORING

A total of 13 cases of SUDEP or near SUDEP have been reported in patients with medically refractory epilepsy undergoing prolonged inpatient continuous video-electroencephalographic (VEEG) recordings scattered among usually isolated case reports.[5,14,22–27] Eight died suddenly and 5 were successfully resuscitated. All had seizures just before the event, GTCS in 12, CPS in 1. Most died during sleep. Other seizures had occurred during the VEEG recordings in all but only 1 triggered the death or near-death event.

Respiratory problems (postictal hypoventilation, apnea, cyanosis, inspiratory stridor, pulmonary edema, or suffocation) heralded the onset of SUDEP in 8 (although the breathing difficulties were confirmed only by visual observation, not comprehensive respiratory monitoring).[22,26–28]

Electrocardiographic (ECG) abnormalities (such as ST-segment increase, peaked T waves, and asystole) usually followed but less often coincided with the respiratory difficulties.[5,22–25] Ventricular tachycardia leading to ventricular fibrillation was observed in 1 patient following a prolonged convulsion lasting 4.5 minutes.[24]

Two patients had prolonged generalized electroencephalogram suppression (PGES) following seizure(s): it followed a seizure in 1, whereas the other showed no movement lying face down and a heart rate of 47 beats per minute before the PGES appeared.[5,23] PGES following a generalized convulsion preceded death in a woman undergoing a home ambulatory electroencephalogram (EEG).[29]

A near-death event in a 20-year-old woman occurred following a convulsion that lasted 56 seconds; her ECG rhythm was normal for 10 seconds after the seizure, then gradually slowed until it stopped 57 seconds later.[25] She had a history of a previous cardiac arrest after a CPS without secondary generalization. The investigators argued that her heart stopped as a result of marked suppression of central respiratory effort after a seizure. She had 3 others during the recording that did not cause such a response, showing the intermittent nature of SUDEP events. After a short time, EEG activity became mixed with progressive flattening of the EEG (without any electrical activity). After the EEG cessation, pulse artifact was seen for 2 minutes.

RISK FACTORS FOR SUDEP

Case-control studies using living people with epilepsy as controls have searched for risk factors for SUDEP.[18,30–32] The most consistently identified risk factor across studies was frequent GTCS. In one study, a history of more than 3 GTCS per year increased the risk of SUDEP 8-fold.[31] Active epilepsy (defined as failure to obtain 5-year seizure remission) was the strongest risk of SUDEP in a prospective longitudinal study of patients with childhood-onset epilepsy followed for longer than 40 years.[8]

A recently published study by Hesdorffer and colleagues[33] pooled data from 4 published case-control studies[18,30–32] to increase the power to identify risk factors for SUDEP. Risk factors for SUDEP in 289 cases and 958 living controls with epilepsy were (1) more than 3 GTCS per year, (2) taking multiple antiepileptic drugs (AEDs), (3) epilepsy duration, (4) onset of epilepsy in childhood, (5) male gender, and (6) symptomatic epilepsy (related to an identifiable cause). Compared with healthy controls, the risk of SUDEP was 37 times greater in persons with epilepsy onset before age 16 years and 8-fold in those whose epilepsy began at age 16 years or older compared with healthy controls.[33] At highest risk of SUDEP were patients with early onset, medically refractory, symptomatic epilepsy with frequent GTCS, and those taking multiple AEDs. Treatment of epilepsy with only 1 drug (called monotherapy) was protective but statistically significant.

One study reported that the risk of SUDEP is increased 8-fold in patients with epilepsy taking 3 or more AEDs (so-called polytherapy) compared with those treated with 1.[30] However, AED polytherapy may represent a surrogate marker for medical intractability, not a causative factor.

In the study cited earlier, Hesdorffer and colleagues[33] found that lamotrigine was associated with a significant increase of SUDEP when prescribed to patients with idiopathic generalized epilepsy (IGE). Another recent study found that 10 (39%) of 26 cases of SUDEP had been treated with lamotrigine (and all but 1 were women).[34] The risk of SUDEP was 5-fold greater in women taking lamotrigine compared with those who were not (2.5 vs 0.5 per 1000 patient-years). This association may only represent selection bias because lamotrigine is a preferred AED for women.

How might lamotrigine increase the risk of SUDEP?[35] Lamotrigine has the potential to induce cardiac arrhythmias by inhibiting rapid, delayed-rectifier, potassium ion, cardiac current.[36] Seizure-induced acidosis, excessively high concentrations of lamotrigine, or concurrent treatment with other drugs that block these potassium currents could add to this risk.[36] Hesdorffer and colleagues[37] reanalyzed SUDEP data from 3 case-control studies and found no increased risk of SUDEP with any particular AED (given alone or in combination) when they controlled for GTCS frequency.

SUDEP risk is significantly greater in patients with longstanding, severe, medically refractory epilepsy, a history of neurologic insult, and cognitive and/or other neurologic impairments. An intelligence quotient (IQ) of less than 75 points greatly increases the risk of early death by secondary or symptomatic epilepsy.[2] The cumulative effects of seizures (GTCS or CPS) on brain structure and function may contribute to this increased risk.[6] Frequent GTCS can progressively damage the brain (especially the hippocampus) and cognition (impairment of short-term memory).[38,39]

Most studies confirm that so-called poor compliance with AEDs can increase the risk of SUDEP in adults with epilepsy 3-fold.[40,41] At least 3 coroner-based forensic studies of SUDEP found subtherapeutic AED level(s) in 57% to 90%.[11,12,42] A study of SUDEP in patients with medically refractory epilepsy enrolled in 112 different AED drug trials found that adding[33] another AED at effective doses reduced SUDEP or near-SUDEP risk 7-fold compared with placebo.[43] **Box 1** summarizes SUDEP risk factors.

POTENTIAL MECHANISMS FOR SUDEP

No single mechanism is likely to explain all (possibly even some) cases of SUDEP. Potential

---

Box 1
Risk factors for SUDEP

Frequent seizures, especially generalized tonic-clonic seizures:

Environment:

  Prone position after seizure

  Postictal breathing difficulty or cardiac arrhythmia

  Lack of nighttime supervision or monitoring

AED therapies:

  Polytherapy

  Frequent or recent abrupt changes in medications

  Poor compliance

  Subtherapeutic AED levels

Epilepsy:

  Long duration (>5–10 years)

  Childhood onset

  Symptomatic

  Mesial temporal lobe epileptic focus

Comorbid conditions:

  IQ <70

  Nonambulatory

  Depression

  Psychotropic use

  Excessive alcohol consumption and/or substance abuse

mechanisms for SUDEP in an individual patient with epilepsy include (1) ictal cardiac arrhythmias (possibly related to the cardiovascular effects of insular cortex); (2) impaired central ventilatory responses, prolonged apneas, or oxyhemoglobin desaturations triggered by seizures; (3) impaired righting responses following a seizure leading to death by suffocation; (4) central nervous system autonomic instability during or after a seizure; and/or (5) postictal dysfunction of serotonin (5-HT) neurons causing depression of breathing, impaired arousal, and repositioning reflexes.

Cerebral Shutdown and Postictal Generalized EEG Suppression

As mentioned earlier, a seizure may lead to, or be associated with, an electrical shutdown of the brain, which may occur with and/or follow brainstem respiratory suppression, central hypoventilation, cardiac standstill, cardiorespiratory arrest, and death.[6,23,27,29] A recent study compared 30 epileptic seizures recorded on VEEG in 10 adults who later died of SUDEP with 92 seizures in 30 matched live controls.[27] They found PGES in 50% of 30 seizures in the 10 who later died of SUDEP and 38% of 92 seizures in the control group. PGES was significantly longer in the generalized motor seizures of the SUDEP group. After adjusting for multiple variables, the risk of SUDEP was significantly increased if a PGES lasted longer than 50 seconds; the risk quadrupled if the EEG suppression lasted longer than 80 seconds. The investigators concluded that a PGES lasting longer than 50 seconds may identify patients with epilepsy at risk of SUDEP.

Another recent study found PGES in 48 (27%) patients who had GTCS when they retrospectively reviewed 470 consecutive VEEG telemetry reports.[44] The mean duration of PGES was 38 seconds (range 6–69 seconds). They then reviewed VEEG ictal behavior in the patients with PGES (analyzing 1 seizure per subject) and compared them with 12 randomly selected controls. They found that patients with PGES were significantly more likely to lie motionless after the seizure and require simple nursing interventions (suctioning, repositioning, supplemental oxygen).

More research and careful monitoring of ECG and respiration (including tidal volume, respiratory rate, pulse oximeter, and carbon dioxide) is needed to discover which factors precipitate witnessed episodes of SUDEP. PGES, central apnea, pulmonary shunting, pulmonary neurogenic edema, suffocation in the prone position asleep, impaired arousal caused by hypercapnea and sleep, and/or respiratory acidosis may combine in varying degrees and cascade with cardiac factors to cause SUDEP.[6]

Fig. 1 shows an episode of PGES lasting 90 seconds that occurred in a 37-year-old woman with left mesial temporal lobe epilepsy (TLE) while undergoing prolonged VEEG monitoring. She had a cluster of 3 CPS that occurred within 6 hours, 72 hours after withdrawing phenytoin. All were CPS that emanated from her left mesial temporal region; 2 secondarily generalized (lasting 45 and 51 seconds). PGES following the CPS without generalization lasted 8 seconds; and 50 and 90 seconds on the CPS that evolved to generalized convulsions. Note how no suppression of the heart rate occurred despite 90 seconds of PGES.

Cardiac Factors Potentially Contributing to SUDEP

Cardiac events have been implicated in some cases of SUDEP.[45–48] Seizure-induced cardiac arrhythmias occur in animals and humans,[46,47] but a malignant cardiac arrhythmia from a partial seizure was the cause of near SUDEP in only 1 of the 13 patients who had SUDEP or near-SUDEP events during long-term VEEG monitoring.[24] Seizure-related hypoxemia or acidosis, and/or abnormalities in cardiac potassium currents, could predispose to cardiac arrhythmias.[36]

Studies in patients with epilepsy show that changes in heart rate and rhythm often accompany or follow seizures, and medically intractable epilepsy over time can be associated with a variety of ECG abnormalities. Interictal and ictal cardiovascular changes have been reported in patients with epilepsy.[46,47] Prolonged corrected QT (QTc) intervals during and following seizures, and shortening of the QTc after seizures, have been reported.[49–51] Ictal asystole occurs in 0.1% to 0.4% of patients during VEEG monitoring.[52–54]

Two studies[55] have reported cardiac structural abnormalities in autopsy studies on patients who died of SUDEP. One prospective study found significant myocardial fibrosis in 6 of 15 SUDEP deaths compared with only 1 control who died of other causes.[55] None had pathologic changes in their cardiac conduction systems. Another case-control autopsy study found perivascular and interstitial fibrosis in 4 of the 7 hearts in the SUDEP group; and none in the 13 controls who died of drug overdose or hanging. The investigators hypothesized that these irreversible cardiac changes result from seizures.

A study by Nei and colleagues[56] found that ictal tachycardia was more severe during sleep in patients who later died of SUDEP. They compared

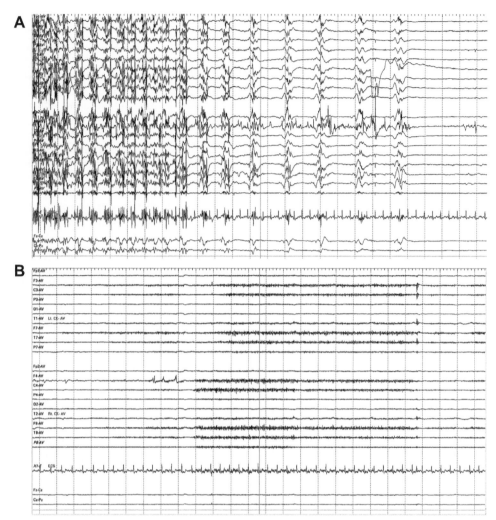

Fig. 1. (*A–E*) An episode of PGES lasting 90 seconds recorded in a 37-year-old woman with left mesial temporal lobe epilepsy (TLE) while undergoing prolonged VEEG monitoring. The duration of each figure is 30 seconds. Note that the secondarily generalized seizure ends in (*A*). Muscle tension artifact is seen in (*B*) but no EEG activity is observed until the brief bursts in (*D*). Predominantly δ EEG activity returns in (*E*). Note how the heart rate continues despite prolonged EEG suppression.

VEEG and ECG data in patients who later died of SUDEP with live controls with epilepsy and found that (1) mean heart rates during seizures that occurred in sleep were 149 beats per minute (BPM) in the SUDEP group and 126 BPM in controls; (2) mean increase in heart rate was higher in sleep compared with wake in the cases of SUDEP (78 BPM in sleep, 47 BPM awake), an effect not seen in the controls (52 BPM in sleep, 43 awake); and (3) ictal cardiac repolarization and rhythm abnormalities (atrial fibrillation, ventricular or atrial premature depolarizations, marked sinus arrhythmia, junctional escape, or ST-segment increase) were found in 56% of cases of SUDEP and 39% of the controls.

Ictal tachycardia accompanies most CPS and GTCS.[52,56,57] Studies have shown that (1) heart rate increases tend to be greater, and other ECG abnormalities more common, with GTCS[57]; (2) ictal tachycardias may be more pronounced with seizures that arise from the temporal lobe[58–60]; (3) increase in heart rate during a seizure correlates with seizure duration.[58]

Other ECG abnormalities are observed in many patients following CPS or GTCS. These abnormalities include longer QT intervals, increased QT dispersion, ST-segment depression, discordant rhythm, and abnormal repolarization.[57,61] These changes were often transient, not present on ECGs repeated 1 to 9 days later.[61] Potentially serious

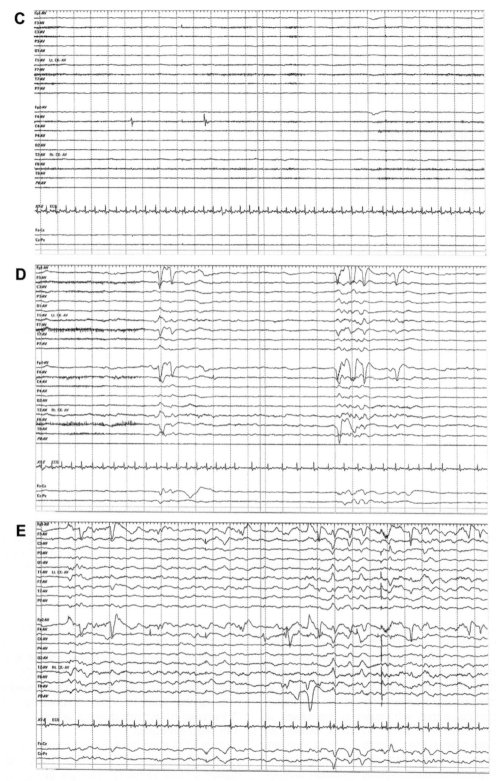

Fig. 1. (*continued*)

ECG changes (ST depression or T wave inversion) were observed in 6% of 102 seizures and 10% of 41 patients undergoing VEEG monitoring, and were more likely to occur in generalized seizures.[57]

Ictal bradycardia or ictal asystole are rare manifestations of typical TLE.[51,52,62–64] Ictal bradycardia was observed in 6% to 8% of patients (and then in only 4%–6% of seizures in an individual patient).[62,63] Ictal asystole is rare. Three large case series reported recording ictal asystole in 0.27% (10/6825),[52] 0.34% (2/589),[53] and 0.4% (5/1244)[54] of patients with epilepsy undergoing VEEG monitoring.

When ictal asystole occurred in 8 patients with TLE undergoing VEEG monitoring, it developed an average of 42 seconds after seizure onset and resulted in a sudden loss of body tone.[52] Sudden atonia is not common in TLE and reports of it in a patient with TLE should prompt concern that some of the seizures may be accompanied by ictal asystole. Ictal asystole was found to accompany seizures in 10 (0.2%, median age 50 years, 9 women) of 4500 patients evaluated in a specialized syncope unit; all were temporal in origin.[65] Eight were subsequently treated with an AED with seizure control; seizures were medically refractory in 2 and required pacemaker implantation. The investigators cautioned that ictal asystole should be considered in patients with recurrent, unexplained, traumatic, and/or convulsive syncope.

Rugg-Gunn and colleagues[66] implanted ECG loop recorders in 20 patients with medically refractory focal epilepsies to determine the frequency of neurogenic cardiac arrhythmias. They found that median heart rates exceeded 100 BPM in 16 patients and ictal bradycardia (<40 BPM) occurred in 8 (2.1%) of 377 seizures. Three patients had ictal asystole, and pacemakers were inserted in 4.

Strezelczyk and colleagues[64] reviewed their experiences and long-term outcome managing ictal asystole or bradycardia in 16 patients with medically refractory TLE from 4 epilepsy centers. Subjects had TLE for a mean of 18 years, a mean age of 51 years, and had a mean of 8 seizures per month. Two-thirds of reported falls, syncope, or trauma were related to their seizures. Ictal asystole (lasting 3–33 seconds) accompanied 30% (28 episodes) of the 92 seizures in the 16 subjects. An additional 17% of seizures had ictal bradycardia. When either occurred, it resulted in an abrupt complete loss of consciousness, and sudden atonia with falls (unless the patient was reclining in bed). Secondary generalization developed following ictal asystole in 2 patients. Treating these patients with AEDs, and/or epilepsy surgery with/without a cardiac pacemaker, led to resolution of these events in 88% of cases.

Why are these cardiac arrhythmias occurring in people with epilepsy, especially those with TLE? The amygdala has efferent connections to cardioregulatory centers in the medulla. Perhaps excessive vagal stimulation in some patients with epilepsy could lead to profound ictal bradycardia, heart block, and potentially SUDEP.[48] Seizure-induced hypoxemia or acidosis could predispose to arrhythmias in some patients. Myocardial fibrosis has been found on autopsy in some patients with epilepsy. Recurrent catecholamine surges related to seizures could be the cause, although more research is needed to confirm this.[55]

Impaired Heart Rate Variability as a Marker of Autonomic Dysfunction

Autonomic instability in the ictal or postictal period could predispose or contribute to SUDEP. Progressive loss of autonomic heart rate variability (HRV) and greater changes in heart rate and rhythm following seizures are observed in patients with medically refractory epilepsy.[37,38,67–69] Reduced HRV is a biomarker of disease in humans, often presenting before overt adverse medical disease, reflecting impaired autonomic nervous system (ANS) function. HRV is an important indicator of health and fitness; it reflects our ability to react and adapt effectively to stress and environmental demands. Impaired HRV (and increased sympathetic tone) predicts negative outcomes in many diseases.

A recent study found that the time-domain components of HRV decreased immediately after seizures in 31 patients with epilepsy undergoing presurgical evaluations.[69] This decrease lasted for 5 to 6 hours and was more pronounced in GTCS than CPS. Low-frequency power decreased in the early postictal phase and high-frequency power of HRV decreased in the late postictal phase. Another recent longitudinal study found progressive reduction in HRV over a mean follow-up period of 6 years in patients with medically refractory TLE, not seen in the patients with well-controlled TLE.[67] A case report of SUDEP showed a progressively significant decrease in HRV before SUDEP in a male patient with medically refractory TLE.[68] Monitoring HRV in patients with epilepsy may prove to be a biomarker of those at increased risk of SUDEP.

Respiratory Dysfunction in Seizures and SUDEP

In 1899, Hughlings Jackson observed that respiratory arrest could occur in humans during temporal lobe seizures originating near the uncus and lead to the patients turning blue.[14,70] Ictal or postictal central apneas or hypopneas were recorded in 10 of 17 patients (20 of 47 seizures) in whom respiration was monitored during VEEG.[71] Seizures were CPS in 16, apneas were usually central in type, lasted a mean of 24 seconds (range >10–63 seconds), and often caused desaturations to less than 85% in 10 patients. In a few, obstructive apneas followed central apneas. Another study of ictal hypoxemia in 56 patients with medically intractable focal epilepsies found that central apneas or hypopneas occurred in 53% and desaturations to less than 90% in 33% of seizures.[72] Seyal and Bateman[73] monitored end-tidal carbon dioxide (etCO$_2$) and oxygen saturation via pulse oximetry (SpO$_2$) in a subset of these patients and reported in a subsequent study that the oxyhemoglobin desaturations in these patients with temporal CPS were caused by hypoventilation. An example of the effects of seizure-related respiratory apnea in a patient following a right temporal CPS with secondary generalization is shown in **Fig. 2**. The etCO$_2$ increased to 64 mm Hg and the oxygen saturation nadir was 78%.

Impaired respiration as a cause of death in SUDEP is supported by reports of difficulty breathing and/or apnea before death in most witnessed cases.[14,19,22,23,25,26,54,71] The most common pathologic finding at autopsy in SUDEP is pulmonary edema.[11,32,74] Seizures can cause pulmonary edema.[75,76] Possible mechanisms for impaired breathing in SUDEP include (1) respiratory problems (respiratory arrest, labored breathing, suffocation in a prone position, laryngeal spasm)[14,71]; (2) prone position after a seizure, which potentially could predispose to airway obstruction and asphyxia; (3) hypercapnea and hypoxia following seizures[19,22,63,77]; and (4) postictal neurogenic pulmonary edema.[6,7,11,32,74]

Another study recorded pulse oximetry in 49 children who had at least 1 CPS or GTCS during VEEG monitoring.[63] They found that (1) 49% had ictal hypoxemia during 27% of 225 seizures and (2) ictal hypoxemia was more likely to occur during generalized seizures, longer lasting seizures, and when tapering AEDs. Another study found that apnea only occurred during CPS that spread to the contralateral temporal lobe.[73]

Postictal depression of serotonin neurons causing depression of breathing and arousal may be shared mechanisms for SUDEP and sudden infant death syndrome

Compared with the general population, people with epilepsy are about twice as likely to have depression, and are 3.6-fold to 5-fold more likely to commit suicide.[63,64,78–81] A history of depression is 2 to 7 times more common in people with newly diagnosed epilepsy.[82,83] An unprovoked seizure is 6 times more likely in people with major depression than in the general population.[82] These data suggest there may be a shared underlying disorder that predisposes patients to

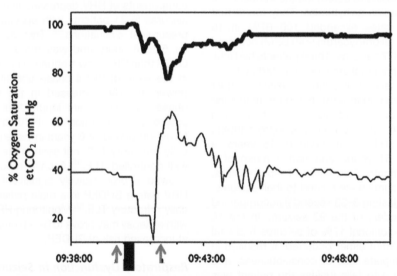

Fig. 2. Seizure-related central apnea in an 18-year-old man with a right temporal onset seizure, which secondarily generalized 40 seconds after onset. The arrowheads mark the start and stop of seizure, vertical bars the apnea. The etCO$_2$ increased to 64 mm Hg and SpO$_2$ decreased to 78%. Increased etCO$_2$ values persisted for several minutes beyond the end of the seizure. (*From* Seyal M, Bateman LM. Ictal apnea linked to contralateral spread of temporal lobe seizures: Intracranial EEG recordings in refractory temporal lobe epilepsy. Epilepsia 2009;50(12): 2561; with permission.)

both seizures and depression (a seizure/depression phenotype).[84]

Defects and/or deficits in the central serotonergic (5-HT) system may explain the shared features of epilepsy and depression.[78,85,86] Neuroimaging data and analysis of resected tissue of epileptic patients, and studies in animal models, all provide evidence that endogenous 5-HT, the activity of its receptors, and pharmaceuticals with serotonin agonist and/or antagonist properties play a significant role in the pathogenesis of epilepsies.[86] Several AEDs increase endogenous extracellular 5-HT concentrations in the brain.

5-HT receptors are expressed in almost all networks involved in epilepsies. Reduced 5-HT$_{1A}$ receptor binding has been shown on positive emission tomography (PET) studies in epilepsy and depression; the decrease is more severe in patients with both.[87,88] Many AEDs increase serotonin levels in the brain and selective serotonin reuptake inhibitors (SSRIs) have anticonvulsant effects.[89] Citalopram reduced seizures by more than 50% in 9 of 11 patients treated in one series.[90]

The caudal brainstem 5-HT system also plays crucial roles in coordinating synchronous homeostatic functions including control of breathing, arousal, respiratory rhythm generation, blood pressure regulation, thermoregulation, upper airway reflexes, chemosensitivity, and synaptic plasticity. It is a critical component of a medullary homeostatic network that regulates protective responses to metabolic stressors such as hypoxia, hypercapnia, and hyperthermia.

Richerson and Buchanan[84] propose that postictal dysfunction of caudal brainstem 5-HT neurons causes depression of breathing and arousal in some patients with epilepsy and could lead to SUDEP. 5-HT neurons affect breathing by (1) stimulating respiratory output, (2) chemoreceptors that respond to hypercapnea by increasing respiratory output, and (3) enabling plasticity of the respiratory network in response to challenges such as intermittent hypoxia.[91] 5-HT neurons project to all the major respiratory-related and autonomic-related nuclei in the medulla. The amygdala has efferent connections to cardioregulatory centers in the medulla. Lesions in 5-HT neurons lead to a decrease in respiratory output, which can be severe. 5-HT agonists stimulate respiratory output and reverse the effects of different respiratory depressants. 5-HT neurons seem to mediate the life-preserving arousal response to hypercapnea.[92] Richerson and Buchanan[84] argue that impairment of this response may contribute to SUDEP, sudden infant death syndrome (SIDS), and sleep apnea.

5-HT neurons respond to hypercapnea by stimulating arousal.[93] When a pillow or blanket obstructs the nose or mouth of a person who is asleep, the person wakes up slightly and turns the head to relieve the obstruction. This life-preserving reflex seems to be regulated by 5-HT neurons.[93] This reflex is absent after genetic deletion of 5-HT neurons in mice.[92] If patients have seizures in bed, face down, covered by pillows or blankets, postical depression (with/without underlying 5-HT deficits) may prevent them from turning their head, increasing their breathing, or both.

Most cases of SIDS are caused by defects in arousal and/or ventilatory response to hypercapnea and/or hypoxia.[94,95] Seventy percent of infants who die of SIDS have abnormalities in caudal brainstem 5-HT neurons.[94,95] Like SUDEP, most such infants are found prone. Prenatal alterations in the maturing 5-HT system weaken the normally robust neonatal respiratory system, increasing the risk of SIDS. Depression of 5-HT neurons in vulnerable infants with SIDS or people prone to epilepsy following seizures may be a shared mechanism for SIDS and SUDEP. In SIDS, the 5-HT defect is likely caused by developmental delay in maturation of 5-HT neurons coupled with environmental threats and decreased 5-HT neuronal firing during sleep. Are the 5-HT neurons in SUDEP stunned postictally and is this threat delivered to a 5-HT–depleted baseline state that is worse in sleep when 5-HT neurons fire less? **Fig. 3** summarizes this cascade of physiologic threats, insults, and conditions that may lead to SUDEP. Would treating people with epilepsy with SSRIs prevent SUDEP as it has been shown to do in a DBA/2 mouse model of SUDEP? Will SSRIs prevent seizure-induced respiratory depression and boost arousal reflexes? These questions require further study.

MEASURES TO REDUCE THE RISK OF SUDEP

There are no prospective or controlled studies on how to prevent or reduce the risk of SUDEP. Because a GTCS precedes most cases of SUDEP, prevention should begin with good control of seizures, compliance with medications, and avoiding frequent changes in AED regimens. It is important to discuss SUDEP and its risks with patients and their families, especially for patients with GTCS, medically refractory epilepsies, and intellectual and/or other neurologic impairments. Counseling should be given about pursuing a healthy lifestyle including avoiding sleep deprivation. Patients with medically refractory epilepsy should be evaluated for epilepsy surgery because

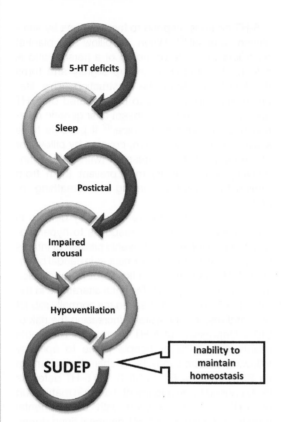

Fig. 3. This cascade of physiologic threats and conditions may lead to SUDEP in some patients.

Labels in figure: 5-HT deficits; Sleep; Postictal; Impaired arousal; Hypoventilation; SUDEP; Inability to maintain homeostasis

Box 2
Strategies to reduce the risk of SUDEP

- Educate patient and family about risks of SUDEP and importance of good compliance with AED medications and observing a healthy lifestyle
- Promote good sleep hygiene; identify and treat insomnia and sleep apnea
- Prescribe higher AED doses at night if seizures occur mostly at night
- Optimize and simplify AED regimen and avoid frequent AED changes
- Evalutate for epilepsy surgery for medically refractory cases
- Advise close supervision when sleeping, particularly in the intellectually or neurologically challenged (audio or audiovisual monitor, bed partner)
- Encourage patient to avoid sleeping prone; reposition supine or lateral after a seizure
- Advise close observation of the patient after a seizure; reposition supine or lateral; stimulate the patient; watch for apnea or severe hypoventilation and, if observed, initiate cardiopulmonary resuscitation and call emergency services
- Avoid drugs that lower seizure threshold (phenylephrine, bupropion, pseudoephedrine)

patients rendered seizure free by surgery have reduced rates of SUDEP with mortality approaching that in the general population.[75,96,97] **Box 2** summarizes preventative strategies for reducing the risk of SUDEP.

Other preventive strategies may include (1) stress reduction, (2) physical activity, (3) knowledge of resuscitation techniques and defibrillator use, and (4) supervision at night, although they have not been studied.[98] Several commercial companies have marketed devices that purport to detect GTCS, but there are almost no data validating their specificity and sensitivity and no evidence that their use prevents SUDEP. A Medpage bed seizure monitor (Medpage Limited T/A Easylink UK, Northamptonshire, UK) is a device placed between the mattress and bed base. One study found that the device detected 5 of 8 GTCS recorded in 64 patients with epilepsy.[99] There were 269 false-positive alarms. The sensitivity, specificity, positive predictive value, and negative predictive value of the alarm were 63%, 90%, 3%, and 100%, respectively. The device needs to be calibrated individually to improve the positive predictive value to less than 3%.

Pulse oximeters and heart rate monitors detect seizure-induced hypoxemia and tachycardia but SUDEP continues to occur in hospitals despite prompt attempts at resuscitation.[28] The use of supplemental oxygen following seizures to reduce the risk of SUDEP has not been studied in humans. However, a study found that mice with sudden fatal audiogenic seizures treated with supplemental oxygen before inducing fatal seizures prevented death, whereas most animals not given it died.[100]

Two studies argue that nighttime supervision, attention to recovery after a seizure, or avoiding sleeping prone or alone might reduce the risk of SUDEP. One study evaluated the circumstances surrounding the sudden deaths of 14 children with severe epilepsy and learning difficulties living at a special needs school.[74] They had died at home; none died when living at school where they were carefully monitored by attendants, sound-monitoring devices, and an on-call nurse. Another case-control study of adults showed that the risk of SUDEP was reduced by a factor of 2.5 if another person older than 10 years was in the room, and by a factor of 10 if frequent nighttime checks or a sound-monitoring device was used.[18]

AREAS FOR FUTURE RESEARCH IN SLEEP AND SUDEP

Research is needed to determine (1) whether patients with epilepsy are at greater risk of SUDEP when sleep-deprived, when seizures occur primarily during sleep, and/or other primary sleep disorders are present (sleep apnea, chronic insomnia, daytime sleepiness); (2) whether treating insomnia, poor sleep hygiene, poorly controlled primarily nocturnal seizures, sleep apnea, and having close supervision when sleeping reduces the risk of SUDEP; (3) whether a progressive loss of HRV identifies those at greater risk of SUDEP; (4) whether loss of central ANS regulation renders patients less capable of buffering rapid changes and maintaining homeostasis when sleeping; and (5) what roles emotional stress, prone body position, impaired arousal and responses, and impaired serotonin functioning have in SUDEP to the final deadly moment.

Sleep, respiration, arousal responses, and caudal brainstem serotoninergic neurons probably play important roles in SUDEP, but more research is needed to understand these complex relationships.

REFERENCES

1. Nashef L, So EL, Ryvlin P, et al. Unifying the definitions of sudden unexpected death in epilepsy. Epilepsia 2011. [Epub ahead of print].
2. Shorvon S, Tomson T. Sudden unexpected death in epilepsy. Lancet 2011;378(9808):2028–38.
3. Duncan JS, Sander JW, Sisodiya SM, et al. Adult epilepsy. Lancet 2006;367(9516):1087–100.
4. Ficker DM, So EL, Shen WK, et al. Population-based study of the incidence of sudden unexplained death in epilepsy. Neurology 1998;51(5):1270–4.
5. Tomson T, Nashef L, Ryvlin P. Sudden unexpected death in epilepsy: current knowledge and future directions. Lancet Neurol 2008;7(11):1021–31.
6. Devinsky O. Sudden, unexpected death in epilepsy. N Engl J Med 2011;365(19):1801–11.
7. Tellez-Zenteno JF, Ronquillo LH, Wiebe S. Sudden unexpected death in epilepsy: evidence-based analysis of incidence and risk factors. Epilepsy Res 2005;65(1–2):101–15.
8. Sillanpaa M, Shinnar S. Long-term mortality in childhood-onset epilepsy. N Engl J Med 2010; 363(26):2522–9.
9. Nashef L, Hindocha N, Makoff A. Risk factors in sudden death in epilepsy (SUDEP): the quest for mechanisms. Epilepsia 2007;48(5):859–71.
10. Shorvon S. Risk factors for sudden unexpected death in epilepsy. Epilepsia 1997;38(Suppl 11): S20–2.
11. Kloster R, Engelskjon T. Sudden unexpected death in epilepsy (SUDEP): a clinical perspective and a search for risk factors. J Neurol Neurosurg Psychiatr 1999;67(4):439–44.
12. Opeskin K, Harvey AS, Cordner SM, et al. Sudden unexpected death in epilepsy in Victoria. J Clin Neurosci 2000;7(1):34–7.
13. Opeskin K, Berkovic SF. Risk factors for sudden unexpected death in epilepsy: a controlled prospective study based on coroners cases. Seizure 2003; 12(7):456–64.
14. Langan Y, Nashef L, Sander JW. Sudden unexpected death in epilepsy: a series of witnessed deaths. J Neurol Neurosurg Psychiatr 2000;68(2): 211–3.
15. Lamberts RJ, Thijs RD, Laffan A, et al. Sudden unexpected death in epilepsy: people with nocturnal seizures may be at highest risk. Epilepsia 2011. [Epub ahead of print].
16. Donner EJ, Smith CR, Snead OC 3rd. Sudden unexplained death in children with epilepsy. Neurology 2001;57(3):430–4.
17. Nobili L, Proserpio P, Rubboli G, et al. Sudden unexpected death in epilepsy (SUDEP) and sleep. Sleep Med Rev 2011;15(4):237–46.
18. Langan Y, Nashef L, Sander JW. Case-control study of SUDEP. Neurology 2005;64(7):1131–3.
19. Terra VC, Scorza FA, Sakamoto AC, et al. Does sudden unexpected death in children with epilepsy occur more frequently in those with high seizure frequency? Arq Neuropsiquiatr 2009;67(4): 1001–2.
20. Terra VC, Scorza FA, Arida RM, et al. Mortality in children with severe epilepsy: 10 years of follow-up. Arq Neuropsiquiatr 2011;69(5):766–9.
21. Ackers R, Besag FM, Hughes E, et al. Mortality rates and causes of death in children with epilepsy prescribed antiepileptic drugs: a retrospective cohort study using the UK General Practice Research Database. Drug Saf 2011;34(5):403–13.
22. Bateman LM, Spitz M, Seyal M. Ictal hypoventilation contributes to cardiac arrhythmia and SUDEP: report on two deaths in video-EEG-monitored patients. Epilepsia 2010;51(5):916–20.
23. Bird J, Dembny K, Sandeman D, et al. Sudden unexplained death in epilepsy: an intracranially monitored case. Epilepsia 1997;38(Suppl 11):S52–6.
24. Espinosa PS, Lee JW, Tedrow UB, et al. Sudden unexpected near death in epilepsy: malignant arrhythmia from a partial seizure. Neurology 2009; 72(19):1702–3.
25. So EL, Sam MC, Lagerlund TL. Postictal central apnea as a cause of SUDEP: evidence from near-SUDEP incident. Epilepsia 2000;41(11):1494–7.

26. Tao JX, Qian S, Baldwin M, et al. SUDEP, suspected positional airway obstruction, and hypoventilation in postictal coma. Epilepsia 2010;51(11):2344–7.

27. Lhatoo SD, Faulkner HJ, Dembny K, et al. An electroclinical case-control study of sudden unexpected death in epilepsy. Ann Neurol 2010;68(6):787–96.

28. Tomson T, Walczak T, Sillanpaa M, et al. Sudden unexpected death in epilepsy: a review of incidence and risk factors. Epilepsia 2005;46(Suppl 11):54–61.

29. McLean BN, Wimalaratna S. Sudden death in epilepsy recorded in ambulatory EEG. J Neurol Neurosurg Psychiatr 2007;78(12):1395–7.

30. Nilsson L, Farahmand BY, Persson PG, et al. Risk factors for sudden unexpected death in epilepsy: a case-control study. Lancet 1999;353(9156):888–93.

31. Walczak TS, Leppik IE, D'Amelio M, et al. Incidence and risk factors in sudden unexpected death in epilepsy: a prospective cohort study. Neurology 2001;56(4):519–25.

32. Hitiris N, Suratman S, Kelly K, et al. Sudden unexpected death in epilepsy: a search for risk factors. Epilepsy Behav 2007;10(1):138–41.

33. Hesdorffer DC, Tomson T, Benn E, et al. Combined analysis of risk factors for SUDEP. Epilepsia 2011;52(6):1150–9.

34. Aurlien D, Larsen JP, Gjerstad L, et al. Increased risk of sudden unexpected death in epilepsy in females using lamotrigine: a nested, case-control study. Epilepsia 2011. [Epub ahead of print].

35. Nashef L, Ryvlin P. Sudden unexpected death in epilepsy (SUDEP): update and reflections. Neurol Clin 2009;27(4):1063–74.

36. Danielsson BR, Lansdell K, Patmore L, et al. Effects of the antiepileptic drugs lamotrigine, topiramate and gabapentin on hERG potassium currents. Epilepsy Res 2005;63(1):17–25.

37. Hesdorffer DC, Tomson T, Benn E, et al. Do antiepileptic drugs or generalized tonic-clonic seizure frequency increase SUDEP risk? A combined analysis. Epilepsia 2011. [Epub ahead of print].

38. Hermann BP, Seidenberg M, Bell B. The neurodevelopmental impact of childhood onset temporal lobe epilepsy on brain structure and function and the risk of progressive cognitive effects. Prog Brain Res 2002;135:429–38.

39. Hermann B, Seidenberg M, Bell B, et al. The neurodevelopmental impact of childhood-onset temporal lobe epilepsy on brain structure and function. Epilepsia 2002;43(9):1062–71.

40. Faught E, Duh MS, Weiner JR, et al. Nonadherence to antiepileptic drugs and increased mortality: findings from the RANSOM Study. Neurology 2008;71(20):1572–8.

41. Pollanen MS, Kodikara S. Sudden unexpected death in epilepsy: a retrospective analysis of 24 adult cases. Forensic Sci Med Pathol 2011. [Epub ahead of print].

42. Lathers CM, Koehler SA, Wecht CH, et al. Forensic antiepileptic drug levels in autopsy cases of epilepsy. Epilepsy Behav 2011;22(4):778–85.

43. Ryvlin P, Cucherat M, Rheims S. Risk of sudden unexpected death in epilepsy in patients given adjunctive antiepileptic treatment for refractory seizures: a meta-analysis of placebo-controlled randomised trials. Lancet Neurol 2011;10(11):961–8.

44. Semmelroch M, Elwes RD, Lozsadi DA, et al. Retrospective audit of postictal generalized EEG suppression in telemetry. Epilepsia 2011. [Epub ahead of print].

45. Dasheiff RM. Sudden unexpected death in epilepsy: a series from an epilepsy surgery program and speculation on the relationship to sudden cardiac death. J Clin Neurophysiol 1991;8(2):216–22.

46. Schuele SU. Effects of seizures on cardiac function. J Clin Neurophysiol 2009;26(5):302–8.

47. Devinsky O. Effects of seizures on autonomic and cardiovascular function. Epilepsy Curr 2004;4(2):43–6.

48. Scorza FA, Arida RM, Cysneiros RM, et al. The brain-heart connection: implications for understanding sudden unexpected death in epilepsy. Cardiol J 2009;16(5):394–9.

49. Brotherstone R, Blackhall B, McLellan A. Lengthening of corrected QT during epileptic seizures. Epilepsia 2010;51(2):221–32.

50. Surges R, Adjei P, Kallis C, et al. Pathologic cardiac repolarization in pharmacoresistant epilepsy and its potential role in sudden unexpected death in epilepsy: a case-control study. Epilepsia 2010;51(2):233–42.

51. Surges R, Scott CA, Walker MC. Enhanced QT shortening and persistent tachycardia after generalized seizures. Neurology 2010;74(5):421–6.

52. Schuele SU, Bermeo AC, Alexopoulos AV, et al. Video-electrographic and clinical features in patients with ictal asystole. Neurology 2007;69(5):434–41.

53. Scott CA, Fish DR. Cardiac asystole in partial seizures. Epileptic Disord 2000;2(2):89–92.

54. Rocamora R, Kurthen M, Lickfett L, et al. Cardiac asystole in epilepsy: clinical and neurophysiologic features. Epilepsia 2003;44(2):179–85.

55. P-Codrea Tigaran S, Dalager-Pedersen S, Baandrup U, et al. Sudden unexpected death in epilepsy: is death by seizures a cardiac disease? Am J Forensic Med Pathol 2005;26(2):99–105.

56. Nei M, Ho RT, Abou-Khalil BW, et al. EEG and ECG in sudden unexplained death in epilepsy. Epilepsia 2004;45(4):338–45.

57. Opherk C, Coromilas J, Hirsch LJ. Heart rate and EKG changes in 102 seizures: analysis of influencing factors. Epilepsy Res 2002;52(2):117–27.

58. Weil S, Arnold S, Eisensehr I, et al. Heart rate increase in otherwise subclinical seizures is different in temporal versus extratemporal seizure onset: support for temporal lobe autonomic influence. Epileptic Disord 2005;7(3):199–204.

59. Garcia M, D'Giano C, Estelles S, et al. Ictal tachycardia: its discriminating potential between temporal and extratemporal seizure foci. Seizure 2001; 10(6):415–9.

60. Marshall DW, Westmoreland BF, Sharbrough FW. Ictal tachycardia during temporal lobe seizures. Mayo Clin Proc 1983;58(7):443–6.

61. Kandler L, Fiedler A, Scheer K, et al. Early post-convulsive prolongation of QT time in children. Acta Paediatr 2005;94(9):1243–7.

62. Odier C, Nguyen DK, Bouthillier A, et al. Potentially life-threatening ictal bradycardia in intractable epilepsy. Can J Neurol Sci 2009;36(1):32–5.

63. Moseley BD, Nickels K, Britton J, et al. How common is ictal hypoxemia and bradycardia in children with partial complex and generalized convulsive seizures? Epilepsia 2010;51(7):1219–24.

64. Strzelczyk A, Cenusa M, Bauer S, et al. Management and long-term outcome in patients presenting with ictal asystole or bradycardia. Epilepsia 2011; 52(6):1160–7.

65. Kouakam C, Daems C, Guedon-Moreau L, et al. Recurrent unexplained syncope may have a cerebral origin: report of 10 cases of arrhythmogenic epilepsy. Arch Cardiovasc Dis 2009;102(5): 397–407.

66. Rugg-Gunn FJ, Simister RJ, Squirrell M, et al. Cardiac arrhythmias in focal epilepsy: a prospective long-term study. Lancet 2004;364(9452): 2212–9.

67. Suorsa E, Korpelainen JT, Ansakorpi H, et al. Heart rate dynamics in temporal lobe epilepsy - a long-term follow-up study. Epilepsy Res 2011;93(1): 80–3.

68. Rauscher G, DeGiorgio AC, Miller PR, et al. Sudden unexpected death in epilepsy associated with progressive deterioration in heart rate variability. Epilepsy Behav 2011;21(1):103–5.

69. Toth V, Hejjel L, Fogarasi A, et al. Periictal heart rate variability analysis suggests long-term postictal autonomic disturbance in epilepsy. Eur J Neurol 2010;17(6):780–7.

70. Jackson JH. On asphyxia in slight epileptic paroxysms. Lancet 1899;153:79–80.

71. Nashef L, Walker F, Allen P, et al. Apnoea and bradycardia during epileptic seizures: relation to sudden death in epilepsy. J Neurol Neurosurg Psychiatr 1996;60(3):297–300.

72. Bateman LM, Li CS, Seyal M. Ictal hypoxemia in localization-related epilepsy: analysis of incidence, severity and risk factors. Brain 2008;131(Pt 12): 3239–45.

73. Seyal M, Bateman LM. Ictal apnea linked to contralateral spread of temporal lobe seizures: intracranial EEG recordings in refractory temporal lobe epilepsy. Epilepsia 2009;50(12):2557–62.

74. Nashef L, Fish DR, Garner S, et al. Sudden death in epilepsy: a study of incidence in a young cohort with epilepsy and learning difficulty. Epilepsia 1995;36(12):1187–94.

75. Pezzella M, Striano P, Ciampa C, et al. Severe pulmonary congestion in a near miss at the first seizure: further evidence for respiratory dysfunction in sudden unexpected death in epilepsy. Epilepsy Behav 2009;14(4):701–2.

76. Swallow RA, Hillier CE, Smith PE. Sudden unexplained death in epilepsy (SUDEP) following previous seizure-related pulmonary oedema: case report and review of possible preventative treatment. Seizure 2002;11(7):446–8.

77. Hewertson J, Poets CF, Samuels MP, et al. Epileptic seizure-induced hypoxemia in infants with apparent life-threatening events. Pediatrics 1994;94(2 Pt 1): 148–56.

78. Kanner AM. Depression and epilepsy: a review of multiple facets of their close relation. Neurol Clin 2009;27(4):865–80.

79. Nilsson L, Tomson T, Farahmand BY, et al. Cause-specific mortality in epilepsy: a cohort study of more than 9,000 patients once hospitalized for epilepsy. Epilepsia 1997;38(10):1062–8.

80. Rafnsson V, Olafsson E, Hauser WA, et al. Cause-specific mortality in adults with unprovoked seizures. A population-based incidence cohort study. Neuroepidemiology 2001;20(4):232–6.

81. Ridsdale L, Charlton J, Ashworth M, et al. Epilepsy mortality and risk factors for death in epilepsy: a population-based study. Br J Gen Pract 2011; 61(586):e271–8.

82. Hesdorffer DC, Hauser WA, Olafsson E, et al. Depression and suicide attempt as risk factors for incident unprovoked seizures. Ann Neurol 2006; 59(1):35–41.

83. Hesdorffer DC, Hauser WA, Annegers JF, et al. Major depression is a risk factor for seizures in older adults. Ann Neurol 2000;47(2):246–9.

84. Richerson GB, Buchanan GF. The serotonin axis: shared mechanisms in seizures, depression, and SUDEP. Epilepsia 2011;52(Suppl 1):28–38.

85. Kanner AM. Depression and epilepsy: a new perspective on two closely related disorders. Epilepsy Curr 2006;6(5):141–6.

86. Jobe PC. Common pathogenic mechanisms between depression and epilepsy: an experimental perspective. Epilepsy Behav 2003;4(Suppl 3):S14–24.

87. Hasler G, Bonwetsch R, Giovacchini G, et al. 5-HT1A receptor binding in temporal lobe epilepsy patients with and without major depression. Biol Psychiatry 2007;62(11):1258–64.

88. Theodore WH, Giovacchini G, Bonwetsch R, et al. The effect of antiepileptic drugs on 5-HT-receptor binding measured by positron emission tomography. Epilepsia 2006;47(3):499–503.

89. Jobe PC, Browning RA. The serotonergic and noradrenergic effects of antidepressant drugs are anticonvulsant, not proconvulsant. Epilepsy Behav 2005;7(4):602–19.

90. Favale E, Audenino D, Cocito L, et al. The anticonvulsant effect of citalopram as an indirect evidence of serotonergic impairment in human epileptogenesis. Seizure 2003;12(5):316–8.

91. Feldman JL, Mitchell GS, Nattie EE. Breathing: rhythmicity, plasticity, chemosensitivity. Annu Rev Neurosci 2003;26:239–66.

92. Buchanan GF, Richerson GB. Central serotonin neurons are required for arousal to CO_2. Proc Natl Acad Sci U S A 2010;107(37):16354–9.

93. Buchanan GF, Richerson GB. Role of chemoreceptors in mediating dyspnea. Respir Physiol Neurobiol 2009;167(1):9–19.

94. Kinney HC, Richerson GB, Dymecki SM, et al. The brainstem and serotonin in the sudden infant death syndrome. Annu Rev Pathol 2009;4:517–50.

95. Duncan JR, Paterson DS, Hoffman JM, et al. Brainstem serotonergic deficiency in sudden infant death syndrome. JAMA 2010;303(5):430–7.

96. Nilsson L, Ahlbom A, Farahmand BY, et al. Mortality in a population-based cohort of epilepsy surgery patients. Epilepsia 2003;44(4):575–81.

97. Sperling MR, Feldman H, Kinman J, et al. Seizure control and mortality in epilepsy. Ann Neurol 1999;46(1):45–50.

98. Scorza FA, Arida RM, Terra VC, et al. What can be done to reduce the risk of SUDEP? Epilepsy Behav 2010;18(3):137–8.

99. Carlson C, Arnedo V, Cahill M, et al. Detecting nocturnal convulsions: efficacy of the MP5 monitor. Seizure 2009;18(3):225–7.

100. Venit EL, Shepard BD, Seyfried TN. Oxygenation prevents sudden death in seizure-prone mice. Epilepsia 2004;45(8):993–6.

Index

Note: Page numbers of article titles are in **boldface** type.

Printed and bound by CPI Group (UK) Ltd, Croydon, CR0 4YY

03/10/2024

01040361-0004